Preparing Deaf and Hearing Persons with Language and Learning Challenges for CBT

Preparing Deaf and Hearing Persons with Language and Learning Challenges for CBT: A Pre-Therapy Workbook presents 12 lessons to guide staff in hospital and community mental health and rehabilitation programs on creating skill-oriented therapy settings when working with people who don't read well or have trouble with abstract ideas, problem solving, reasoning, attention, and learning. Drawing from the worlds of CBT, current understandings of best practices in psychotherapy, and the emerging clinical specialty of Deaf mental health care, the workbook describes methods for engaging people who are often considered poor candidates for psychotherapy.

Neil S. Glickman, PhD, is a former psychologist with Advocates Deaf Services in Framingham, Massachusetts, and a former unit director and psychologist with the Mental Health Unit for Deaf Persons at Westborough State Hospital in Westborough, Massachusetts. He is faculty at the University of Massachusetts Medical Center in Worcester, Massachusetts. He teaches and consults on the subjects of Deaf mental health care and cognitive behavior therapy and pre-therapy.

Books by Neil Glickman

Glickman, N. & Harvey, M. (Eds.). (1996). *Culturally affirmative psychotherapy with Deaf persons*

Glickman, N. & Gulati, S. (Eds.). (2003). *Mental health care of Deaf people: A culturally affirmative approach*

Glickman, N. (2009). *Cognitive-behavioral therapy for Deaf and hearing persons with language and learning challenges*

Glickman, N. (Ed.). (2013). *Deaf mental health care*

Preparing Deaf and Hearing Persons with Language and Learning Challenges for CBT

A Pre-Therapy Workbook

NEIL S. GLICKMAN

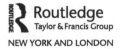

Routledge
Taylor & Francis Group

NEW YORK AND LONDON

First published 2017
by Routledge
711 Third Avenue, New York, NY 10017

and by Routledge
2 Park Square, Milton Park, Abingdon, Oxon OX14 4RN

Routledge is an imprint of the Taylor & Francis Group, an informa business

Library of Congress Cataloging-in-Publication Data
Names: Glickman, Neil S., author.
Title: Preparing deaf and hearing persons with language and learning challenges for CBT : a pre-therapy workbook / Neil S. Glickman.
Description: 1 Edition. | New York : Routledge, 2016. | Includes bibliographical references and index.
Identifiers: LCCN 2015049698 | ISBN 9781138916913 (hardback : alk. paper) |
    ISBN 9781138916937 (pbk. : alk. paper) | ISBN 9781315686851 (ebook)
Subjects: LCSH: Deaf—Mental health. | Hearing impaired—Mental health. | Language disorders—Treatment. |
    Learning disabilities—Treatment.
Classification: LCC RC451.4.D4 G58 2016 | DDC 617.8/06—dc23
LC record available at http://lccn.loc.gov/2015049698

ISBN: 978-1-138-91691-3 (hbk)
ISBN: 978-1-138-91693-7 (pbk)
ISBN: 978-1-315-68685-1 (ebk)

Typeset in Minion
by Apex CoVantage, LLC

Contents

Acknowledgments xii

Introduction xv
The World of Cognitive Behavior Therapy xv
Best Practice xviii
Deaf People 101 xix
Language and Learning Challenges xxiii
Many Hearing People Have Language and Learning Challenges xxvi
CBT, Evidence-based Treatment and Best Practice xxvii
What is Pre-therapy? xxvii
A Workbook for Staff xxix
The Lessons xxx
Tools Incorporated into This Workbook xxxiii
Conclusion xxxv
Notes xxxv
References xxxvi

LESSON ONE   Coping Skills 1
Introduction 1
A Coping Skills Story 1
Key Teaching Strategies 3
What Are Coping Skills? 4
A Strength-based Approach 4
Common Coping Skills 5
Summary 16
Lesson 1 Skill Sheet 17
Lesson 1 Quiz 17
Lesson 1 Questions for Discussion 18

Lesson 1 Quiz Answers. 19
Note. 19
Bibliography. 19

LESSON TWO   Conflict Resolution Skills. **20**
Introduction. 20
Conflict and Conflict Resolution Skills 21
Pictures of Common Conflicts 24
More Complicated Conflicts 28
Cross-cultural Conflicts 29
Common Conflict Resolution Skills. 30
Attitude Is Everything. 39
Advanced Conflict Resolution Skills 41
Lesson 2 Skill Sheet 44
Lesson 2 Quiz. 44
Lesson 2 Questions for Discussion 45
Lesson 2 Quiz Answers. 46
Note. 46
References. 46

LESSON THREE   Strength-based Work. **47**
Introduction. 47
Changing Expectations. 48
Four Key Strategies 48
Asking Strength-based Questions. 61
Lesson 3 Skill Sheet. 64
Lesson 3 Quiz. 64
Lesson 3 Questions for Discussion 65
Lesson 3 Quiz Answers. 66
References. 67

LESSON FOUR   Empathy. **68**
Introduction. 68
Acceptance and Change. 68
The Role of Empathy. 68
The Purpose of Unhealthy Behaviors. 70
Balancing Change and Acceptance. 70
The Power of Relationships 71
The Importance of Gathering Feedback. 81
What Should You Ask?. 82
Wrap-Up. 84
Lesson 4 Skill Sheet. 85
Lesson 4 Quiz. 85
Lesson 4 Questions for Discussion 86
Lesson 4 Quiz Answers. 87
References. 87

LESSON FIVE   The Power of Working "One-Down"..88

Introduction..88

Using Power and Authority in a One-Up Stance 88

The Role of Control in Mental Health Programs 90

Behavior Modification and Other Rationales for Behaving One-Up with Clients 93

Drawbacks to a One-Up Stance..94

The Awesome Power of Working "One-Down" 97

One-Down: Humility in Action 100

Benefits to Providers..101

Common Examples of One-Up and One-Down Stances 101

Lesson 5 Skill Sheet 109

Lesson 5 Quiz..109

Lesson 5 Questions for Discussion 110

Lesson 5 Quiz Answers..111

Sample Answers to Practice Exercise 5.2 111

Bibliography..112

LESSON SIX   Questions Are Better than Answers..113

Introduction..113

The Role of Questions in CBT..113

Using Questions as Part of Behavioral Analysis 115

Summary: Common Questions and Considerations When Conducting a Behavior Analysis 126

Lesson 6 Skill Sheet 130

Lesson 6 Quiz..130

Lesson 6 Questions for Discussion 131

Lesson 6 Quiz Answers..131

References..132

LESSON SEVEN   Promoting Self-Assessment 133

Introduction..133

Quick Review..133

Reality Therapy 134

Adapting WDEP 145

Self-Monitoring..145

Lesson 7 Skill Sheet 154

Lesson 7 Quiz..154

Lesson 7 Questions for Discussion 155

Lesson 7 Quiz Answers..156

References..156

LESSON EIGHT   Thoughts and Self-Talk 157

Introduction..157

The Connection between Thinking and Feeling..157

Notice Your Own Thoughts 168

Lesson 8 Skill Sheet 173

Lesson 8 Quiz..173

Lesson 8 Questions for Discussion 174
Lesson 8 Quiz Answers 175
Answers to Practice Exercise 8.1 175
References 175

LESSON NINE   The Connection between Thoughts, Feelings, and Behaviors **177**
Introduction 177
The Challenge of CBT 177
Cognitive Behavioral Pre-therapy 178
The Links between Thoughts, Mood, and Behavior 180
Lesson 9 Skill Sheet 199
Lesson 9 Quiz 199
Lesson 9 Questions for Discussion 200
Lesson 9 Quiz Answers 200
Note 201
Bibliography 201

LESSON TEN   Changing Self-Talk **202**
Introduction 202
Externalizing Problems 202
Creating Mood Monsters 203
Recovery Creatures 205
Creating Recovery Scripts 208
Modeling and Role Playing 212
Questions to Help People Think Differently 214
Lesson 10 Skill Sheet 218
Lesson 10 Quiz 218
Lesson 10 Questions for Discussion 219
Lesson 10 Quiz Answers 219
Note 220
Bibliography 220

LESSON ELEVEN   Deaf Mental Health Care and Relapse Prevention I **221**
Introduction 221
Five Key Strategies 221
Introduction to Relapse Prevention 222
Teaching and Counseling Strategy 1: Mindful Attention to Language and Communication 224
Teaching and Counseling Strategy 2: Using Stories and Examples 230
ASL and Building from Specific to Abstract 232
Back to Relapse Prevention 235
Summary 240
Lesson 11 Skill Sheet 241
Lesson 11 Quiz 241
Lesson 11 Questions for Discussion 242
Lesson 11 Quiz Answers 243

Notes 243
Bibliography 243

LESSON TWELVE   Deaf Mental Health Care and Relapse Prevention II 244
Introduction 244
Teaching and Counseling Strategy 3: Using Pictorial Aids and Drawing 244
Teaching and Counseling Strategy 4: Role Playing 250
Teaching and Counseling Strategy 5: Have the People You Serve Become Helpers and Teachers 255
Lesson 12 Skill Sheet 262
Lesson 12 Quiz 262
Lesson 12 Questions for Discussion 263
Lesson 12 Quiz Answers 264
Note 264
References 264

Acknowledgments

This workbook emerges out of more than three decades of work in what I now call Deaf mental health care. When I entered then Gallaudet College in 1981, this field had no name. The number of books on the subject of counseling deaf people could be counted on one hand, and the number of qualified mental health counselors for work with deaf people was not that much higher. Like many mental health workers with "the deaf" from my generation, I began as a vocational rehabilitation (VR) counselor. At the time, VR counselors and interpreters were the all-purpose helpers for deaf people. There were a few specialized mental health services, mostly inpatient units, and a few pioneers (Edna Levine, Hilde Schlesinger, Allen Sussman, Larry Stewart, Barbara Brauer, Eugene Mindel, McCay Vernon, to name a few in the U.S.) beginning the conversation about specialized mental health care for deaf people.

Over the course of my career, I've had the good fortune to work with hundreds of deaf clients and colleagues in a variety of inpatient- and community-based outpatient programs and to see this Deaf mental health field begin to take shape. It would be impossible to identify all the deaf and hearing colleagues who have influenced me, but I want in this acknowledgment section to note people who have been particularly influential and helpful in the development of this manual.

The approach developed here began to take place at Westborough State Hospital in Massachusetts which had a Deaf inpatient unit from 1987 to 2010. I was the director or co-director of that program for 17 years. Two books emerged from that experience. The first was *Mental health care of Deaf people: A culturally affirmative approach*, which I co-edited with Sanjay Gulati, the unit psychiatrist. The second was *Cognitive behavioral therapy for deaf and hearing persons with language and learning challenges*. I see this workbook as the companion piece to that second work. It covers a lot of the same territory, but the ideas and strategies have been further refined in a variety of community, as opposed to hospital, programs. It is also designed as a workbook, not an academic text, with a series of lessons presenting the key ideas and treatment strategies in an organized fashion.

In that second book, I acknowledge the talented staff who worked there and contributed to the development of this approach. This included Susan Jones, who read some of the chapters of this workbook and continues to inspire me, and Michael Krajnak, who contributed nearly 2000 illustrations and pictures which are now used in programs around the world, some of which are found here, including on the cover.

In 2010, Westborough State Hospital closed, and I moved to a community agency called Advocates, which provides psychiatric rehabilitation services and which has a large Deaf services program. I was able to refine and test out many of these practices there with persons who live in group homes as well as their own apartments and with dozens of talented Deaf services staff. I particularly want to acknowledge the support and skillful work of these Advocates colleagues: Dara Baril, Ellen Berger Vershbow, Sara Dugas, Shane Fuller, Robert Harris, Brittney Kleinemas, Jena Kohashi, Jonathan Lejeune, Sharon MacLean, Sandy Martins, Amy Morgan, Christina O'Neill, Ronda O'Neill, Paul O'Rourke, Anthony Petrowicz, Jenna Richmond, William Stratemeier, and Lisha Weeks.

During the fall, winter and spring of 2014–2015, each of these lessons was piloted at PAHrtners Deaf Services in Glenside, Pennsylvania. I can't imagine this project being completed without the active support I received from PAHrtners' mega-talented COO Wendy Heines as well as her dedicated leadership staff of Alesia Allen, Melissa Watson, and Amy Lagleder.

When it comes to the emergence of Deaf mental health care as a specialty, no one has done more to advance this than Robert Pollard at the Deaf Wellness Center of the University of Rochester Medical Center. He and the staff, which includes Robyn Dean, Lori DeWindt, Sharon Haynes, Amanda O'Hearn, and Denise Thew, have pioneered the emergence of culturally affirmative (Deaf-friendly) assessment and treatment interventions. I've borrowed in particular from them their emphasis on storytelling as a teaching technique that is found throughout this workbook and especially in Lesson 11. More deeply, I've borrowed from their thoughtful explorations of what it takes to adapt behavioral and public health information and techniques for culturally Deaf people.

In the larger mental health field, I've been most influenced by the work of Allen Ivey, Marsha Linehan, Ross Greene, and, especially, Donald Meichenbaum. I studied closely with Allen Ivey when I was a doctoral student at the University of Massachusetts. Ivey taught me to break interventions down into "microskills," which is one source for the interest in specific coping and conflict resolution skills found in this book. Ivey helped people learn by breaking down approaches into smaller skills. One builds from small skills to larger skills; that is, skills develop from simple to complex, and we can often help people by focusing on the developmentally simpler skills.

Ivey also taught me that different therapies match different cognitive developmental abilities of clients. In other words, one couldn't (or shouldn't) just expect that any client can immediately understand and apply any counseling or psychotherapy approach. Rather, one has to work to match each treatment intervention to what each person can readily understand and use. I have found Ivey's insight about this to be profoundly true, especially when I came to focus on work with persons who have language and learning challenges. Finally, he emphasized the multicultural context of mental health work. Cultural frameworks, beliefs, expectations, and ways of learning have great impact on an enterprise like counseling. These three ideas from Ivey are guiding assumptions of this workbook.

The greatest teacher of psychotherapy I've been exposed to in my life is unquestionably Donald Meichenbaum, one of the originators of CBT. Indeed, if I hadn't studied his work intensely, I don't think I'd be as strong a CBT fan. That's because he emphasizes best practices, used creatively, and not the kind of formulaic procedure that CBT often becomes in the hands of less skillful practitioners. I cite in the Introduction specific techniques I've borrowed from Meichenbaum, but overall I've been impressed with the artistry with which he used these strategies based on a very close attention to how people use metaphor and stories. He develops an empathic understanding of people by listening expertly to how they use words and construct meaning. It's brilliant and it keeps the art in psychotherapy. In addition, I've also found that Meichenbaum's early CBT framework, with its emphasis on coping skills and self-talk, is more useful for persons with language and learning challenges that that of his CBT colleagues Albert Ellis and Aaron Beck, which works, according to Ivey's taxonomy, at a higher cognitive developmental level.

From Marsha Linehan, I learned about the importance of balancing skill building with acceptance/validation in a "dialectical" way. This dialectic is reflected in, on the one hand, the emphasis here on helping people develop skills and, on the other hand, the importance of empathy, skillful listening, and mindful "stopping and noticing" to what is already present. Without this exposure to Linehan's framework, I might have made the mistake of talking about skills without talking about empathy and validation. As she has noted, that's probably the biggest mistake that cognitive behavioral therapists make. You can find that dialectic in the shift from skill building found in Lessons 1 to 3 to empathy and relationship building found in Lessons 4 and 5.

From Ross Greene, I learned about the importance of working with staff to build skill oriented treatment environments. I see the kind of environments I want this workbook to foster to be very compatible with the environments using his collaborative problem-solving approach. The basic idea I got from him was that students and clients were struggling because they lacked key cognitive and psychosocial skills, and that what they needed were treatment milieu in which everyone engaged them in the process of skill development, especially the skill of problem solving. I also took from him this importance of working closely with program staff, especially direct care workers. Thus, this is a workbook aimed at primarily at the staff providing services in treatment milieu.

At Advocates, I was introduced to the recovery movement in mental health with its emphasis on changing the traditional power relationships between mental health providers and persons receiving services as well as the game changing strategy of bringing persons with lived experience on as colleagues and treatment providers. The recovery movement reinforced ideas I had already embraced about helping staff move away from controlling strategies. For instance, at Westborough State Hospital we were very focused for over a decade on reducing our use of restraint of patients and on creating a safer treatment milieu for everyone. We made great strides in that effort primarily by teaching staff to work one-down, and stop trying to force people to behave in the way we wanted them to.

Learning to work one-down means learning to skillfully invite, not compel, participation. It is consistent with the recovery movements emphasis on collaboration in mental health care and of empowerment of consumers. It is also consistent with what we know about best practices in psychotherapy. We know that best practices emphasize doing everything you can to engage, motivate, and empower clientele. We know that engaged consumers are far more likely to recover, as they define recovery. Thus, this workbook of pre-therapy, designed to bring persons who can't readily use standard counseling techniques to the starting gate of this work.

All the leadership at Advocates embraces this recovery philosophy, but I've been most guided here by Naomi Pinson, Keith Scott, Brenda Miele-Soares, and Amy Morgan. You will find these themes woven into this workbook, especially in Lessons 4, 5, and 12.

As I was writing these lessons, several colleagues were kind enough to read sections and give me invaluable feedback. These include Susan Jones, Melissa Anderson, Wyatte Hall, and John Gournaris. As mentioned, the whole workbook was piloted at PAHrtners Deaf Services in Pennsylvania where I received live feedback about what does and doesn't work. Margaret Endres provided me with a close reading and skillful editing assistance, always working to make my language simpler, clearer, and better organized.

I want to thank Deaf interpreter Raylene Lotz for her willingness to be photographed signing some of the key ideas. I also want to thank Michael Krajnak, whose wonderful pictures illustrate my CBT book as well and for his willingness to prepare numerous pictures again for this workbook. I love the WORD illustration provided by Phillip Martin and encourage readers to check out his website at www.phillipmartin.com to see his astonishing collection of useful illustrations and clip art.

I've received enormous support for this project from my Routledge editor Anna Moore who immediately "got" what this workbook was about and helped me turn it into a reality. She was more than ably assisted by Zoey Peresman who walked me through the countless details of creating a workbook, including managing hundreds of pictures with different file formats and navigating the intricacies of Dropbox. Zoey and Anna were very hands-on, in a constructive way, always eager to help. They didn't put obstacles in my way, but rather helped me overcome obstacles to make this workbook happen.

Finally, I acknowledge and thank my terrific husband, Steven Riel, who keeps our small ship of state steady and even, so we both can focus and dream.

Introduction

This is a workbook for staff working in educational, rehabilitation and mental health programs that serve deaf and hearing people who have language and learning challenges. It was created to give staff a set of tools and strategies that they can use to help people with language and learning challenges build the key skills they need in order to participate in conventional counseling and therapy. In other words, it is a *pre-therapy* workbook.

Because many of these individuals lack critical reading skills, this workbook is designed to teach staff to use these core strategies, and, in turn, introduce them to the people they are serving. These strategies are intended to bridge the gap between the mental world of the language- and learning-challenged people you serve and the mental world of conventional cognitive behavioral therapy (CBT).

This workbook emerges out of a new clinical specialty called Deaf mental health care (DMHC) (Glickman 2013). While the deaf population is an enormously diverse group, it is more common to encounter individuals with significant language and learning challenges when you are working with deaf people than it is when you are working with hearing people. This is especially true for DMHC practitioners working in public sector hospitals and clinics.

Those who specialize in DMHC recognize the profound impact that language and learning deficits have on the way mental health services are provided. They have learned the importance of adapting standard mental health practices to make them more clear, engaging, and relevant to people with language and learning challenges. When working with individuals with language and learning challenges, it is not uncommon to discover that many of them are not ready for counseling or therapy. The problem is not necessarily that an individual is resistant to change or isn't ready emotionally. Rather, language and thinking problems can make it difficult for a person to use the verbal, problem-solving strategies that counseling and therapy require.

This pre-therapy workbook draws on the creative adaptations made by DMHC specialists in order to make cognitive behavioral therapy accessible to individuals, deaf or hearing, who have difficulty understanding and using common CBT techniques.

In order to use this workbook effectively, it is important to understand some key things about counseling, psychotherapy and CBT, the most widely used and evidenced-based form of therapy available today. It is also necessary to understand something about "best practice" in mental health care as it is currently understood.

The World of Cognitive Behavior Therapy

You may be familiar with *The Big Bang Theory*, a popular television comedy about a group of very intelligent but socially awkward scientists. Some people might refer to them as "nerds." The main character is Sheldon, the most socially awkward of them all. He lives with Leonard who has a girlfriend named Penny, who lives across the hall.

Penny is the opposite of Sheldon. She is fun-loving, outgoing, and uninhibited. She is definitely not a genius. She sings and dances in the apartment, laughs out loud in a squeaky voice, and doesn't even try to be quiet during sex. All of this grates on Sheldon. In a wonderful episode called "Behavior Modification," Sheldon comes up with a plan to change Penny's behavior.

The first step occurs when Penny graciously agrees to move out of the spot on the sofa that Sheldon has claimed as his own. To Leonard's astonishment, Sheldon says "thank you" to her in an overly sweet voice, and then offers her a chocolate. Later, she makes a silly comment about a cartoon that he likes. He looks at her with disapproval and she pantomimes zipping up her lips. He then offers her another chocolate. When a friend calls her on the phone, Penny begins chatting with her loudly. Sheldon gives her another disapproving look, and she offers to take the phone call into the other room. He then gives her another chocolate.

Leonard, who has been studying the whole interaction silently, finally turns off the television and confronts Sheldon.

Leonard: *"OK, I know what you are doing."*
Sheldon: *"Really?"*
Leonard: *"Yes. You are using chocolate as a positive reinforcement for what you consider correct behavior."*
Sheldon: *"Very good."*
           Sheldon offers Leonard some chocolate.
Leonard: *"No, I don't want any chocolate. And Sheldon, you can't train my girlfriend like a lab rat."*
Sheldon: *"Actually, it turns out I can."*
Leonard: *"Well, you shouldn't."*
Sheldon: *"There's just no pleasing you, is there, Leonard? You weren't happy with my previous approach to dealing with her, so I decided to employ operant conditioning techniques, building on the works of Thorndike and B.F. Skinner. By this time next week, I believe I can have her jumping out of a pool, bouncing a beach ball on her nose."*
Leonard: *"No, this has to stop now!"*
Sheldon: *"I'm not suggesting we really make her jump out of a pool. I thought the 'bazinga' [joke] was implied. I'm just tweaking her personality, sanding off the rough edges, if you will."*
Leonard.   *"No, you are not sanding Penny!"*
           Sheldon looks puzzled.
Sheldon: *"Are you saying that I am forbidden from applying a harmless, scientifically valid protocol that will make our lives better?"*
Leonard: *"Yes, you are forbidden!"*
           Sheldon turns around, grabs a spray bottle of water and sprays Leonard in the face.
           "Bad Leonard!" he exclaims. (Lorre et al. 2009)

This is a wonderful parody of behavior therapy, one of the oldest approaches psychology has to help people change. Behavior therapy is based on the idea that people are motivated to behave because of reinforcements. Sheldon is using a form of behavior therapy called "operant conditioning." In operant conditioning, you attempt to change someone's behavior by offering a positive reinforcement when the person shows the behavior you want. This is Sheldon's strategy for changing Penny's behavior by using chocolate as a reward. You can also try to punish behaviors you don't want. This is Sheldon's strategy when he sprays Leonard with the water bottle and exclaims, "Bad Leonard!"

Nowadays, behavior therapy has, in most places, been updated with something called cognitive behavior therapy, or CBT. CBT is different than the older behavior therapy in at least two important ways. First, much more attention is paid to cognition or thinking. It's unlikely, for instance, that Penny would be so easy to influence if she realized that Sheldon was not being nice to her. He was trying to manipulate her. If she realized this—that is, if she *thought* differently—she'd probably have a different reaction.

The second way is a shift of emphasis away from rewards and punishments towards skills. In traditional behavior therapy, rewards and punishments are used to help someone change their motivation. In CBT, we are more likely to assume that people are doing the best they can. If they don't behave in the most skillful way, it's not because they aren't motivated. It's because they don't know *how* to behave better. Sometimes the skills they are lacking are thinking or problem-solving skills. Rather than focus on motivation per se, we more often focus on skill training. We use a variety of strategies to help people learn new skills.

In CBT, the kinds of skill we focus on are called "psychosocial skills." These skills go by different names. Some examples can be found in Table I.1. The categories of skills overlap with one another.

If you are helping someone learn these psychosocial skills, it is probably safe to say you're working in the CBT world. Once a person has agreed to learn skills to address a problem, CBT has hundreds of techniques and strategies to offer.

Ah, but getting people to the point at which they say, "I want to learn these skills," is a very different matter!

Within the CBT world, most of the problems people face are understood to be due, in some way, to a *lack of skills* or *skill deficits*. For example, the emotion of anger becomes a problem when a person lacks sufficient

TABLE I.1 Psychosocial Skills Developed in CBT

Skill	Purpose	Examples
Coping skills, also called **distress tolerance skills**	To cope with distressing situations and emotions	Talking to oneself in a soothing way
Emotional self-regulation skills	To maintain a fairly even emotional state	Sleeping and eating well
Social skills	To form and maintain relationships and deal with conflicts	Greeting people Making friends Handling disagreements
Stress management skills	To cope with stressful situations and emotions	Deep breathing Mindfulness Prioritizing and problem solving
Symptom management skills	To manage symptoms of depression anxiety, anger, substance use, etc.	Noticing and changing the thinking patterns that support these symptoms and emotions
Problem-solving skills	To identify ways to manage or solve problems	Making lists Prioritizing Pros and cons
Communication skills	To communicate feelings and thoughts and listen well	Reflective listening I-statements
Independent living skills	To help an individual be more independent	Making and following a budget Cooking
Self-care skills	To take care of one's body and one's environment	Cleaning oneself Setting up and following a laundry schedule
Skills for managing medications	To understand the risks and benefits of medication, making informed choices and following doctors' orders	Knowing the name, purpose, dosage, administration and side effects of medications
Skills for working with mental health providers	To participate and benefit from mental health interventions	Asking good questions about diagnosis and treatment plans
Relapse prevention skills	To prevent a problem symptom or behavior from happening again	Understanding triggers, risk factors and warnings signs

skills to manage or cope with anger. People who show behavioral problems like harming themselves or others lack sufficient skills for managing emotions and environmental stressors safely. People who struggle with anxiety and depression need skills to manage and decrease these symptoms. In all of these situations, a central therapeutic task is to engage people in the work of learning these crucial life skills.

There are different sub-schools within the CBT world. The form of CBT that we're discussing has been most influenced by CBT founder Donald Meichenbaum, the person who shifted the emphasis in behavior therapy from motivation to skills. Many of the strategies described in this workbook were first articulated and developed by Meichenbaum (Meichenbaum 1977a, 1977b, 1994, 1996, 2001, 2012; Meichenbaum & Biemiller 1998), such as:

- The focus on coping skills (Lesson 1).
- The concern with being strength-based (Lesson 3).
- The use of a "one-down" stance (Lesson 5).
- The art of questioning (Lessons 3, 6, and 7).
- The use of self-monitoring (Lesson 7).
- The focus on changing how we talk to ourselves (Lessons 8, 9, and 10).
- The attention to drawing out of people their story about resiliency and recovery and helping them develop these stories further (Lessons 9 and 10).
- The idea of having the people who receive services help and teach others (Lesson 12).

The world of CBT is increasingly becoming the non-medication part of mental health care. Today, most mental health and rehabilitation programs use some variant of CBT or strive to do so. If you are a staff person working in a mental health program, you need to know the basics of CBT to do your job well. It also will help you to understand the basics of CBT if you are a person receiving mental health or rehabilitation services.

When we talk about counseling or therapy in this workbook, we are referring to a CBT approach developed by Meichenbaum that places emphasis on teaching psychosocial skills and changing person's stories about themselves. You could summarize these two themes as "skills and stories." This approach includes a variety of best practices that enable counselors to engage people in the process of learning skills. It emphasizes influencing the way people talk to themselves, their "self-talk," and the stories people tell themselves about their own abilities. It also places great emphasis on "resiliency," or noticing, labeling, and building on the skills and strengths that people already have. In this model of CBT, we work to engage people in learning skills; but at a deeper level, we use strategies to help them change the way they think and talk about themselves. At this deeper level, we are helping them change not just their skills, but also their story about themselves, their core beliefs, and identity.

CBT places emphasis on helping people use thinking skills to change their behaviors. Yet people with language and learning challenges often lack the skill with language that this approach appears to depend on. This presents some obstacles. Can we use CBT with people who have significant language and learning challenges? The answer is "yes." This workbook outlines an approach that we refer to as "pre-therapy" and provides a toolbox of strategies for engaging persons who, because of language and learning challenges, are often written off as "poor candidates for psychotherapy."

Best Practice

Whether you use CBT or some other form of psychotherapy, it's crucial that the people providing and receiving services have a shared language and model for what they are doing. The process of counseling can be mysterious. Exactly how does it work? Recent research into what works in psychotherapy found that client understanding and valuing of the process has a major impact on whether or not it will be successful (Duncan, Miller, Wampold, & Hubble 2010). "Best practice" may not be a particular approach to therapy but rather a series of strategies that engage and empower people so they want to participate in treatment. That is to say, there may be many ways to help people "get better," but what matters is that the client and clinicians understand and agree on what they are doing, and the client says, "I want this."

Thus, you will find in this workbook a lot of attention to presenting a simple, clear, and empowering model for "what we are doing together." You will also find a continuing concern with being strength-based; that is, engaging people by helping them discover what they already do well, and then inviting them to consider whether they could do better.

Research into best practices has also found that that the nature of the therapeutic relationship has a huge impact on treatment outcome (Duncan et al. 2010). All too often, when the people receiving services have language and learning challenges, staff who work with them use a controlling, "one-up" style of work that actually makes things worse. Thus, you will also find here a lot of attention to changing how staff and clientele interact. In a nutshell, the change is one of moving from directing and controlling, to questioning and inviting. It is a change from telling people what they should do to asking helpful questions that promote engagement and the development of problem-solving skills.

The model of CBT that Meichenbaum developed aligns very nicely with current understandings of best practice. It turns out that the strategies he recommends to engage people in the process of skill development are best practices. Most importantly, Meichenbaum is concerned with helping people become active agents in their own self-development. That is our focus here as well.

Deaf People 101

Before we explore these pre-therapy strategies, it is important to understand a few important things about Deaf people. Then we must elaborate on what we mean by "language and learning challenges."

Hearing adults who find themselves involved with signing Deaf people learn a few important lessons very quickly. Some of these lessons could be considered "Deaf People 101," like the introductory, overview classes offered at universities, including the following.

Not All deaf People Are Deaf

There are Deaf communities that have their own history, language, and culture. "Big D Deaf" refers to the culture of Deaf people, Deaf culture, and the Deaf community. "Little d deaf" refers to hearing loss. A Deaf person is a person who is culturally Deaf, a member of the Deaf community, whereas a deaf person is a person with a severe hearing loss. To a culturally Deaf person, being Deaf is about identity, not hearing loss.

Signing Deaf people are a linguistic and cultural minority, a disempowered group comparable to other minority groups. The relationship between Deaf and deaf people is represented in Figure I.1. The culturally Deaf group can include some hearing people, such as hearing children raised in culturally Deaf families (though this is sometimes debated), as well as some people who are hard of hearing who sign well and identify with the Deaf Community.[1]

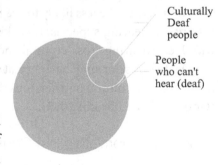

Culturally Deaf people

People who can't hear (deaf)

Figure I.1 The relationship between Deaf and deaf people

American Sign Language Is Not English on the Hands

American Sign Language (ASL) and sign languages used in other countries and regions are real languages. They are not shorthand codes for spoken languages and are not elaborate, non-grammatical gestures, as many used to think. Although sign languages have grammatical rules and structures, they may be very different from the spoken language of the community. In the hands of skilled signers, sign languages are rich, complex, subtle, and beautiful. The grammar and vocabulary of ASL has important implications for mental health care, as we will see in Lessons 11 and 12.

Deaf People Face Common Forms of Prejudice and Discrimination, As Well As Some Unique Challenges

Throughout history, deaf people have faced, and indeed still face, prejudice and discrimination that are as destructive as any faced by other oppressed groups. The most dramatic form of oppression occurs when deaf children are deprived of access to sign language, a trend that has been sadly accelerated by the development of cochlear implants and educational policies that promote mainstreaming, regardless of the needs of individual deaf children. Throughout their lives, deaf people are routinely deprived of information. This means that gaining access to information and having full communication inclusion is often one of their primary concerns.

Creating real communication inclusion is, therefore, the first and major challenge and focus of any service for deaf people. Most programs and services are not accessible even when the Americans with Disabilities Act is followed and modest attempts are made to provide interpreter services. This is because interpreter services are often offered for only a small percentage of the time they are needed and, when these services are provided, they are of very uneven quality. Often, interpreting is not even attempted because, frankly, it is expensive and providers argue, self-servingly, that it isn't needed. In addition, not all communication challenges can be overcome by providing interpreters.

Hearing people also vary in how effectively they use language. To interpret clearly from one language to another, interpreters depend on an individual being able to use his or her native language well. It is one challenge to interpret between two people who are fluent in their respective languages; it is an entirely different challenge to interpret for people who can't communicate clearly in their native language. Think about this. How could you interpret something into a different language for someone who isn't making sense in his or her native language? How do you interpret if you don't understand what the person is saying?

Deaf Culture Is Real

Signing Deaf people have a community and culture that goes well beyond a shared language. In addition to language differences, Deaf and hearing people often have cultural differences. There is a rich Deaf history, many Deaf organizations, and many forms of Deaf art. Deaf and hearing people also sometimes have different beliefs and thought worlds, at least in some domains. Because hearing people typically understand deafness as a disability, they are less likely to see the cross-cultural dynamics that can separate them from Deaf people. For instance, a hearing supervisor working with a Deaf counselor may not appreciate all the baggage that comes with Deaf–hearing cross-cultural encounters. The hearing supervisor might not understand, for instance, why the Deaf counselor may be angry at something that was said or has difficulty trusting hearing people. Deaf–hearing cross-cultural partnerships require a great deal of self-awareness, knowledge, and skill to be successful (Gournaris & Aubrecht 2013).

Language Deprivation Is a Continuing Problem for Many deaf People

If you can't hear or see the language being used around you, you will not learn it with anything approaching native language abilities. This is the main reason why there are many deaf people with normal intelligence who are poor language users. Some Deaf people sign beautifully but don't use the spoken language of the larger community well. These persons are fluent language users but struggle in a second non-native language. There are other deaf people who, because of language deprivation, can't be said to have native abilities in any language. At the extreme, there are deaf people who have no formal language skills at all (Schaller 1991).

When deaf people who have been language deprived develop emotional or behavioral problems, they may be referred to the local mental health program. Typically, these programs are unprepared for the communication challenges and make a lot of what could be considered beginner's mistakes. For instance, they may assume that communication through speech reading or writing will be adequate, or they may assume that someone who has taken a sign language class can interpret. Once they learn that sign languages are real languages, they may make a more advanced mistake in assuming that every deaf person they encounter is a fluent signer.

Language deprivation results in *dysfluent* or poor language skills in both signed and spoken languages. Without strong language abilities, including the ability to read and write, deaf people also may have an impoverished "fund of information" (Pollard 1998) about the world. They have not heard or seen a lot of things that hearing people have been exposed to. The result is a complex set of "language and learning challenges" that have direct bearing on their ability to make use of common mental health practices, such as counseling.

Identifying and Matching the Communication Needs of deaf Individuals Is Much Harder Than It Seems

If you are running a mental health clinic in America, you expect to face a communication challenge if a recent immigrant from Ghana, who speaks a dialect of Twi and no English, is referred to your clinic. You may not have anyone on staff who speaks that dialect of Twi, but you can be reasonably confident of one thing: the person is a native speaker of her own language. Although you don't know how skilled a user of Twi the person is, you can assume with reasonable certainty that the person has full, intact, native language abilities in Twi.

However, when a signing Deaf person comes into your hearing clinic, you can't make a similar assumption. The extent of communication diversity among deaf people is far greater than it is among hearing people. The Deaf person may well be multilingual, knowing several sign and spoken languages. He may be alingual, knowing no language at all, a situation that is extremely rare among hearing people. The person's language skills may fall anywhere in between. Unlike the situation with the Twi speaker, it is difficult to know exactly what *kind* of communication challenge you are facing.

In Lesson 11 of this workbook, you will learn about the importance of asking the question, "Am I clear?" and how it differs from the question, "Do you understand?" "Am I clear?" is about the *speaker*, whereas "Do you understand?" is about the *recipient*. When working with deaf or hearing persons with language and cognitive compromises, you must ask the question, "Am I clear?" over and over. Then, you must work on becoming clear—that's the hard part.

When working with deaf people, especially those with severe language problems, you cannot rely on your own judgment about whether or not you are communicating clearly. Neither can you necessarily rely on assurances from a deaf consumer that they understand what you are communicating. This is because the language problems that emerge from language deprivation vary enormously. If you don't sign like a native user, you can easily miss these language problems. It is also because there is a great pull on all parties in the conversation to pretend that communication is fine. American Sign Language even has a sign for pretending to understand. There is no one English word that captures the meaning of this sign. (Indeed, there are many concepts like this that are expressed more clearly in ASL than in English.)

I remember an incident that highlighted for me the dangers of imagining that you are communicating more effectively than you actually are. I was part of a Deaf Unit team that included very linguistically sophisticated native signers and interpreters. We were having a conversation about our difficulty communicating with a deaf person in the program who was nearly alingual. He knew hardly any ASL or English. He communicated using a smattering of familiar signs and some "home signs" that were known only to him and his family. Most of the time, he communicated through gestures. While we were having this conversation, a new hearing staff person came by. Filled with enthusiasm after his first sign language class, this staff announced confidently that *he* had no difficulty communicating with this deaf person.

We all looked at each other and sighed. *A little knowledge is a dangerous thing.*

You need expert help if you are hearing and have anything less than native sign language abilities yourself, especially when you are working with deaf persons with language and learning challenges. In many situations, this expert help will come from sign language interpreters. Using an interpreter may create the illusion that the communication challenges have been overcome but it is important to talk to the interpreters, and to the consumer if possible, about the language and communication challenges. Search for people who can assess the person's language skills in sign and spoken languages. Ask, with an open mind, what resources are needed to bridge the communication challenges. If there is a Deaf service program that can do a better job with communication access, advocate for your Deaf consumer to have the option of going there. Here are two true stories from my experience that illustrate this dynamic.

Scenario I.1

A Deaf young woman with a mild developmental disability was living in a group home funded by the Department of Developmental Services. The young woman had some difficulties with independent living skills. She was also occasionally aggressive with her staff and peers. She was the only Deaf person in the program and staff had taken sign language classes and could communicate with her with a vocabulary of maybe 50 signs and sign phrases. Her family and DDS case worker all said she was placed appropriately because "staff could sign."

Fortunately for her, the program manager recognized that the staff could not sign any more than a person who has taken one semester of French could speak French. The program manager realized that this person needed a sign language rich communication environment that could only occur if there were Deaf staff and peers. The program manager advocated tirelessly for her to be transferred to an agency that offered Deaf-run group homes and programs. Eventually, the transfer happened. In the new Deaf-centered signing environment, the woman's behavioral problems disappeared and she started learning skills that her protective family never imagined she could acquire.

Scenario I.2

A Deaf patient named Joe was hospitalized on a Deaf inpatient unit after telling staff in his hearing day program and group home that he wanted to kill himself. Joe was mildly developmentally delayed, a graduate of a Deaf residential school, and a functional user of American Sign Language.

Joe was living and working in environments exclusively with hearing people who signed poorly, if at all. As a graduate of a Deaf school, he knew what good sign communication looked like. He missed it. He missed being around deaf people. This contributed to his depression. Each day, he faced incident after incident where he was misunderstood and left out and, in response, his depression, frustration and anger increased. Joe didn't have the language sophistication to say, "I'm frustrated because no one here communicates with me well. I want to be around other signing Deaf people." Even if he could have expressed this, no one around him would have understood him and his concerns would not have been validated. Instead he said, "I want to kill myself." This was treated as a psychiatric emergency that caused his outpatient psychiatrist to wonder if he had a major depressive disorder.

On the Deaf inpatient program, staff immediately understood the communication isolation that Joe faced. The team saw that whatever depression he had disappeared once he was surrounded by signing Deaf people. His behavior also miraculously improved. The team was sophisticated enough to not approach this as a medical problem but, rather, as a problem of social isolation. The treatment with Joe consisted of helping him say to people, "I don't understand you. I need Deaf people. I need an interpreter." Just as important, the team was able to advocate for him to live and receive services in a more appropriate setting.[2]

Working with Deaf People Requires Cultural Competence

Because Deaf people have cultures and languages of their own, the hearing people who work with them need to develop Deaf cultural competence. Cross-cultural misunderstandings between Deaf and hearing people are common. Indeed, they are powerful enough to destroy a program or service or create treatment failures. Here are some more stories from the author's experience.

Scenario I.3

There is one Deaf person working in a hearing mental health agency and setting. That person has been hired to work with the program's few Deaf participants. The Deaf staff person is routinely left out of agency trainings and inter-agency communications. Deaf participants communicate with the Deaf staff person about their isolation and frustrations, but the Deaf staff person has the same experiences and feelings. Her requests for support go largely ignored by her busy supervisor who makes, at best, token efforts to obtain interpreters. The supervisor doesn't really want to be bothered to address the special considerations of Deaf people in the agency.

Scenario I.4

A Deaf therapist working in a mental health clinic has a Master's degree but needs additional hours of supervision to apply for her licensure. She works with a hearing supervisor and finds that she has to spend most of the supervision sessions educating her supervisor about Deaf people and advocating for her clients. She feels that she isn't getting the type of clinical supervision and training she needs. She asks the agency to support her request to receive supervision from an experienced signing clinician outside the agency. The agency's management responds that there is no funding and doesn't seem to understand why the current supervisory relationship isn't adequate. The Deaf therapist starts to get a reputation for thinking she is "entitled" and being "demanding" and "difficult."

Scenario I.5

A mental health program that serves both Deaf and hearing people has posted a promotional opportunity for line staff. Some of these staff are Deaf and some are hearing. About a third of the program's caseload are Deaf people. Both Deaf and hearing staff apply for the promotion. Agency managers express concerns about having Deaf staff supervise hearing people. However, they have never been concerned about having hearing people supervise Deaf people.

Deaf staff argue that the supervisor needs to be able to sign competently and that a Deaf person should be offered this rare promotional opportunity. They point out that hearing people have far more job opportunities, especially for supervisory positions. The managers respond that the supervisor must have native abilities in written English so they can complete all the necessary paperwork, and that the supervisor must be able to communicate effectively with everyone. They argue that only the hearing applicants have those abilities. They ignore the protests from Deaf staff that the hearing applicants don't really have those communication abilities when working with Deaf staff and clients. Deaf staff argue that there is a double standard. The hearing supervisors complain that the Deaf staff don't appreciate the agency's efforts to serve and employ them.

Scenario I.6

Every year a local district recognizes a "mental health worker of the year." An agency that serves mainly Deaf people is asked to submit nominations. Someone in the agency nominates a hearing employee who is a very good worker. Others object that only a Deaf person should be nominated by the agency. This opportunity to recognize an employee became a crisis for the agency because it revealed underlying tensions about the roles and status of Deaf and hearing people. Agency leadership was forced to face some difficult questions head on: When evaluating an employee for hire, promotion or an award, how important is it that the employee be deaf or Deaf? How should they weigh the relative importance of identity and communication abilities against other aspects of work performance? Who decides?

These kinds of cross-cultural conflict are found in programs that serve Deaf persons. They are often handled badly, with Deaf participants and staff feeling oppressed and hearing persons feeling misunderstood. Needless to say, it is hard to create a healing mental health environment if the minority participants, both staff and people receiving services, perceive that the same oppression that they face in the larger world is occurring in the treatment program where they are supposed to receive help.

Language and Learning Challenges

The material and approach presented in this workbook was first developed on the Westborough State Hospital Deaf Unit in Massachusetts, a Deaf psychiatric inpatient unit where the author worked for 17 years. The approach was presented in the book, *Cognitive behavioral therapy for deaf and hearing persons with language and learning challenges*, which was published in 2009. Since then, the material and approach have been refined, clarified and systematized in a variety of community and educational settings where the author has worked.

The Westborough Deaf unit staff understood and were committed to the idea, new at the time of the unit's founding, of Deaf cultural affirmation within a mental health setting (Glickman 1996). We understood that the unit's primary clientele were people who used American Sign Language. The Unit opened in 1987 but it wasn't until after the millennium that we began to pay serious attention to the fact that most of our signing Deaf patients were not fluent users of ASL. Spurred on by the pioneering research of psychology intern Patricia Black, and with the aid of detailed communication assessments done by our communication specialist Michael Krajnak who was assisted by an interpreting team of Wendy Petrarca and Susan Jones, we began to pay much closer attention to the sign language abilities and deficits of all our deaf patients. We discovered that in about two-thirds of our patients, foundation language skills were weak or missing. We also began to connect language problems with the emotional and behavioral problems that brought these individuals into the unit.

Some of the language problems we saw were:

1. Very limited vocabulary with many signs used incorrectly.
2. Absence of or weakness in using time and tense structures. A tendency to mix up events that happened or were happening in the past and present; and also difficulty clearly distinguishing them from events that one hoped to see happen in the future. Staff continuously sought clarification: When did that happen? Did it happen or is it something you imagined or is it something you wanted to happen? Some of our deaf patients could not reference day, week, month or years. They could not use a calendar and certainly didn't use ASL grammatical structures like THREE-MONTHS-FUTURE and FIVE-YEARS-PAST.[3]
3. An inability to establish topics clearly. Clients frequently omitted subject and object, or mixed them up, leaving staff to continuously seek clarification: Who are you talking about? Who did what to whom? Sometimes signing with a person who has been language deprived feels like joining a conversation in the middle. One can't follow along because one never hears a clear statement of the topic.
4. Limited ability to indicate transitions from one topic to another. Information was jumbled together. It's very common when working with deaf people with language deprivation to spend an enormous amount of time trying to figure out what happened. Even very skilled Deaf communicators can struggle to understand what a very language-deprived deaf person means to say.
5. Difficulty identifying cause and effect. For instance, while many patients could say they were angry, they had enormous difficulty identifying what came before the anger. This certainly made discussions about "triggers" and "stressors," a cornerstone of CBT, difficult. This is also one reason why questions that help people sequence events are taught in this program (Lesson 6).
6. Sign language uses space and movement for grammatical purposes, such as establishing who is where, who did what to whom, and how people are relating to each other (e.g., who helps, teaches, supports whom). Common grammatical space and movement structures were not used well or consistently. You need to be raised in an ASL-rich environment to learn these features, which have no equivalent in spoken language.
7. A great deal of sign language occurs not on the hands but on the face and body, yet these basic structures were also used poorly or inconsistently (Glickman 2009).

These and other language problems contribute to broader thinking and learning problems.

For instance, many patients had difficulty with abstract thinking. In the past, psychologists and educators working with deaf people often drew the wrong conclusion by generalizing that all deaf people were "concrete" thinkers. This isn't true of deaf people as a whole, but it is true of people who have had significant language deprivation. In addition, many people, deaf and hearing, served in mental health settings are, in fact, concrete thinkers. They may have difficulty with hypothetical situations (e.g., if you do this, what might happen?). The inability to anticipate consequences also makes learning difficult and makes a treatment strategy such as relapse prevention especially challenging.

Many of the typical conversations that go on in mental health settings are highly abstract. Many mental health concepts such as coping, symptom, hallucination, conflict solving, relapse, cycle, pattern, trigger, warning signs, bipolar disorder, recovery, treatment, therapy may not be easy for concrete thinkers to understand.

Abstract thinking also includes the ability to see patterns: how what you are doing now relates to how you feel and think; how your current behavior is related to your past behavior and experiences; how your behavior with your counselor is related to your behavior with other people, etc. Indeed, one can consider insight to be the ability to make new connections, to relate things in a new way. Therefore, it is easy to take the next step and conclude that people who have difficulty making these connections lack insight. It is, indeed, more difficult for concrete thinkers to make these connections, to show insight. This can be frustrating for the counselors working with them.

Poorly developed language skills also seem to make it difficult to stop and notice one's thinking—in other words, to think about thinking. Asking questions like "What were you thinking?" leads to blank stares. In CBT, after a person identifies a belief, such as "I'm stupid," the counselor may respond by asking, "What is the evidence for that belief?" This is a very abstract question that assumes the person has had prior exposure to science and understands the concept of evaluating evidence. How can you answer this question if you lack this experience or you can't identify what a thought is?

Consider the complex thinking and language skills that would be required to respond to these other common requests that a cognitive behavioral therapist might ask:

- Categorize your thoughts. Is this "all or nothing" thinking?
- Think in "shades of grey" or consider other perspectives to help you respond to your thoughts more rationally.
- Evaluate the pros and cons of thinking a particular way or evaluate the pros and cons of *not* thinking this way.
- Do a "behavioral experiment" to evaluate whether or not a thought is true or helpful. For example: The thought "no one likes me" could be tested by asking various people if they like you. The person is asked to gather and evaluate evidence supporting or contradicting the belief.

How does one do CBT with people who have difficulty with these kinds of abstract question? How does one ask questions pertaining to thoughts to people who can't readily identify a thought, much less analyze it?

As we paid more attention to these language and cognitive problems, we couldn't help but notice something else. A great many of our deaf patients were admitted to the hospital because of severe behavior problems, especially aggression towards others. In a medical context, it is common to assume that some form of mental illness caused these behavior problems and that the appropriate intervention is medication. However, we increasingly began to question this assumption. These behaviors seemed more related to poor language development than to mental illness. After all, how do you learn concepts like coping, emotional self-regulation or conflict resolution when you have poorly developed language? How do you learn to express emotions in language, not behavior, if your language is itself poorly developed?

To make matters worse, we also found that that our deaf patients had experienced very high levels of developmental trauma: neglect, physical, and sexual abuse. Almost all had experienced the trauma of lifelong communication isolation. Some may have been born with neurological compromises, but with so many subsequent bad life experiences, it was often difficult to tease out whether bad biology or bad environments were more harmful to how they interacted.

Regardless of the causes, the result is a group of people who:

- Didn't use sign or spoken language well.
- Couldn't read or write beyond simple words.

- Had enormous gaps in their knowledge of the world.
- Often showed challenging behaviors, like aggression.

Given these challenges, many were not prepared to sit and use a language-based helping procedure, such as counseling. Even when counselors signed very well, it was difficult to make much headway and it often seemed like we were trying to lay the foundation for future counseling. In fact, that is *exactly* what we were doing. It just took us a while to realize it. Since coming to this realization, I've tried to better organize these "pre-therapy" experiences and draw on the collective wisdom of the many Deaf mental health care counselors with whom I've worked.

Many Hearing People Have Language and Learning Challenges

The Westborough Deaf Unit was located adjacent to two units for hearing adolescents with severe behavioral and emotional problems. We often talked with the staff from these programs throughout the day and found something surprising when we compared notes. Even though the adolescent units worked almost exclusively with hearing people, the staff there said their patients seemed to have the same profound language and learning challenges as the people we were serving. While they knew spoken language, their language skills were so poor that their reasoning abilities were also compromised. Staff there would also talk about patients who:

- Had small vocabularies.
- Were very concrete thinkers who had difficulty seeing patterns, making connections, or understanding concepts they couldn't immediately see, feel, or touch.
- Could not organize space. For instance, the task of cleaning a room would be overwhelmingly difficult or they wouldn't be able to complete a simple jigsaw puzzle.
- Had poor attending abilities. In order to learn anything, one has to attend. If a person is too sleepy, excited or isn't able to manage their emotions, the result is often an inability to attend and, therefore, an inability to learn and remember.
- Had poor short- and long-term memory. Poor memory contributes to poor learning.
- Showed poor reasoning skills. They didn't see cause and effect. They couldn't consider possibilities ("if this, then that"). They couldn't consider other points of view. They couldn't talk to themselves or coach themselves through a difficulty.
- Had limited ability to read and interpret the facial expressions and emotions of other people. In fact, they often couldn't identify their own emotions.
- Had poor reading, writing and other academic skills. They were teenagers, yet their academic abilities were well below middle school level (Gaines, Meltzer, & Glickman 2009).

Later, we discussed our experiences with staff that worked with adult hearing persons who had severe and chronic mental illnesses. Again, we found some striking similarities. We often heard that these hearing adult patients had many of the same problems. While language deprivation appears to be a particular problem for many deaf persons, we realized that:

1. Severe language and learning challenges are very widespread in clinical populations.
2. Staff everywhere seem to have difficulty getting these persons to use the evidence-based practices, such as CBT, which they are constantly being told work so well.

Considering all of the developmental challenges, skill deficits and weaknesses that these deaf and hearing individuals exhibited, is it any wonder that many were not ready for a highly verbal, problem-solving oriented activity like mental health counseling?

CBT, Evidence-based Treatment and Best Practice

Most current evidenced-based counseling practices are some variant of CBT. This is largely because you can put CBT procedures into a manual, have people read, study, or follow the manual, and then test for results. It is also because CBT procedures can be formalized into a set of steps, and that you can evaluate the progress of people who follow these steps. It may well be, then, that CBT isn't necessarily better; it's just easier to put into a structure that lends itself to empirical research. How can one find evidence for the effectiveness of treatment approaches with people who can't or won't follow this structure?

In practice, individuals who have the kind of language and learning challenges that are the focus of this workbook would not make it into trials of therapy effectiveness. They would be screened out or would drop out early. Just being unable to read and write will make these persons unsuitable for any treatment procedure that requires following a workbook, reading, or writing. Their poor thinking skills would lead to dropping out of research that requires strict obedience to a treatment protocol. Indeed, many would not qualify because they would not be able to easily understand all the consent forms they must sign to qualify. Yet the evidence-based practices that are touted in the psychology literature and by insurance providers are presumed to be applicable to everyone.

For these reasons, I can't present you with empirical evidence that the strategies presented in this workbook work. With regard to deaf people with language and learning challenges, there is really no scientific evidence that anything works. There's no research and therefore there is no evidence (Glickman & Pollard 2013). This doesn't mean that nothing works. It just means that the evidence we have comes mainly from stories.

Nonetheless, CBT, especially the variant developed by Meichenbaum, coincides with much of what we know about best practices. We know that best practices are focused on eliciting informed, client engagement. We know that it's vital that clients and staff share a map for what they are doing, and that the clients find value in following this map. We know that people in a therapeutic relationship with clinicians/staff who they feel understand and support them, do better. We know that it is vital to work from client strengths and to develop their belief in their own capacity for change and growth. We also know that any treatment method has to be adapted for individual and cultural considerations (Duncan et al. 2010). You will find these themes well addressed in this workbook.

What is Pre-therapy?

There are many reasons why a person may not be ready to participate in counseling and psychotherapy, regardless of the therapeutic approach used. The concept of "pre-treatment" or "pre-therapy" routinely comes up in mental health literature. It comes up when people talk about "stages of change," and readiness for change, as with Motivational Interviewing (Miller & Rollnick 2002; Prochaska, Norcross, & DiClemente 1994). In that case, people are helped to become more ready to make use of change-oriented treatment, such as psychotherapy. Pre-therapy also occurs:

- When people receive psychoeducation about mental health and mental illness. This psychoeducation is designed to teach people how to use mental health services. It often is designed to teach people how to be mental health consumers, including how to talk to psychiatrists about medication risks and benefits.
- When people discuss the stigma associated with mental health care. Campaigns to overcome stigma by emphasizing how common it is for people to struggle with mental health problems are designed, in part, to make it easier for people to make use of mental health interventions.
- When people are oriented to the procedures and expectations associated with particular styles of psychotherapy, such as the pre-therapy orientations in dialectical behavior therapy (Linehan 1993). Pre-therapy orientations have also been used with minority communities where the concepts of mental health, mental illness, counseling and psychotherapy are new (Acosta, Yamamoto, & Evans 1982; Dolgin, Salazar, & Cruz 1987; Sue & Morishima 1982).

- In Allen Ivey's developmental therapy. Ivey showed how various psychotherapy styles work for people with different cognitive abilities. Ivey contributed the important and powerful idea that counseling and therapy styles have to match the thinking abilities and belief systems of the consumer (Ivey, 1986, 1991). As a doctoral student, I worked closely with Ivey. The most valuable idea he taught me was that counseling and psychotherapy must fit the cognitive developmental abilities of the client. That idea is a guiding assumption of this workbook.
- In the precursors model associated with Fred Hanna where psychological attributes (e.g., a sense of necessity, a willingness to experience anxiety, self-awareness, the ability to confront a problem, will and effort, hope and social support) are developed to prepare people for the emotional demands of psychotherapy (Hanna 2002).

All of these pre-therapy approaches can be helpful and applicable, but the approach presented in this workbook is designed to tackle the particular challenges created by poorly developed language and thinking skills.

In this pre-therapy approach, we engage these individuals in counseling by providing them with a simple, clear, and non-stigmatizing way to think about "getting better." We help them discover their own abilities and capacity for change and we help them develop foundation problem-solving skills. We interact with them in a way which challenges their learned helplessness and dependency and helps them construct a self-story of "I can do it."

When does pre-therapy work become therapy? The line in practice is blurry. Here is a helpful way to think about this.

Many people are referred to mental health programs and providers because someone else is worried about them, usually because of their challenging behaviors. Mental health programs, especially government funded programs, are tasked with the job of engaging these persons to become, at the least, safer. When something bad happens, like a suicide or a school shooting, and it is done by someone who appears to be mentally ill, people ask the staff of mental health programs why they didn't prevent it. When someone commits suicide, for instance, people look around and ask why the treatment providers didn't prevent it from happening.

People like to imagine that mental health providers have some kind of magic, that we can force people to behave differently. In reality, mental health providers don't have that kind of power. We perform at our best when we form helping relationships and, in that process, engage people in the process of their own growth and recovery. The best tool we have for preventing bad things from happening always boils down to the quality of our relationships and our ability to draw people into a collaborative process of problem solving with us.

At the end of the day, mental health treatment has to be understood and chosen to be effective. The resources should be there and they should be tailored to different communities so that people will want to use them. We should aim to offer quality services that people want, not force them to accept services they don't want. In any case, mental health providers aren't particularly good at forcing people to change, neither should we be. We are at our best when we can skillfully *invite* people to change and, once the invitation is accepted, provide them with tools tailored to their own abilities and mental world. This workbook is written with this awareness and in this spirit.

The line, then, between pre-therapy and therapy is essentially the moment of informed consent. Many of the techniques presented in this workbook, such as helping people learn coping skills and develop more helpful self-talk, are staples of CBT. The real difference between pre-therapy, or pre-CBT, and CBT is this issue of informed consent. Pre-therapy is about the work of creating informed, motivated consumers of mental health care. Pre-therapy is best practice because it is about engaging people so they see purpose in working with us in a particular way. Once they become informed, motivated participants, they become people who are "good candidates for psychotherapy," who can use this process to achieve important life goals. Pre-therapy, then, becomes therapy when the individual understands and chooses it. It's at that point that it becomes fair to use the word "client" to describe the person receiving services.

There are many workbooks available on CBT. However, this is a cognitive behavior *pre-therapy* workbook, designed to help you bring individuals with language and learning challenges to the starting gate where counseling and psychotherapy can help them. Because many of the people you serve are not prepared to use a therapy manual, this workbook is designed:

- For *staff*, especially line staff with whom the "patients," "clients," "consumers," "members," or "persons served" spend most of their time.[4]
- For *clinical* and *administrative leaders* who are presumed to have a solid foundation in CBT and other therapy approaches but who need assistance translating these to line staff and the people served in their programs.
- To be used in places where there is a team of mental health workers, such as psychiatric hospitals, partial hospitals, day programs, residential schools, rehabilitation facilities of different stripes, and community outreach programs. Some of these workers have professional degrees and licenses in fields like psychiatry, psychology, social work, counseling, occupational therapy, and nursing. Many, however, do not.
- To foster a seamless treatment context where all staff, in their own disciplines are helping the people they serve learn the life skills they need to advance towards their goals.

This workbook presents a framework and language that is useful for both the people providing services and the people receiving them. There is no assumption that staff members have a broad range of coping and conflict resolution skills while the people receiving services do not. In fact, it is far safer to assume that everyone needs help in these areas. Thus, discussions of skills should be raised with staff as well as clientele. For example, we ask the staff, "When you are angry, nervous, depressed, stressed, etc., how do you cope? How do you manage conflicts? What skill, or lack of skills, do you model each day?" If you hope to be a good teachers/counselors, you need to be able to practice what you preach, to "walk the walk," to demonstrate how to cope and solve problems effectively.

This program asks a lot of staff. It asks them to give up some of the power that comes with their roles. It asks them to see themselves as skill coaches, providing more support and less management of the people being served. It teaches them the fundamentals of best practice in mental health settings, and it also asks them to work with humility. Not all program staff will embrace this. Many will feel too vulnerable. They may hold unhelpful beliefs such as the following:

> "I'm staff so I'm in charge."
> "As a staff person, I can't show any weakness or vulnerability."
> "It's not safe for me to admit I have problems also."
> "If I allow myself to be vulnerable, to work in the one-down way you recommend, both the clients and the administration will walk all over me."

There is a great deal of emphasis in this program on changing the usual power dynamics between staff and clientele and working from a humbler one-down stance. Because assuming this stance may make people feel more vulnerable, it is vital that supervisors and administrators show that this is, indeed, a safe, acceptable and recommended way to work much of the time. The pre-therapy approach presented here will not work if staff feel that they are responsible for fixing client problems or, at the least, controlling client behaviors. If you are convinced that mental health providers must always maintain the posture of experts in human behavior and must always remain in control, this is not the program for you.

This approach is often therapeutic for staff as they learn how to:

- Recognize their own abilities.
- Develop their own coping and conflict resolution skills.
- Become more empathetic.
- Improve their own moods and behaviors by changing what they say to themselves.
- Develop more comfort with "sharing the dilemmas" they face as staff people with the persons they are trying to help.
- Recognize that they can't fix someone against their will, and that instead they need to become more skilled at partnering with people in their recovery or growth process.
- Appreciate that their job is to teach psychosocial skills and that to do so they need to model these skills themselves.

In addition, having a simple schema for "what we do together" brings coherence to a program. The schema is that we work together to develop skills. At a deeper level, we work to change stories. Skills and stories.

The Lessons

The domains of the pre-therapy model presented in this workbook are summarized in the pyramid presented in Figure I.2. Remember, these are the recommended practices *for staff* to bring their clientele into the world of meaningful CBT.

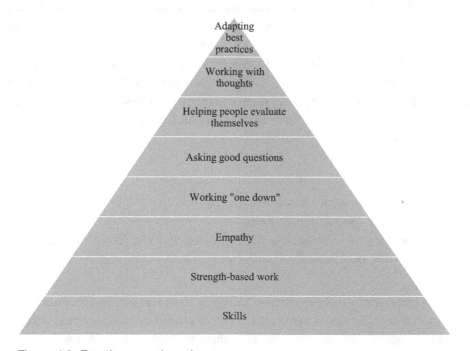

Figure I.2 Pre-therapy domains

Let's look at each lesson more closely.

Skills (Lessons 1 and 2)

The first pre-therapy issue is finding a way to talk about what we are doing. We need a simple, clear, non-stigmatizing way to explain "how we propose to help you." This model is our map or, more technically, our "schema."

Drawing on the essence of CBT, we find this map by discussing skills. What we are doing together is developing skills. It doesn't matter if you think of this work as counseling, psychotherapy, recovery, pursuing goals, or making a life worth living. We discuss our work by referring to skills; both those you already have and those you might want to develop. The language or *schema* of skills is the territory of this work. It is a map showing where you've come from and where you can go.

This simple, straightforward map takes the mystery out of mental health work. The schema of "skill building" is also very practical. You can accomplish quite a lot by engaging your clientele in the process of developing skills.

Lessons 1 and 2 lay out a vocabulary for two kinds of essential skill. The first relate to skills for managing one's inner life (e.g., emotions, thoughts, sensations, experiences, and symptoms). The second concerns skills for managing one's outer life (e.g., relationships and conflicts with other people). In both cases, skills are considered from a developmental model. That is, we recognize that skills develop from simple to complex. This workbook focuses on assisting people with developmentally simpler skills.

Strength-based Work (Lesson 3)

A second important pre-therapy concept is working in a strength-based way. People who sometimes behave badly or function poorly are used to getting a lot of criticism and correction from others. If their experience in a treatment program is that staff focus on what they do wrong or on problems that staff believe they have, then it is understandable that they will resist treatment and find counseling unappealing. An important engagement strategy is making the conversation affirming to them. This is easy to say but difficult to do. Lesson 3 presents four strategies for doing strength-based work with individuals who function poorly and/or have challenging behaviors. These strategies focus on ways to stop, notice and talk about skills that are already present, including asking questions that *pull for* the skills and strengths people have.

Empathy (Lessons 4)

Lesson 4 addresses empathy. It is widely recognized in mental health care that the single most important tool we have to help people is our ability to develop a therapeutic relationship with them. Nothing is more important in our ability to work well with people than our capacity to communicate to them an empathetic understanding of their world. The most effective mental health counselors lead with empathy. That is, the first thing they do is to empathize. Before we can ask anyone to change or learn skills, we need to convey a full, deep appreciation of who they are and what they struggle with. As a general rule, people will not engage in skill building if they don't feel understood and accepted. When a person isn't willing to work on skills, the most likely problem is that the counselor or team has not shown enough empathy.

I find this to be a good rule of thumb: *When all else fails, strive to better communicate an empathetic understanding of what the person you are serving is experiencing.* In other words, always *lead (begin) with empathy.*

Working One-Down (Lesson 5)

Lesson 5 addresses how staff uses power in their relationships with the people they serve. Typically, people with language and learning challenges find themselves in disempowered roles. People tell them how they should behave, what they should do, and use behavior plans, like Sheldon did with Penny, to get them to respond in certain ways. This sometimes creates behavior change, but the controlling environment also provokes resistance and distorts staff-client relationships.

The people with language and learning challenges that we are trying to engage are typically *acted on.* They find themselves in settings where there is a very fine line between efforts to help them and efforts to control them. As a result, they usually don't develop a strong sense of themselves as capable of managing their own lives. They become dependent on others. When they do assert themselves, they often do so in socially unskilled ways, such as bullying.

Our pre-therapy efforts are designed to reverse this pattern. We want to help people discover their own abilities and motivate them to develop their abilities further. This requires a very different way of working with them than what they, and most staff in mental health programs, are used to.

A more effective way to engage people is to use a one-down style that reverses the usual power structure and is consistent with our strength-based focus. When staff works one-down, they learn how to skillfully *invite*—not compel—client participation. Under this new way of working, one-up interventions, where you directly try to influence or control people by telling them what to do, become last choice interventions.

Asking Good Questions (Lesson 6)

Consistent with a one-down style of work, our counseling style shifts to one where we mainly ask good questions. For many programs, this is a dramatic shift from a style where staff usually direct or tell people what they should do. Generally speaking, when it comes to engaging people in these skill-building efforts, asking good questions works better than telling people what they should do. Asking good questions promotes more skillful thinking and problem solving. Good questions help people become active *agents* in their own development.

Three types of question are discussed in this workbook. Strength-based questions are discussed in Lesson 3. Lesson 6 presents questions that are more problem based but that help to answer the questions, "Why did the problem occur?" and "What will help you do better?" These questions are formally referred to as "behavior analysis." The third style of questions is discussed in Lesson 7.

Self-assessment (Lesson 7)

In Lesson 7, we draw on the excellent structure for asking questions that is presented in William Glasser's reality therapy. Glasser's WDEP (**w**ant, **d**o, **e**valuate, **p**lan) format is immensely practical and useful and should be in every counselor's toolbox (Wubbolding 2000).

By asking good questions, you help people evaluate themselves. Lesson 7 also presents self-monitoring, another commonly used CBT procedure that promotes self-assessment. Self-monitoring forms and procedures provide a user-friendly way to determine whether or not something one does is helpful. These tools enable people to become their own judge, to decide whether or not to proceed or back off, to measure whether or not they are making progress towards their own goals. They are very useful for pre-therapy and can help move the person from pre-therapy to therapy.

Working with Thoughts (Lessons 8–10)

Lessons 8 through 10 address the cognitive, or C, part of CBT. Many people with language and learning challenges have difficulty working with thoughts and beliefs. They have difficulty with abstract thinking, including the ability to actually think about thinking. The cognitive part of CBT offers a wealth of interventions designed to help people think better, *provided they are able to notice how they think*. This is a big "if." These three lessons present simple ways to help people pay attention to their thoughts. We focus on self-talk, the simplest form of cognitive therapy, and help people learn the skill of talking to themselves with a friendlier voice.

It's very useful for staff to understand how thoughts, feelings and behaviors reinforce each other even when the people you are working with have difficulty making these connections. Lesson 9 is devoted to this topic. It is important to understand, for instance, the kind of thoughts that accompany depression, anxiety, anger, and substance use, as well as the kind of thoughts that accompany recovery. This will help you to search for opportunities to help the people you serve make these connections.

These lessons also outline activities that help people "externalize" their thoughts; that is, to put their thoughts outside of themselves, much like characters in a comic strip do with thought bubbles. One technique is to create creatures that talk to you, promoting different moods and behaviors. Another technique is to develop scripts for practicing helpful self-talk.

Treatment Adaptations from Deaf Mental Health Care (Lessons 11 and 12)

On the surface, the final two lessons may appear to be about relapse prevention. However, their real focus is on the issue of adapting counseling and teaching approaches to the unique needs of this clientele. Specialists in DMHC commonly adapt standard counseling practices in predictable ways. Some adaptations, as you will see, have to do with the structure of American Sign Language and the way ASL *pulls for* certain kinds of conversation. Some have to do with the fact that Deaf mental health care is so obsessively focused on good communication, including finding ways of helping that are less dependent on sophisticated language abilities.

These adaptations are examples of what is now being called "Deaf gain" (Bauman & Murray 2014). The opposite of "hearing loss," "Deaf gain" refers to aspects of the experience of Deaf people that provide a benefit or gain for hearing people. In this workbook, we're focused on five kinds of "Deaf gain" adaptation:

- Paying close attention to communication skills and process.
- Working with examples and stories.
- Using pictorial aids.
- Role playing.
- Putting the people who receive services into helper or teacher roles.

Tools Incorporated into This Workbook

All 12 lessons also use true stories, pictures, activities, quizzes, and discussion questions to help you understand the content.

Pictures and Illustrations

Wherever possible, pictures are used to illustrate key points. Some of these pictures were drawn by Deaf artist Michael Krajnak and were originally found on the CD that accompanied my 2009 book. These pictures are now available at the Routledge website (http://routledge.com/9781138916937. Look up this book and click on the E-resources tab.). Stock photos, purchased from iStock.com, are also used. A few photos of Deaf interpreter Raylene Lotz signing key concepts are also included.

Tips, Questions, and Definitions

You will also find these elements included in the lessons:

 Bright idea: Concise statements of key learning points.

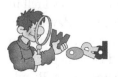 **Definition:** Key vocabulary is presented with definitions and examples.

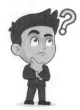

Questions to ponder: Questions posed to you, the reader, to help you apply lessons to your own life.

Practice Exercise: Each lesson contains exercises that provide opportunities to practice the techniques introduced.

Skill Learned

The skills taught in each lesson are summarized in a series of bullet points at the end of each lesson.

Quizzes and Answers

Each lesson concludes with a short multiple-choice quiz, designed to reinforce key points. An answer key with explanations is also included.

Questions for Discussion

A series of open-ended questions is included to guide further consideration and group discussion of the ideas presented.

References

References in this workbook are intentionally kept to a minimum. I include references to specific works or authors if I am discussing a particular work or if a theme, approach or idea was clearly developed by other people. The researchers, clinicians and other people who have influenced this approach are documented in this introduction and in the acknowledgments.

Confidentiality

The workbook contains many stories. A few of the stories are from television or movies, but most are from real-life experiences, mainly those that took place in Deaf mental health educational, mental health, and rehabilitation settings. Some of these are my personal experiences, but others are based on stories other people have told me. Having done this work for over three decades, I've collected a lot of stories.

Almost everyone likes stories and learns from clinical examples but this practice has its drawbacks. On one hand, storytelling is a particularly "Deaf-friendly" way of teaching, as discussed in Lesson 11. On the other hand, personal stories could violate an individual's privacy. The Deaf world is notoriously small and confidentiality is an enormous concern.

I couldn't write this workbook without stories, but I am very aware of the dangers of violating people's privacy. The only way to handle this is to disguise the identity of the people involved in the stories by changing, not only names and sometimes gender, but other non-essential details. The more one changes a story, the more one can be accused of making it up, of it not being true. However, I'm reasonably confident that the stories I tell in the lessons that follow will ring very true for deaf and hearing readers alike. They are often stories of day-to-day problems that occur in treatment settings. It's typically very mundane stuff. People argue over what television show to watch. They argue because someone took food out of the refrigerator that belonged to someone else. People get upset because staff members say "no." People want something and can't immediately get it. People are frustrated, anxious, angry, or afraid, and don't handle it well.

There are stories about staff as well. The more I've consulted with different programs, the more I've found that pre-therapy challenges are universal. I'm counting on the fact that if you do this work, you will recognize your own colleagues, clients/students, and work challenges in these stories. I'm betting you will see yourself in the stories also. If you think you know who a particular person is, that is only because you have met people like this before and the situations are familiar.

I welcome feedback on any aspect of the approach presented here. I'd also love to hear stories about tools that you have used to teach and counsel persons with language and learning challenges as well as your ideas about other strategies (besides those discussed in Lessons 11 and 12) from Deaf mental health care that seem effective for deaf and hearing people. You can reach me through my website, www.neilglickman.com.

Conclusion

Robert Fulghum famously wrote that, "All I really need to know I learned in kindergarten" (Fulghum 2003). He means that when people develop normally, they learn basic life lessons very early on. The lessons become more sophisticated as you grow older. "Play fair," for instance, develops into a more complicated appreciation of justice and social harmony.

I think he's very right . . . when people develop normally. But what happens when they don't develop normally? What happens when so many basic rules for life are *not* learned in kindergarten?

Children who never learned these basic life rules become adults who struggle to manage their emotions, deal with other people, stay safe, and function independently. They may or may not develop formal mental illnesses with names like schizophrenia, bipolar disorder, and posttraumatic stress disorder, but they get in trouble. Some end up in jail; others end up in mental health and rehabilitation programs.

This book is for you if you work in a program that serves people who never learned these life lessons. When people are deaf and language deprived, they may have these kinds of problems, but there are plenty of hearing people who have language, cognitive, and other developmental deficits that make it hard for them to function well and benefit from standard mental health practices.

In a mental health setting, we may want to provide therapy, but what we often end up providing, or struggling to provide, is pre-therapy. We might want to provide the "evidence-based practices" like CBT that insurance providers and others insist are the marks of quality treatment, but find we spend all of our time getting people ready for such work. My own stress levels went way down when I finally understood this. Many of the people we were trying to help never learned foundation skills in kindergarten, and now they are adults in trouble. We need to build this developmental understanding into our treatment model. We need to help people learn now what they should have learned long ago.

Notes

1. Thus, in this book. "Deaf is used to indicate a culturally Deaf person or the Deaf community and culture. When "deaf" is used, we are referring to people who can't hear, whether or not they are culturally Deaf. If the distinction between culturally and auditorally deaf people isn't important, we use the lowercase "deaf."
2. See Glickman, *Deaf Mental Health Care*, pages 61–63.
3. Throughout this book, words written in capital letters represent glosses for the American Sign Language signs. ASL does not have a widely used written form, but it is conventional to gloss or tag particular English words to represent specific signs. These glosses are approximations, not translations. Glossing often appears to make ASL look like simple, non-grammatical versions of English. There are conventions for representing ASL grammar, but it is not essential to present them in this workbook.
4. Most of the time in this book, we refer to "people receiving services," or "people we serve." Occasionally, we will use other terms. "Patient" is a term appropriate for medical settings. "Client" assumes the person has chosen to make use of services. "Resident" or "member" can describe people who live in group homes or attend programs. The term "people we serve," while awkward, seems to best fit the spirit of this work, but we vary somewhat the words used to create a smoother, easier to read text.

References

Acosta, F., Yamamoto, J., & Evans, L. (1982). *Effective psychotherapy for low-income and minority patients*. New York: Plenum.

Bauman, H.-D. L., & Murray, J. J. (Eds.). (2014). *Deaf gain: Raising the stakes for human diversity*. Minneapolis, MN: University of Minnesota Press.

Dolgin, D., Salazar, A., & Cruz, S. (1987). The Hispanic treatment program: Principles of effective psychotherapy. *Journal of Contemporary Psychotherapy, 17*(4), 285–289.

Duncan, B. L., Miller, S. D., Wampold, B. E., & Hubble, M. (Eds.). (2010). *The heart and soul of change: Delivering what works in therapy* (2nd ed.). Washington, DC: American Psychological Association.

Fulghum, R. (2003). *All I really need to know I learned in kindergarten*. New York: Ballantine.

Gaines, J., Meltzer, B., & Glickman, N. (2009). Language and learning challenges in adolescent hearing psychiatric inpatients. In N. Glickman (Ed.), *Cognitive behavioral therapy for deaf and hearing persons with language and learning challenges*. New York: Routledge.

Glickman, N. (1996). What is culturally affirmative psychotherapy? In N. Glickman & M. Harvey (Eds.), *Culturally affirmative psychotherapy with deaf persons*. Mahwah, NJ: Lawrence Erlbaum Associates.

Glickman, N. (2009). *Cognitive behavioral therapy for deaf and hearing persons with language and learning challenges*. New York: Routledge.

Glickman, N. (Ed.). (2013). *Deaf Mental Health Care*. New York: Routledge.

Glickman, N., & Pollard, R. (2013). Deaf mental health research: Where we've been and where we hope to go. In Glickman, N. (Ed.), *Deaf mental health care*. New York: Routledge.

Gournaris, M. J., & Aubrecht, A. L. (2013). Deaf/hearing cross -cultural conflicts and the creation of culturally competent treatment programs. In N. S. Glickman (Ed.), *Deaf mental health care*. New York: Routledge.

Hanna, F. J. (2002). *Therapy with difficult clients: Using the precursors model to awaken change*. Washington, DC: American Psychological Association.

Ivey, A. (1986). *Developmental therapy*. San Francisco, CA: Jossey-Bass.

Ivey, A. (1991). *Developmental strategies for helpers: Individual, family and network interventions*. Pacific Grove, CA: Brooks/Cole.

Linehan, M. (1993). *Cognitive behavioral treatment of borderline personality disorder*. New York: Guilford Press.

Lorre, C., Prady, B., Ferrari, M., Aronsohn, L, Rosenstock, R. (Writers), & Cendrowski, M. (Director). (2009). "The Gothowitz Deviation" (Television series episode). In L. Aronsohn (Executive Producer), *The Big Bang Theory*. Los Angeles, CA: Warner Brothers Television.

Meichenbaum, D. (1977a). *Cognitive-behavioral modification: An integrative approach*. New York: Plenum Press.

Meichenbaum, D. (1977b). *Stress-inoculation training: Cognitive-behavior modification*. New York: Plenum Press.

Meichenbaum, D. (1994). *A clinical handbook/practical therapist manual for assessing and treating adults with post-traumatic stress disorder*. Waterloo, Canada: Institute Press.

Meichenbaum, D. (1996). *Mixed anxiety and depression: A cognitive-behavioral approach*. The Newbridge assessment and treatment of psychological disorders series. New York: Newbridge Communications, Inc.

Meichenbaum, D. (2001). *Treatment of individuals with anger-control problems and aggressive behaviors: A clinical handbook*. Clearwater, FL: Institute Press.

Meichenbaum, D. (2012). *Roadmap to resilience: A guide for military, trauma victims and their families*. Clearwater, FL: Institute Press.

Meichenbaum, D., & Biemiller, A. (1998). *Nurturing independent learners: Helping students take charge of their learning*. Newton, MA: Brookline Books.

Miller, W. R., & Rollnick, S. (2002). *Motivational interviewing: Preparing people for change* (2nd ed.). New York: Guilford Press.

Pollard, R. (1998). Psychopathology. In M. Marschark & M. D. Clark (Eds.), *Psychological perspectives on deafness*. Mahwah, NJ: Lawrence Erlbaum Associates.

Prochaska, J. O., Norcross, J. C., & DiClemente, C. C. (1994). *Changing for good*. New York: William Morrow.

Schaller, S. (1991). *A man without words*. Los Angeles, CA: University of California Press.

Sue, S., & Morishima, J. (1982). *The mental health of Asian-Americans*. San Francisco, CA: Jossey-Bass.

Wubbolding, R. (2000). *Reality therapy for the 21st century*. Bridgeport, NJ: Brunner-Routledge.

Coping Skills

Introduction

In Lesson 1, we begin talking about skills. We focus on skills that are very important for mental health, the ability to handle or cope with strong emotions. We attend to a large array of behaviors that human beings engage in to help themselves cope and function, with the goal of understanding that all these behaviors are skills. We attend especially to skills that are developmentally simpler; that is, skills that people normally learn and use as children. Our intent is to help the people we serve recognize and name the skills they already have. This is a first step to engaging them in the work of strengthening these skills and learning new skills.

A Coping Skills Story

While I was traveling through Costa Rica, my traveling group decided to go on a zip-line canopy tour. These are tours of the jungle from the treetops. You put on a harness and climb up a wooden tower to the top of the trees. Then a guide attaches the harness to a cable connected to another tower. You put one hand in a thick glove and hold it behind you, letting the cable wire slip through your grip while you hold onto the harness with the other. On this particular zip line tour, the cable hung several hundred feet above the forest floor. The platforms were built around the top of the tree trunks. These platforms were about 10 square feet with no railings. Hundreds of feet separated the 12 treetop platforms. I have had a fear of heights my whole life. I couldn't believe I was about to leap off of a tower, hundreds of feet above the jungle floor, in the middle of Central America. How did I let myself be talked into doing something so completely against my nature?

As the group members climbed up the first tower, I learned that other group members had also experienced panic attacks in the past. A few members of the group started to hyperventilate. They turned back. The tour guides told us that we shouldn't worry because we could practice on the first few cables. I thought that meant these cables might be 10 feet off the ground. It actually meant that you could get off after the fourth platform; there was no turning back until that point. All of the platforms were at the treetop level. The "practice" platforms were just as high up and just as scary as the ones that followed.

Before we set out, the guides provided an orientation. The main thing I remember was a guide telling us that "speed is your friend." He meant that once you left the platform, you should travel as fast as you could to the next one. If you clutched the cable to slow yourself down, you might not make it to the next platform. I knew I would want to clutch the cable. I had images of myself dangling on the cable, suspended hundreds of feet above the jungle floor. My anxiety soared.

The walk up the wood steps to the first treetop platform was the most frightening part of the experience. I had no idea we would climb so high so quickly. Standing on top of the tower, I was so terrified that my legs buckled underneath me. I could not stand up. Many of the other group members appeared nervous but excited and happy. They were having fun. The really nervous members, besides me, had already turned back. As the other tour members lined up to be hooked up to the cable, I hung back and sunk to my knees, terrified. I saw the other tour members leap from the platform and hurtle themselves off into the distance. Because of the tree canopy, I couldn't see where they landed. The cable made a whirling, whizzing sound, and some of the participants hollered and cheered and screamed in delight. I was dead silent. I didn't know how I would survive this.

Fortunately, I had one thing going for me. I knew about coping skills. I had studied coping skills, knew my own coping skills, and was prepared to use them. Five coping skills came in especially handy.

First, and perhaps most important, I knew how to breathe slowly and fully from the diaphragm, the way babies do . . . the way I practiced in relaxation and meditation exercises. I began to breathe slowly and fully.

Second, I knew about self-talk. I knew how to think comforting but believable thoughts. I said to myself, "This may be a big deal to me, but to these tour guides, I'm just another scared American tourist, and we are just the morning tour group. They probably have an afternoon tour group. They are probably focused mostly on getting tips. If tourists died in these activities, they wouldn't be in business. Besides, I'm sure the government inspects these cables . . .

(Then I remembered that I was in Central America and that I wasn't confident that the United States government inspected zip-line cables in America. Drop that line of thinking, I thought.) I then told myself that the whole activity would be over in two hours, and I'd have a story to tell. I reminded myself that "This too shall pass."

Third, I was kneeling beside a tree in the middle of the platform. I moved my hand up and down the rough bark of the tree. I knew this sensory experience would be grounding. I let myself really feel the rough texture of the tree trunk. I let the sensory experience settle me.

While doing this, I noticed a stream of black ants marching up one of the crevices in the tree trunk. I realized this was something I could focus my attention on. I knew that having a focus, like looking at a candle flame or reciting the sound "om" or attending to one's breathing, was a common meditation technique. I focused my attention on the marching ants. I meditated on the ants. I watched the ants as I breathed slowly and slid my hands up and down the tree bark.

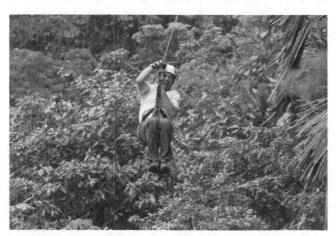

Figure 1.1 The author using his coping skills

Used with permission

Finally, I made a joke. I told my companions, "You know, I stopped praying years ago. Do you think God will give me credit if I make up for it now?" I laughed a little. I thought, "A lame joke, but I'll take it."

Then my turn came. I walked slowly up to the edge of the platform and the guide hooked me up. He told me to jump, but I couldn't. I was frozen. Finally, he lifted me up and pushed me off the edge. As I hurtled forward, I looked ahead and kept repeating to myself, "Speed is your friend. Speed is your friend."

In about a minute, I was on the next platform. I had made it. There were 11 platforms to go but once I had conquered one, I knew I'd survive. The rest were easier. As I was reaching the final platform, a photographer took this picture of me. He charged me $30. He didn't know that I would have paid $100 for it.

Practice Exercise 1.1

I'm aware that I used five coping skills to survive this experience:

1. Breathing.
2. Self-talk.
3. Sensory grounding.
4. Focused attention.
5. Humor.

Before going on, take a few minutes to reflect on your own coping skills. This is critical. Please don't jump ahead until you do this exercise.

What do you do to help yourself feel better when you are sad, anxious, angry, stressed or overwhelmed? Write down three to four specific actions or activities that you use to calm yourself in difficult situations. These are some of your coping skills:

_____

_____

_____

_____

Did you do the exercise? If you didn't, please don't go on. This is important because the first step in strength-based work is *noticing* and *labeling* the coping skills people already have. You will be able to notice these skills more easily in others if you are able to notice and label the skills *you* already have.

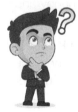 **Questions to ponder 1.1:** How hard is it for you to identify your own coping skills? How many could you identify? Are you satisfied with your ability to handle stress and unpleasant emotions or would you like to be more skillful at this?

Key Teaching Strategies

You might notice that I:

- Began Lesson 1 with a story.
- Included a picture.
- Introduced the idea of coping skills by giving examples, not offering a definition.
- Asked you to do a self-assessment and to consider whether your own abilities are adequate.

We will return to and build on these key teaching strategies throughout this workbook.

What Are Coping Skills?

Coping skills are behaviors that people use to manage unpleasant situations and emotions. In this program, coping skills focus on one's "inner world" of feelings, sensations, thoughts, and symptoms. They involve noticing what you are experiencing, then doing something to feel different.

The purpose of a coping skill is to feel better. People often cope by doing something to their environment, such as seeking out a different, more pleasant experience. In contrast, social skills involve interactions with other people. Social skills, including the important social skill of conflict resolution, will be discussed in the next lesson. Although coping skills and social skills sometimes overlap, coping skills are more inner focused while social skills are more outer focused.

In cognitive behavior therapy (CBT), coping skills are sometimes distinguished from emotional self-regulation skills. These are the things we do to keep ourselves as healthy and emotionally stable as possible. Emotional self-regulation skills include things like:

- Following regular sleep habits.
- Eating well.
- Developing interests and hobbies.
- Exercising.
- Connecting with other people, animals or a "higher power."

The term also refers to recognizing and naming what is going on in our bodies and doing things to feel less upset and happier.

The distinction between coping and self-regulation is not important to this program because we are aiming for simple vocabulary. It will be easier for your clients to understand these concepts if you use simple language and fewer, smaller, and easier words. Thus, we will use the term "coping skills" very broadly to refer to all of the activities people do to keep themselves as healthy and happy as possible, including what they do to manage distress. In this workbook, the term will include a broad range of human behaviors, including very common and simple activities.

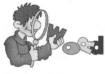

Coping skills

Definition 1.1: Coping skills: Activities that people do to keep themselves as happy and healthy as possible, including what they do to manage distress.

Example of coping skills: Eleanor loves all kinds of needlework. She doesn't think of needlework as coping skills but more as a hobby and recreation. Nonetheless, when she is stressed and upset, the first thing she does to cope and feel better is to pick up her needlework.

A Strength-based Approach

This workbook is designed to help you recognize and build on the skills that people already have. However, many people with language and learning challenges don't function at high skill levels. For instance, they may be poorly educated, unable to read and write well, unemployed, or unable to live independently. In addition, they are most likely in a structured program because of problem behaviors that have gotten them in trouble and caused other people to worry about them. How can a strength-based approach work with people who seem to function poorly and/or behave badly?

A strength-based approach can be very effective if you recognize that many common, everyday behaviors can be considered skills. If you understand that skills develop from simple to complex, even simple actions can be labeled as skills that you can then point out to a person as something he or she already does well. This also sets the stage for inviting the person to do better and to learn more skills.

The world of CBT is filled with skills that a person can use to manage their inner and outer worlds. You want to invite the people you serve into this world. The best way to do this is to recognize and celebrate what skills they already have rather than fault them for what they lack. After doing that, you can wonder out loud, and invite them to consider: *Is this enough? Could you do even better?*

The focus of Lesson 1 is on noticing and labeling skills that people already have, no matter how poorly developed these skills may be. The search for existing skills is at the core of a strength-based program. The larger strategy is not to fix problems but to *invite* people to further develop their existing skills or to learn new skills. You will explore strategies to do this in Lessons 4 through 7. But, before we introduce any strategies to help people change their behavior, you need to become an expert at noticing and labeling skills that a client already has.

 Bright idea 1.1: We begin to create strength-based programs by noticing and labeling skills that people already have. To do this, we need to see a great many everyday activities as skills and have a large vocabulary to name them.

Common Coping Skills

Now, let's consider different kinds of coping skill. As you learn about each one, ask yourself: Which are important to you? How are they important? Why are they important?

Some of the most common coping skills are:

1. Distraction.
2. Sensory-based Movement.
3. Controlled Breathing.
4. Humor and Laughter.
5. Creative Expression.
6. Religious and Spiritual Practices.
7. Thinking Skills and Positive Self-talk.
8. Mindfulness and Meditation.

Distraction through Activities

Distraction is a superficial but widely used skill. It gets your mind off of what is bothering you by shifting your attention to doing or thinking about something else. Distraction skills are so commonly used for coping that people may not realize other skills work at a deeper level. Distraction is helpful at times when you are not really prepared to deal with a feeling or a stressor. It puts off more profound and helpful ways of coping until later.

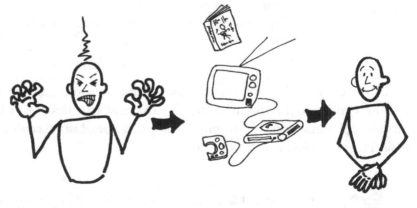

Figure 1.2 Distraction

You will often find that it's easy to identify when a client is using distraction skills. When you recognize the skills, you should name them, being as specific as possible. The names are the common ways the skills are talked about, everyday language.

Here are some examples:

"You seemed angry, but you went to your room and listened to music."

"I notice that when you are stressed, you use some of the game apps on your cell phone. What are your favorites? Do you notice how you feel when you use them?"

"It seems like it is just too painful to talk about that now, and you'd rather watch television. I'm impressed by your ability to distract yourself when you aren't ready to talk about some painful stuff. You have some great skills at distraction. I hope you will keep doing that until you feel ready to talk about it."

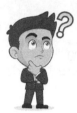

Questions to ponder 1.2: All of us use distraction skills. I used distraction while waiting for my turn to zip line by focusing on the rough tree bark and the moving line of ants. These were sensory-based distraction skills. When and how do you use distraction? What specific distraction skills do you use?

Distraction skills apply to any activity, even activities that are self-destructive. For example, a person might get into fights, race wildly, or do other dangerous things to distract themselves from pain. It is widely recognized that there are many unhealthy ways to cope with distress and pain. Substance use is a prime example. For the moment, we are not concerned with judging, or helping others to judge, whether or not a particular skill is healthy. We'll address that in Lessons 5 through 7. Rather, our focus is on getting people to talk about skills and establish the common understanding that *what we do here is develop skills*.

Developing a shared understanding for *what we do here* is especially important with people who have language and learning challenges. It's very likely they may not have a map in their heads for *how I get better*. In psychology, the word *schema* is used to describe a conceptual framework, a way of thinking about things. We want to establish in our work that our way of thinking about things, our schema, is to talk about skills. This will give us a concrete language for describing what people already do well and how they can do better.

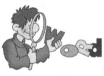

Schema

Definition 1.2: Schema: A conceptual framework, a way of thinking about things.

Example of a schema: Joe explained to people in his program that "the way we think about our work here is to talk about skills. We're very interested in skills. We're especially interested in skills you already have, so we spend a lot of time looking for those skills. Then we explore whether there are other skills you might want to learn that will help you in your life."

A distraction coping skill is any activity that a person engages in to distract themselves from unpleasant emotions and thoughts. Because these are concrete activities, it isn't hard to find or create pictures of them. Including pictures is one of our core teaching strategies. Lists of coping skills involving distraction are also easy to find (McKay, Wood, & Brantley 2007).

Bright idea 1.2: Everyone uses coping skills to help with distress but people rarely identify them as "skills." Distraction is the most common and easiest coping skill to identify. This is often where the conversations about skills begin.

Sensory Movement-based Skills

Sensory strategies help people to cope with distress through physical movement and using their senses. Sensory-based coping skills are very powerful for all people and may be the primary coping strategies for people with significant cognitive impairments. The effectiveness of a sensory-based coping strategy is well illustrated in the movie *Temple Grandin* (Jackson 2010) about a woman with autism who used her disability to gain insight into how animals see the world and, ultimately, create more humane strategies for slaughtering cattle.

When Temple was a young woman, she spent the summer on her aunt's farm. In the film, she observes how the cowboys get cows to calm down for injections by placing them in a metal contraption that contracts to hold them tightly in place. A bit later on, she goes to her room, but quickly becomes overwhelmed by sensory stimuli. Things are out of order. A piece of paper has fallen off the door onto the floor. The curtains are rustling. The fan is rotating, making a grating, metallic sound. Temple runs screaming from the house, followed by her frightened aunt. She runs to the contraption for the cows and puts herself in it. She begs her confused aunt to close it on her so that it holds her tightly. Only then can she calm down. This is a powerful illustration of how she used a sensory-based strategy to help her cope. Temple later uses this insight to create a "squeeze machine," which is used to help children with autism when they have tantrums. The machine allows the person to feel tight pressure on each side of their body and works in the same way that tight swaddling calms an infant.

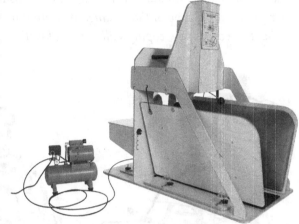

Figure 1.3 Temple Grandin's Squeeze Machine
Reprinted with permission from the Therafin Corporation

As with distraction, it is easy to illustrate sensory coping strategies. Recognizing how often sensory strategies are used as coping skills enhances your ability to have strength-based conversations with everyone, especially children and persons with intellectual challenges. For instance, a client might be using movement as a coping strategy when he or she:

- Rocks in a chair
- Walks or does any kind of exercise
- Interacts with a real or stuffed animal
- Rubs or pounds something
- Uses hearing, sight, smell, touch, and taste to feel better.

Eating pretzels is a good example of how a sensory experience can be used as a coping skill. Suppose you bring a bag of pretzels or carrots or a pack of chewing gum to keep your mouth moving while driving on a long trip? You are using the sensory principal that the experience of crunching and chewing can cause you to be more alert. If you struggle with anxiety, crunching and chewing also can be grounding. Chewing gum may even help avoid a panic attack.

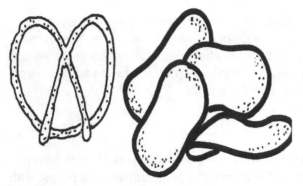

Figure 1.4 Can crunching pretzels or chips be a coping skill?

Of course, people overeat or eat unhealthy food as a way of coping. This wouldn't be a recommended healthy coping skill. Neither would drinking alcohol or engaging in cutting oneself to self-soothe. Nonetheless, they are coping skills. We start the conversation by recognizing that they serve a function for people even if they have a serious downside.

Scenario 1.1

On a psychiatric inpatient unit, the nursing staff watched in alarm as a patient with autism marched up and down the unit hall, pounding on the walls. They assumed he was escalating into an assault. The unit's astute occupational therapist recognized that he was using a sensory-based coping strategy and needed more of it. She approached him with a heavy medicine ball and tossed it to him. He tossed it back. She soon had him jumping rope and doing push-ups. The nursing staff caught on and cheered him on. Within a very short time, a potentially dangerous situation was diffused, and everyone was praising the patient for his excellent use of his new coping skills: "pound wall," "medicine ball," "jump rope" and "push-up."

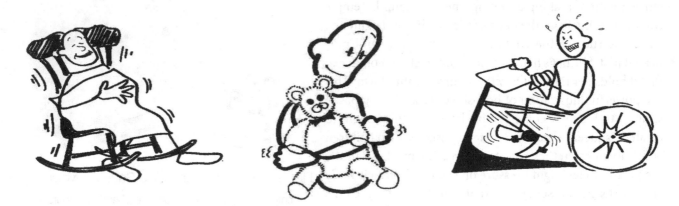

Figure 1.5 Sensory-based coping skills

Sensory-based coping skills are not just for children or people with language and learning challenges. Participating in sports or exercise, going to the gym, taking a long hot bath, going in the hot tub, etc., are all common examples of sensory-based coping strategies. People who spend a lot of time in intellectual pursuits are especially in need of sensory-based coping skills.

Scenario 1.2

Sal loves basketball. He talks about it all the time. He plays it whenever he can. He wears his team's jersey and colors. He has a collection of caps from every basketball team. Every day he sits and makes up statistics for actual or make-believe basketball games. When asked about his coping skills, Sal responds immediately by talking about basketball. Sal relates to his staff as coaches and referees and his housemates as team members. Staff quickly discovers that the way to connect with Sal and to introduce a discussion about skills is by framing things in terms of basketball.

Sensory and body-based coping skills also may be more important than thinking and problem-solving skills for people who have experienced serious childhood trauma. Practices such as yoga teach body and sensory self-awareness and that unpleasant emotions and sensations come and go. People practicing yoga learn how to self-regulate through breathing and turning inward. They may also learn the profound coping skill of observing their inner experience without judging. Trauma expert Bessel van der Kolk argues that these kind of body-based practices are more useful than conventional CBT in recovery from childhood trauma (Kolk 2014).

Diaphragmatic Breathing

Breathing well is an essential skill for everyone of all levels of ability, including clients and staff.

Breathing well is a core strategy for managing stress, anxiety and anger. Just about every book or workshop devoted to coping skills will address diaphragmatic breathing, especially to help manage anxiety and anger. When I was preparing for my zip-line experience, breathing well was the skill that was most helpful in coping with the overwhelming anxiety I felt.

The good news is almost everyone can learn to control their breathing. Strong language skills aren't needed for this.

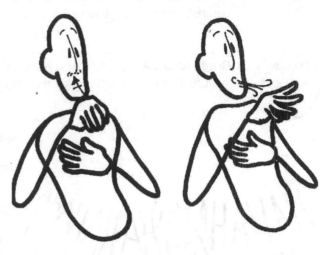

Figure 1.6 Deep breathing

Scenario 1.3

Joleen has severe cerebral palsy and cannot walk or stand independently. She is strapped into a wheelchair because her arms flail about when they are not restrained. Joleen sometimes has outburst of temper during which she thrashes around in her chair. She has learned the key coping skill of abdominal breathing. Staff and she have worked out a plan whereby a staff member stands in front of her and breathes slowly, deeply and obviously, modeling what they hope she will do. Importantly, they don't tell her to breathe. They don't say, "You should use your breathing skills now." Instead, they model it and she takes the cue. This is a much more subtle and respectful way of making a suggestion.

When Joleen stops and breathes, she usually settles down. Because she is strapped into her chair and unable to do much harm to other people, staff members can wait for her to breathe and calm down, then re-engage with her. Joleen's mobility and cognitive impairments limit her repertoire of coping skills, but she can breathe as skillfully as anyone. Staff members are quick to praise her for using this wonderful coping skill.

Practice Exercise 1.2

1. Sit comfortably in a chair.
2. Relax your head and neck.
3. Put your dominant hand gently on your stomach. Place your non-dominant hand on your chest.
4. Breathe in slowly through your nose. Notice that your dominant hand rises and falls with your breathing. Your non-dominant hand resting on your chest should barely move. As you inhale, it may help to gently think to yourself "in." As you exhale, you may say to yourself "out." Keep repeating the words "in" and "out," along with your breathing. Eventually, make your inner voice quieter and quieter.
5. Continue this gentle breathing for at least five minutes.

Deep, abdominal breathing is natural for babies, but adults often have to relearn what they once knew. There are many variations on this theme and many resources are available to help you learn more.

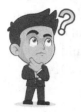

Questions to ponder 1.3: Don't assume that you breathe skillfully. If you are a "normal" adult in our society, you have probably forgotten the breathing skills you knew as a baby and you probably need to retrain yourself on this core coping skill. Chances are good that when you are angry, anxious, or stressed, you breathe in a short, shallow way that makes your symptoms worse. Ask yourself honestly whether you need to practice diaphragmatic breathing so you can help others with this skill. Do you need to breathe better to help your own coping?

Bright idea 1.4: Everyone who works in human services should be able to model proper abdominal breathing. We need these breathing skills to manage our own stress and teach clients.

Humor and Laughing

Laughter is another natural coping strategy.

Scenario 1.4

George was a Deaf program member who was frequently assaultive. As a result, it was difficult for staff to identify George's coping skills. It seemed like he was quick to anger whenever he didn't immediately get what he wanted. He also laughed quite a lot and his laughter was infectious. Staff began the search for his coping skills by commenting on his wonderful laughter and discussing with him how he felt after a good laugh. They said he was a LAUGH PERSON CHAMP and EXPERT FUNNY.[1] George loved those comments, and they created a good opening for discussing other skills he has or could develop.

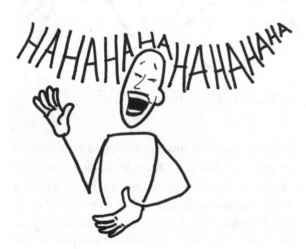

Figure 1.7 Laughing

Scenario 1.5

Calvin was another Deaf client who loved to laugh. He was a special fan of old Three Stooges movies. He collected these movies and watched them regularly. He loved the slapstick falls and pranks. He was a Three Stooges expert and especially loved the stooge, Curley. Staff would tease Calvin and call him Curley, which never ceased to make him laugh. Staff identified his 3 STOOGES COPING SKILL referring to his easy ability to laugh.

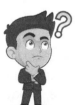

Questions to ponder 1.4: What role does your sense of humor and ability to laugh play in your own coping?

Bright idea 1.5: Sometimes, you really need to search to find another person's coping skills. It may be someone's sense of humor, especially if the person is able to laugh at him or herself. People can usually recognize that they feel better after laughing. Talking to someone about how laughter helps them can help to show them that they can do something to feel better.

Creative Expression

Any means of expressing oneself creatively can be considered a coping skill. This includes writing or drawing about one's experiences. Many deaf people with language and learning challenges cope with distressing situations by drawing or using other forms of art. Many programs that serve people with language or learning challenges have art-related activities. Artistic activities can be used to open up a dialogue about skills.

Scenario 1.6

Alesandro came to his group home from a hospital setting. He is a Deaf person who was very language deprived and signs at a very simple level. However, he loves to draw, paint, and make collages. He could keep himself busy and happy for hours at a time while engaged in art activities. Staff embraced these activities as the main way to form relationships with him and also to give him a toolbox of coping skills. They went to the art store with him and bought a variety of art supplies. They also began using the word "skills" when talking to him about art. They discussed his DRAW SKILL, PAINT SKILL, and PICTURE COLLAGE SKILL. Soon after, they elaborated on how these art skills were EXPRESS SELF SAFE SKILLS. From there, they eventually introduced the more abstract concept of COPING SKILL.

The ability to express oneself well in language is considered a key sign of maturity in children. It is also an important skill we want to promote in treatment programs with adults who struggle with language. Indeed, a treatment goal may well be for the person to express himself well in words or signs, rather than with behaviors. Expressing yourself through art can work just as well. It's vital to realize that a person is using coping skills any time that they express themselves safely—whether through words, signs, or actions. These are key moments to investigate. Broadly speaking, the skills could be called EXPRESS SELF SAFE skills.

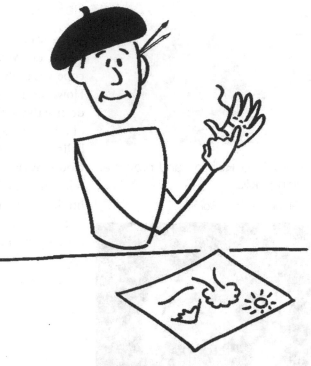

Figure 1.8 Art as a coping skill

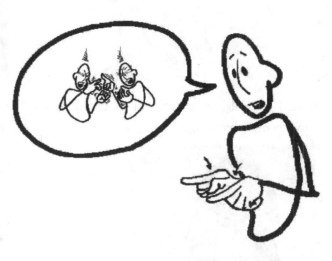

EXPRESS FEELINGS SAFELY

Figure 1.9 Expressing yourself safely as a skill

 Bright idea 1.6: Don't overlook the skills involved in using language to express yourself. It may seem so natural to you that you don't consider it a skill, but in many persons with language and learning challenges, the ability to express oneself safely in language represents an important step in skill development.

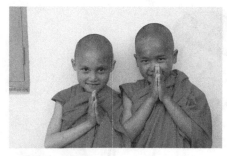

Figure 1.10 Religion and prayer as coping skills

©iStock.com/beemore

Religious and Spiritual Practices

Religious and spiritual practices can help or hurt. If it were possible to survey everyone in the world about the top three things that help them cope with adversity, religious practices would certainly make the list. However, from a psychological standpoint, religious practices can be destructive at times. For instance, a person who believes in the presence of a loving, supportive, forgiving God will probably be helped by this belief; whereas someone who believes in a harsh, critical, judgmental God may suffer unnecessarily (Griffith 2010). Exploring how clients' religious and spiritual beliefs, or beliefs in a "higher power," help or hinder their coping abilities is often a very useful dialogue.

Sometimes discussing faith, religion or spirituality with a client can start a conversation about coping and self-care.

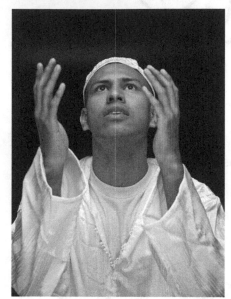

Figure 1.11 Religion and prayer as coping skills

©iStock.com/Juanmonino

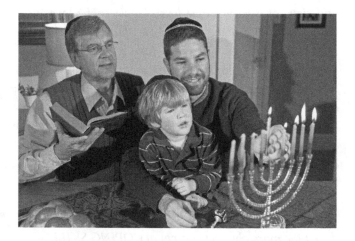

Figure 1.12 Religion and prayer as coping skills

©iStock.com/Kai Chiang

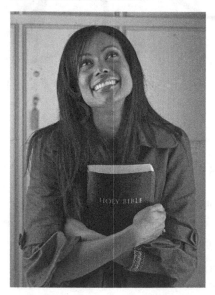

Figure 1.13 Religion and prayer as coping skills

©iStock.com/Juanmonino

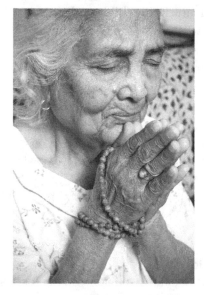

Figure 1.14 Religion and prayer as coping skills

©iStock.com/Vikram Raghuvanshi

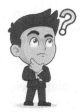

Questions to ponder 1.5: Religious beliefs that promote self-acceptance and love (for instance, the idea "God loves me") are likely to be psychologically helpful. If a person's concept of God and religious practices can be used to promote a kind, forgiving, accepting, and loving view of self and others, this is likely to contribute to psychological growth and healing. Do the people you work with use religious or spiritual beliefs or practices that could be considered helpful coping skills?

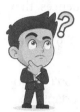

Questions to ponder 1.6: Consider your personal religious or spiritual beliefs. How do they help you? What aspects of your religious or spiritual beliefs give you the most comfort and support in your daily life?

Thinking Skills and Positive Self-Talk

What you think is directly related to what you feel and how well you cope. It can be especially difficult for people with intellectual challenges to notice and change how they think. The simplest way to do this is by trying to help people pay attention to their "self-talk." Self-talk is what a person says to himself or herself. People are often unaware of their self-talk, but they may reveal it to you if you know how to listen for it.

Scenario 1.7

Joanne is a hearing patient on a psychiatric inpatient unit. Susan is a mental health worker and a direct care provider who works as part of the nursing staff. Joanne has a history of self-harm through cutting herself. While Susan was doing "ward checks," she found Joanne in her bedroom with a pair of sharp scissors. Susan asked Joanne to give her the scissors. Joanne became angry and threw the scissors at the wall. This was actually an improvement over her usual behavior of cutting herself or hitting people. Susan used a strategy of noticing skills when behavior is less bad than normal. (This strategy will be discussed further in Lesson 3.) She began with empathy, commenting that Joanne seemed angry with her. When Joanne agreed, Susan thanked her for not throwing the scissors at her and wondered out loud how Joanne was able to do that. Joanne thought for a moment and then said, "Well, I didn't want to get in trouble." That was Susan's opportunity to comment on Joanne's self-talk.

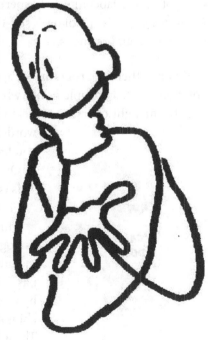

Figure 1.15 Thinking as a coping skill

"Oh, so if I understand right, you were angry, but you talked to yourself. You said, 'If I throw the scissors at Susan, I'll get in trouble. I don't want to get in trouble, so I'll throw them at the wall instead.' Is that right? Do you know what skill you were using?"

Joanne didn't know. The first time staff members ask this question, clients often don't know how to respond. They will know how to respond after the question has been asked enough and the schema for coping skills is established.

After a back and forth discussion, Susan told her, "Well, first you were talking to yourself, being a kind of coach to yourself. You were thinking. You were using skills we call 'self-talk.' You were also thinking about possible consequences. So, really, you were doing some problem solving. Very nice work."

Joanne took that in. Susan then wondered out loud if there was another reason she didn't throw the scissors at her. Joanne thought for a while and responded, "Well, I could have really hurt you if I did that. I was mad, but I didn't really want to hurt you."

Susan recognized that this was an even more impressive and skillful response. "Wow, so even though you were angry, you still thought about me. You showed empathy for me. You talked to yourself and reminded yourself that you didn't really want to hurt me. That's really impressive. I also appreciate it and thank you for it."

People also cope through the more sophisticated skill of rational problem solving. People think about their problems, then think about and evaluate possible solutions. Whenever you see any skillful problem solving, try to point out to the person that they are thinking skillfully. They may just be *thinking about consequences* but that is an important problem solving skill. If they adjust their behavior to avoid unwanted consequences, they are using a cognitive form of coping.

You will learn more about the connection between thoughts, feelings and coping abilities in Lessons 8, 9, and 10.

 Bright idea 1.7: Rational problem solving is a sophisticated strategy for coping. Don't fail to notice simple versions of this, such as when people identify a consequence then adapt their behavior to pursue or avoid a consequence. You almost always want to promote a client's abilities to think and solve problems rationally.

Stopping and Noticing (Mindfulness)

Mindfulness is one of the most profound coping skills. Mindfulness is the ability to pay attention to one's thoughts, feelings, sensations and behaviors in the present moment *without judging them*. Marsha Linehan's dialectical behavior therapy (DBT) turned the mental health world's attention onto the importance of mindfulness. There are now entire psychotherapies based on it (Linehan 1993).

Mindfulness is powerful because it fosters the ability to experience feelings without the interference of damaging self-talk. It allows you to experience sadness, anger, anxiety, and pain without an internal monologue saying how awful and unbearable these experiences are. Mindfulness can be life changing for those who can develop this skill.

But not everyone can do it. The concept of mindfulness is very abstract. It requires the ability to:

- Notice and label internal experiences.
- Monitor and control one's self-talk, including judgments.
- Let it go and re-focus.

In this pre-therapy program, we approach the concept of mindfulness through the practice of stopping and noticing. We help people notice what they do, feel, and think. Initially, we say, "just notice."

A traffic light offers a concrete representation of this skill. The *red light* means "stop and notice." In other words, stop and think. What are you doing? What are you about to do? What are you feeling or sensing? What are you thinking?"

Once you have stopped and noticed it, calm yourself down (the *yellow light*). This is usually accomplished through a sensory movement skill.

Finally, consider your options (the *green light*).

Mindfulness is often taught through movement and breathing activities, such as yoga. While practicing yoga, participants are asked to notice what they feel, including discomfort, breathe, and let it go. They learn "this sensation also will pass." Mindfulness also can be taught through slowly eating a raisin or grape, or by walking slowly while paying full attention to all the sensations. In tai chi and chi gong, mindfulness is taught through movement, breath, and self-awareness. The addition of a movement or activity, or the use of food, can make this experience more approachable, yet very concrete thinkers are still likely to miss the point and find it boring.

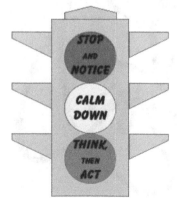

Figure 1.16 The red, yellow, green light skill

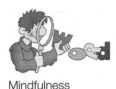

Mindfulness

Many of the people we serve in our programs are impulsive. They act, often in destructive ways, with very little thought. Your goal is to help them develop the ability to "stop and notice" what they are feeling (red light), slow down their response (yellow light), and choose the best plan going forward (green light). You want to support development of any skill that interrupts impulsive behavior, whether it be stopping and noticing internal cues, slow breathing, or helpful self-talk.

Whenever you see someone intentionally using a skill to manage his or her feelings, you can infer that the person had a "stop and notice" moment. In order for the person to *not* harm themselves or other people, *not* take an alcoholic drink, *not* act on impulse, they must have

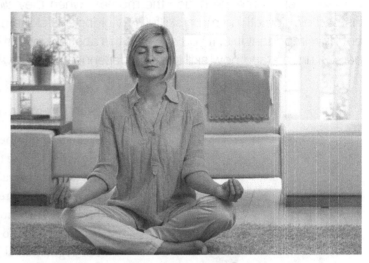

Figure 1.17 Mindfulness meditation as a coping skill
©iStock.com/nyul

had a brief moment where they noticed that they were headed in that direction and changed their path. This moment is often brief and fleeting. Can you help them discover that they did, in fact, stop and notice, that they did show a moment of mindfulness?

Bright idea 1.8: Whenever a person takes a step to manage a feeling, impulse, or thought, they must have first noticed that feeling, impulse, or thought. By recognizing this experience, and proactively taking a step, the person is demonstrating the ability to take some control over his or her life. You want to promote this ability to notice, step back, and reflect. The "stop and notice" moment, however small, indicates that a person is beginning to feel capable of managing his or her behaviors. The task for staff is to help people notice this crucial empowering first step.

Scenario 1.8

Selina was angry. She wanted Bill's attention. Bill, a staff person, was busy with another matter. Usually, Selina screams or breaks something if she doesn't get immediate attention. Today, however, she saw that Bill was busy, and when she couldn't get his attention, she went to watch television. Bill talked to her later. He helped her notice the WATCH TELEVISION distraction skill. But, even more important, he helped her notice that she had felt frustrated and then made a decision to not scream and to watch television instead. He then asked her, "Did you notice how you used the 'red light, stop and notice' skill? Did you notice that you felt frustrated, then made a decision to use a healthy coping skill, watching television." He engaged her in a role play of that moment, intentionally slowing it down and replaying it. This helped to make that very subtle moment of dawning awareness more obvious to her.

Bill is also using a particular style of questioning to help Selina figure something out. He asked a strength-based question, asking her to notice something she did successfully. He also guided her to discover what she did well. Bill then followed up with a question he knew was abstract and that Selina would not initially be able to answer. He asked, "How did you do it?" Selina looked confused, but she started to think.

Practice Exercise 1.3

Can you help someone notice the moment when they *didn't react* as he or she normally would and instead did something more skillful? Try giving this skill a name such as "stop and notice" and pointing out how important it is. If you can root this abstract insight into the person's behavior, you may help the person understand how skill building depends on self-awareness.

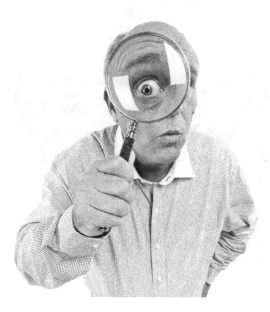

Figure 1.18 Stop and notice. What coping skills are being used?

©iStock.com/ranplett

Summary

As a staff member, your job is to "stop and notice" when clients use skills, to give these skills names, and to find ways to encourage the person to practice the skills further.

When you are working with people with severe behavioral problems, or whose abilities to live independently are poor, it can be challenging to find skills and strengths. Broadly speaking, any self-regulation skill that a client uses to manage his or her inner world is a coping skill. It is essential to have a broad framework for understanding simple and more complex skills, and to have a large vocabulary for skills. This framework includes an appreciation of developmentally simpler skills, such as the kind of skills that a child might show. These skills might be found when a client does a puzzle, laughs, or rocks in a chair.

In the next lesson, we'll review and name some of the foundation skills needed to manage one's outer world, especially the part that involves conflicts with other people. In Lesson 3, you'll explore other strength-based methods for identifying skills such as how to find skills when a problem behavior *doesn't* happen or occurs in a more manageable way. You'll also learn to find skills when a person is recovering from a destructive episode.

Lesson 1 Skill Sheet

- Participant recognizes these kinds of coping skill:

  a. Distraction skills.

  b. Sensory and body-based skills.

  c. Self-expression skills though art, language or other means.

  d. Humor and laughter.

  e. Religious and spiritual practices.

  f. Self-talk and cognitive problem solving.

  g. Self-awareness and mindfulness.

- Participant recognizes and labels the coping skills of the people (both clients and coworkers) they work with.

- Participant seeks to develop their vocabulary for skills and identifies more and more behaviors as skills.

- Participant recognizes and labels some of their own skills and strengths.

Lesson 1 Quiz

1. Which of the following could be considered coping skills? Check all that apply:

   a. Deep breathing.

   b. Taking a time out.

   c. Going for a walk.

   d. Having a cigarette.

   e. Telling yourself to calm down.

   f. Thinking of consequences.

   g. Sleeping.

   h. Praying.

   i. Playing a game.

   j. Yelling to let your feelings out, no matter what you say.

   k. Petting a cat.

   l. Cutting yourself on purpose.

2. David is a Deaf person who experienced extreme language deprivation in childhood. As a result, he has a limited sign vocabulary and virtually no spoken language vocabulary. David never went to school and cannot read or write. He was raised on a farm and spent most of his time interacting with and taking care of animals. David is usually quiet and calm, but he has occasional temper outbursts. Where would you be likely to find some of David's coping skills? Check all that apply:

   a. David is good at distracting and entertaining himself.

   b. David has a very strong rapport with animals, which he seems to prefer over people.

   c. David likes to watch television.

   d. David is good at coaching himself to calm down.

   e. David expresses himself well through art.

3. Why is it important to notice and label skills that the person is already using? Check all that apply:

    a. It puts the focus on the person's strengths, on what they do well.

    b. It encourages the person to get more involved in his or her own growth and development.

    c. It promotes strength-based work.

    d. It is easier to get a person to do more of what they do well then it is to fix what they do badly.

    e. It can lead to a discussion of how they could use even more skills.

    f. This is a bad idea because it means we don't confront a person about bad behaviors.

4. A person gets angry and walks out of the room. While walking out, the staff person observes the person signing to himself: "Calm down. If you blow up again, you will get in trouble. Go sit under the tree." What skills has the person just used?

    a. Positive self-talk.

    b. Stopping and noticing.

    c. Red, yellow, green light.

    d. A sensory-based relaxation technique.

    e. Prayer.

5. Julien, a staff person in a residential program, thinks about his own coping skills. He realizes that he uses a combination of healthy and unhealthy strategies for coping with stress. Which of the following might be considered *unhealthy* or *unhelpful* coping skills?

    a. Smoking cigarettes.

    b. Drinking alcohol.

    c. Taking his frustration out on other people.

    d. Screaming.

    e. Scratching himself till he bleeds.

    f. Tuning out completely from what is going on around him.

Lesson 1 Questions for Discussion

1. What do you do to help yourself when you are distressed? What are your own emotional self-regulation or coping skills?

2. What are the natural coping skills of the people (both clients and coworkers) you work with? What do they already do to help themselves feel better?

3. Do religious or spiritual practices appear to help the people you serve? How do they help? Do you have any concerns that these practices may be unhelpful or harmful to them?

4. Do you see clients using physical or sensory-based strategies for coping? What do you see?

5. Do you notice the people you serve saying things to themselves as a way of coping with a situation?

6. Do you notice that the people you serve use any rational problem solving?

7. How can you promote the use of rational problem solving?

8. How could you help the people you work with to better understand the concept of mindfulness?

9. In your program, do recovery discussions include identifying the coping skills that people already have?

10. Would your clients be more engaged if there were more conversations about coping skills, especially about skills that people already have?

Lesson 1 Quiz Answers

1. All of these behaviors could be considered coping skills, but clearly not all of them are *healthy* coping skills. In this lesson, we focused on identifying what people do to help themselves cope with distress and labeled these as skills. In Lesson 5, we will take the next step of helping people evaluate how helpful or healthy these skills are.

2. All of these could be coping skills. An obvious place to look for David's skills is in his interactions with animals (*b*). Because David has weak language skills, he may well have learned to entertain himself rather than depend on other people (*a*). He might, in fact, talk to himself (*d*) although it could be difficult to understand what he is saying. You would need time to determine if he finds television entertaining (*c*) or whether he likes to draw or do any other form of artistic expression (*e*).

3. The correct answers are *a*, *b*, *c*, *d*, and *e*. All of these are good reasons to notice and label skills. Using this approach does not mean that you can't address negative behaviors so *f* is incorrect. In later lessons, you'll learn ways to address negative behaviors. At this point, however, you want to engage people in the process of self-evaluation. If they can identify behaviors as unhelpful, they will be much more likely to work on changing them.

4. The correct answers are *a*, *b*, *c*, and *d*. The person did stop and notice his anger (*b*) and chose to leave the situation. This stopping and noticing is the red light of the "red, yellow, green light" skill. Walking out and sitting under the tree could be a yellow light skill; and the self-talk (*a*) could be a green light of the red, yellow, green light skill (*c*). Sitting under a tree is a sensory-based relaxation technique (*d*). We don't know whether or not he used prayer (*e*).

5. All of these behaviors could be considered unhealthy or unhelpful coping skills. Although each may have a positive side in that they help Julien cope or feel better in the moment, they all have significant costs. At this point in the program, we are not concerning ourselves with whether or not a person's coping skills are healthy. We want to start by recognizing the skills that a person uses, even if a skill is unhealthy. Recognizing a specific coping skill is a way to begin the conversation. In subsequent lessons, you will learn to ask questions that help people evaluate their skills and decide if they want to develop new ones.

Note

1. The capital letters reflect the fact that these are "tags" or "glosses" for common signs. The writing may appear odd and ungrammatical, but in sign language, it is perfectly grammatical and clear.

Bibliography

Glickman, N. (2009). *Cognitive behavioral therapy for deaf and hearing persons with language and learning challenges*. Chapter 5. New York: Routledge.

Griffith, J. L. (2010). *Religion that heals, religion that harms: A guide for clinical practice*. New York: Guilford Press.

Jackson, M. (Writer). (2010). *Temple Grandin* [DVD]. S. Ferguson (Producer): HBO Films.

Kolk, B. V. D. (2014). *The body keeps the score: Brain, mind, and body in the healing of trauma*. New York: Viking.

Linehan, M. (1993). *Cognitive behavioral treatment of borderline personality disorder*. New York: Guilford Press.

McKay, M., Wood, J., & Brantley, J. (2007). *The dialectical behavior therapy skills workbook*. Oakland, CA: New Harbinger Press.

Conflict Resolution Skills

Introduction

In Lesson 1, you learned about some important coping skills that people can use to deal with one's "inner world." Lesson 2 will focus on some of the key *social skills* that help people deal with their "outer world" by helping them to manage interactions and conflicts with other people. The structure of Lesson 2 is the same as that of Lesson 1. We will explore some common scenarios in educational and residential settings where there is conflict between people and then we will look at—and name—the skills needed to resolve them.

Scenario 2.1

A doctor has an appointment with a Deaf patient named Angelo who lives in a group living environment run by Agency X. Monica, a staff member, brings Angelo to the appointment. Monica, who is hearing, has studied and practiced sign language for three years. She's enthusiastic about sign language and supporting people who are Deaf. Unfortunately, she doesn't always recognize the limits of her signing skills. She and Angelo were told that the doctor would provide an interpreter for the appointment. However, when Monica and Angelo arrive, they discover that no one has arranged for an interpreter. The doctor assumed that because Agency X served Angelo, they would bring the interpreter, or at least a staff member would help out. He says, "I don't have time to be arranging for interpreters." The doctor is impatient, gives Monica an annoyed look, and asks her to interpret for them. He talks directly to Monica, not to Angelo who is his patient.

"Just sign what I say," the doctor says.

Even though Monica has been told not to interpret, she has a hard time saying "no" to the doctor. Monica uses her signing skills to explain the situation to Angelo, who tells her to go ahead and interpret.

Once they start, it becomes clear to Monica that the doctor is asking technical questions that she isn't trained to interpret. For instance, he asks whether there is any history of COPD in Angelo's family. Monica doesn't know what COPD is or how to sign it so she just signs HISTORY and fingerspells C-O-P-D. Monica can see that Angelo is getting restless and isn't really paying attention.

As the appointment goes on, Monica becomes more and more overwhelmed with the complexity of the interpreting task. Is she supposed to tell Angelo that the doctor is annoyed and complaining about her? Should she point out to the doctor that he keeps talking to her, not to Angelo? She doesn't fully understand the doctor herself and, truth be told, she doesn't always fully understand Angelo!

She fumbles on, interpreting as the best she can. Angelo is starting to appear tense and angry. Fortunately, the appointment is almost over. When she and Angelo arrive back at the program, she tells her supervisor that there was no interpreter.

"I know I wasn't supposed to interpret, but what could I do? The doctor didn't want to reschedule and Angelo told me to go ahead," Monica explains.

The supervisor responds by reprimanding her for having "poor boundaries" and Angelo complains that she is a "lousy signer." When a deaf coworker learns about the incident, he complains that Monica is "oppressing deaf people" by forcing them to accept "lousy interpreting."

When you read this story, your first reaction may have been "Poor Monica! She is in a no-win situation." And, you're right. Monica encountered conflict from all sides in this situation. She needed to call on some heavy-duty conflict management skills but it appears she didn't have them.

Lesson 2 is about conflict resolution skills. Most of the skills we will explore are developmentally simple. This is because the focus of this program is on helping people with language and learning challenges. These simpler skills typically develop in childhood. We are not trying to develop the sophisticated conflict resolution skills required in international negotiations or business. Instead, our focus is on helping people learn how to deal with common conflicts that arise in the daily lives of people who receive services in schools and treatment programs.

As we will see, many conflict resolution skills are really communication skills, especially the skills of expressing oneself in a way that helps others listen and then listening to them well in return. Our primary goal is to help people learn to resolve day-to-day conflicts in safe, respectful ways using simple communication skills. As part of this process, we need to help people who have usually depended on others for problem solving discover that they have these abilities themselves. Indeed, developing this belief in one's own capacity for problem solving can be more difficult than teaching the skills themselves.

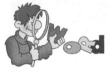

Communication skills

Definition 2.1: Communication skills: the ability to express, receive, and process information effectively.

Example of communication skills: Seymour is angry at his counselor Mary Beth and screams at her. Rather than defending herself and fighting back, Mary Beth focuses on listening well. She really wants to understand what is bothering him. She maintains eye contact, nods to indicate she is following him, and responds, "I can see you are really angry at me. I wasn't here when you needed me and you felt abandoned by me." Seymour stops yelling and starts to cry.

People with language and learning challenges struggle to communicate well which means they usually also struggle in their social relationships. Commonly, their conflict resolution skills are weak. Even if they live with additional challenges, such as mental illness, trauma, and addictions, much of your day-to-day work with them focuses on helping them develop and use these foundation communication, social, and coping skills. For example, your ultimate goal may be to help a person cope with trauma or learn to manage an addiction. But, if the person lacks the basic language and cognitive skills needed for such work, you have no choice but to work on building this foundation first. Thus, much of the pre-therapy work with persons with language and learning challenges can be considered developmental. We're helping them to learn skills that they likely would have already mastered if their development had followed a more typical pattern.

Conflict and Conflict Resolution Skills

In this workbook, a conflict is any disagreement or argument between two or more people that requires the parties involved to work together to resolve the situation. Unresolved conflicts can cause serious emotional distress. Over time, they can lead to aggressive behavior, cause or increase mental health problems, and damage personal relationships among other things.

Conflicts can happen anywhere, at any time, even between people who usually get along well. People need social skills to resolve conflicts. We will look at some common conflicts that occur in schools and treatment programs where people with learning and language challenges receive services.

Conflict resolution skills can take many forms. The simplest skills, the ones that the people you serve likely lack, include being able to:

- Accurately label their internal experiences (e.g., feelings) and communicate them to other people in a safe, non-threatening way.
- Listen and consider what others have to say.
- Understand other people's feelings and viewpoints.
- Communicate safely (e.g., avoiding threats, insults, bullying).
- Stay physically safe by avoiding aggressive behaviors.
- Accurately read other people's facial expressions and body movements.
- Wait patiently.
- Take turns.
- Identify a problem and possible solutions.
- Evaluate possible solutions and choosing one.
- Negotiate and compromise.

When people lack these skills, or have weak skills, we say they have a "skills deficit."

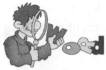

Skills deficit

Definition 2.1: Skills deficit: A term used to describe a missing or weak skill or skill that a person has but is unable to access when needed.

Example of a skills deficit: Brian thinks that communicating well is saying whatever he feels even if he is rude and insulting. He doesn't realize that to communicate well, he has to stop insulting people so that they are willing to listen to him and consider what he has to say. He has a skill deficit in expressing himself safely.

Practice Exercise 2.1: Conflicts in Agency Settings

Let's look at some conflict scenarios that commonly occur in a school, residential, or other treatment settings. This exercise has four parts.

Part A

1. Review each of the following scenarios.
2. Identify the skills needed to help solve the conflict. Consider *skills that both the client/student and the staff person need*.
3. Write your answers in the space provided.

Scenario 2.2

Joe is a 16-year-old Deaf student who doesn't like to get up in the morning. School begins at 8:00. A staff person flashes the bedroom light and then shakes the bed to wake him up. He responds by screaming at the staff person. When the staff person persists, Joe finally gets up, pushes her away, kicks her, and then returns to bed.

Skills that Joe needs:

_____

_____

Skills staff need:

_____

_____

Scenario 2.3

Shatira is a 25-year-old woman with a developmental disability who lives in a group home. It's 3:00 in the afternoon and she wants the staff person to drive her to the mall. The other staff person on the afternoon shift has called in sick and the program's remaining staff person has to stay on site to attend to other matters. He asks Shatira to wait until there is a second staff on duty. She demands to go NOW!

Skills that Shatira needs:

_____

_____

Skills staff needs:

_____

_____

Scenario 2.4

A program has only one television. Several people begin arguing over what show to watch. One pushes another, then knocks over the television. Tyrian, a staff person, comes over to help.

Skills the client need:

_____

_____

Skills staff person Tyrian needs:

_____

_____

Scenario 2.5

Jonathan, a program resident, enters the room while staff members are talking with another resident. Jonathan interrupts and says he needs help. A staff member asks Jonathan to wait but he is unable or unwilling to do so. Instead, Jonathan insists on being helped immediately. The other resident pushes Jonathan out of the way and they begin to argue. When staff members try to separate them, the second resident pushes a staff person.

Skills the residents need:

_____

_____

Skills staff need:

_____

_____

Scenario 2.6

Sebastian has trouble interpreting other people's non-verbal expressions. When a staff person politely asks him to help with cleaning up, Sebastian misinterprets the staff member's facial expression and body language and decides the staff member is "mean." Sebastian then complains to the human rights officer who, in turn, contacts the staff member to discuss the situation. The staff person is surprised to hear of Sebastian's complaint.

Skills Sebastian needs:

_____

_____

Skills staff need:

_____

_____

Pictures of Common Conflicts

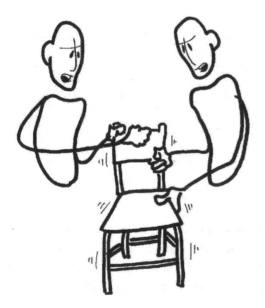

Figure 2.1 "This is mine!"

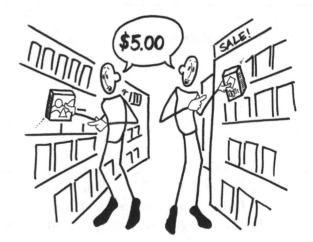

Figure 2.2 "I want this!"

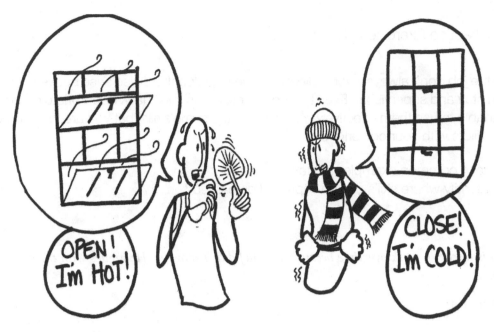

Figure 2.3 Window open or closed?

In Lesson 1, you learned that using pictures and images to explain and reinforce important skills can be an effective way of teaching people with learning and language challenges. These simple drawings are a good example of this technique. You will find others throughout this workbook. All these pictures, and many more, are available at the Routledge website associated with this book (http://routledge.com/9781138916937). Click on the E-resources tab for this book.

Practice Exercise 2.1, Part B

Review the necessary skills that you identified for each scenario. Did you list any of the basic skills identified earlier? These basic skills include:

- Accurately labeling one's internal experiences (e.g., feelings) and communicating them to other people in a safe, non-threatening way.
- Listening and considering what others have to say.
- Understanding other people's feelings and viewpoints.
- Communicating safely (e.g., avoiding threats, insults, bullying).
- Staying physically safe by avoiding aggressive behaviors.
- Accurately reading other people's facial expressions and body movements.
- Patience and waiting.
- Taking turns.
- Identifying a problem and possible solutions.
- Evaluating possible solutions and choosing one.
- Negotiation and compromise.

Practice Exercise 2.1, Part C

Conflicts on the job don't always involve clients. Sometimes, conflicts also arise between staff members and between staff and supervisors. Even trained professionals might lack appropriate conflict resolution skills or be unable to use them effectively. You can use the same skills that you are teaching your clients to resolve conflicts with your coworkers:

1. Review these common examples of staff conflicts.
2. Can you identify where skills can be improved or learned?

Scenario 2.7

A staff person is forced to work overtime because his relief didn't show up. He argues with the supervisor, swears at her and quits.

Possible skills needed:

_____

_____

_____

Scenario 2.8

Two staff members argue over who is responsible for driving a client to an appointment.

Possible skills needed:

_____

_____

_____

Scenario 2.9

A staff member complains that a supervisor is showing favoritism. The supervisor denies any favoritism and responds by saying the staff person isn't doing her work properly.

Possible skills needed:

_____

_____

_____

Scenario 2.10

A signing Deaf person and a non-signing hearing person work together in a Deaf program. The signing Deaf staff member complains about having to do all the work with the Deaf clients because he is the only one with communication skills. The hearing staff person complains that he is asked to do all the physical chores in the program. He thinks the Deaf staff should help with the chores.

Possible skills needed:

_____

_____

_____

Practice Exercise 2.1, Part D

1. Review your responses to the scenarios presented in Parts A and C of this exercise.
2. Did you notice any similarities between the skills that staff need and the skills that people receiving services need?
3. Write down any similar skills that you identified.

_____

_____

_____

Practice Exercise 2.2: Identify Your Conflict Resolution Skills

In this exercise, you will assess your own conflict resolutions skills:

1. Identify at least one conflict that occurred among or with the people you serve.

_____

_____

2. Identify at least five skills that would have helped you to resolve or manage the conflict more effectively:

- _____

- _____

- _____

- _____

- _____

3. Identify one work-related conflict that you have been personally involved in with clients, peers or supervisors:

_____

_____

_____

4. Identify at least five skills that you think were relevant to solving this conflict:

- _____
- _____
- _____
- _____
- _____

More Complicated Conflicts

The conflicts we explored at in Practice Exercise 2.1 were pretty straightforward. Someone did or said something and another person reacted. Simple. However, many conflicts are not straightforward. This was evident in the story that began this lesson. As you'll recall, Monica was faced with unexpected, complicated conflicts related to Deaf culture, miscommunication, unclear expectations, and trouble dealing with authority figures.

More complicated situations require a more complex response that draws on multiple skills and being sensitive to many different issues and points of view.

Let's consider some examples of more complex conflicts.

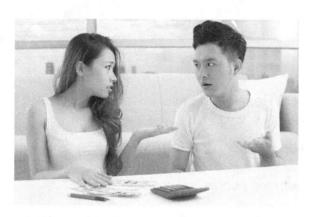

Figure 2.4 Couple argues about money
©iStock.com/DragonImages

Arguments About Money and Finances

Money and finances are very emotional subjects and arguments often arise when the people involved have different perspectives on saving, spending, and investing. It's not surprising, then, that many couples argue about money. They may have grown up in families with very different income levels and very different styles of dealing with money. Spending or saving money may also hold different, intensely personal meanings for each of them (e.g., "If you really loved me, you'd spend money on me," or "I need to save money in order to feel safe in the world."). As you can imagine, these arguments may not be easily resolved without getting to the deeper roots of the issue.

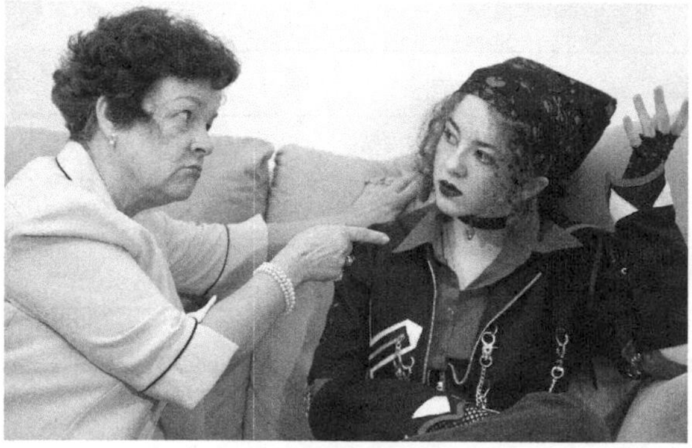

Generational Conflicts

Conflicts in values between a parent and child are very common. For example, conflicts can occur when a strict mother tries to set rules for her rebellious adolescent daughter. The stricter the mother becomes, the more defiant the girl becomes. Eventually, they are barely able to talk with one another.

Handling a Car Accident

Following an automobile accident, the two parties involved will have to complete a number of complicated tasks: Make sure everyone is okay; obtain medical, police, or automotive

Figure 2.5 Mother/daughter values conflict
©iStock.com/Lisa F. Young

assistance; handle their own emotions, and physical and psychological reactions; respond to the other party's behavior; and exchange insurance and other important information. This conflict is stressful enough but imagine how complicated the interaction will become if they use different languages; there are more than two parties involved; or one or both drivers lack insurance; or one or both are too hurt to participate in problem solving.

Parent Conflicts Affecting Children

Children are affected when parents argue. Parents who are at odds need skills to handle their own conflicts, as well as skills to take care of their children and protect them from possible emotional and physical harm related to their interpersonal conflicts.

Cross-cultural Conflicts

Cross-cultural dynamics often complicate conflicts as happened in the story that began this lesson. This type of conflict can occur in settings where people who are raised or live in one culture are supported by individuals who are raised or live in a different one, such as a Deaf program staffed by hearing staff members. In this situation, conflicts can arise because cultural norms are misunderstood, language barriers stand in the way, and people don't recognize the cross-cultural dimensions of their work.

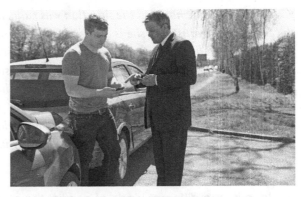

Figure 2.6 Handling a car accident

©iStock.com/monkeybusinessimages

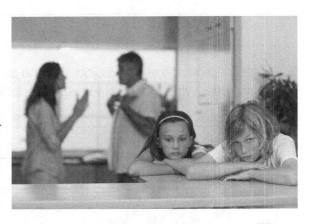

Figure 2.7 Children react to parental conflict

©iStock.com/Wavebreakmedia

Practice Exercise 2.3: Cross-cultural Conflicts

1. Read the following story from the Westborough Massachusetts State Hospital Deaf Unit.[1]

Scenario 2.11

A hearing nurse, who doesn't sign and is new to working with Deaf people, approaches a Deaf patient with development delays and speaks to him as she would a hearing person. She also approaches a Deaf-blind client and, to the astonishment of Deaf staff, speaks to the client as if he could see and hear her. One of the Deaf mental health workers interrupts the nurse and tells her, through sign, gestures and unclear speech, that she can't do that. He is visibly annoyed and impatient with her. He gets an interpreter and tells her very bluntly that she is not communicating respectfully with Deaf people.

The nurse takes this as a scolding from someone who, in this setting, reports to her and is therefore, in the organization, her "inferior." She responds by complaining about his rudeness, then writes him up for disciplinary action. This triggers an angry response from the Deaf mental health worker who feels that multiple forms of hearing oppression are occurring. He complains that this nurse is culturally insensitive and unsuitable to work with Deaf people. He doesn't appreciate that while he is right about the nurse's ignorance about communicating with Deaf and Deaf-blind persons, the way he handled the situation was rude, insulting and, yes, insubordinate. When the nurse hears about the complaint against her, she is also enraged. She is not willing to be scolded by someone she supervises.

Her personal life is also complicating her response. He coworkers are not aware that she's in the middle of a difficult divorce and custody battle with a "bossy" husband. The behavior of the Deaf male staff person triggers the feelings of anger that she has toward her husband. She feels victimized as a woman and has been telling herself that she would not permit men to bully her again.

The male Deaf mental health worker also feels victimized. He feels he is being singled out because he is a Deaf person. He can't believe that someone so culturally insensitive would be allowed to work in a Deaf program. Even worse, this person is his supervisor!

2. Identify the different kinds of conflict the story contains:

    _____

    _____

    _____

3. Identify some of the skill deficits that the supervisor and the deaf staff member either lack or need to improve. What skills would help them both resolve this conflict?

    _____

    _____

    _____

 Bright idea 2.1: Life's day-to-day conflicts require foundation communication and conflict-solving skills. Effective mental health and substance abuse treatment depends on these same foundational skills. When these skills are not in place, they must become a focus of the pre-therapy work, no matter the other problems the person has. You can't get to B (for instance, treating depression), without going through A (teaching people to recognize and communicate feelings).

 Bright idea 2.2: Conflict resolution is a more complex task than coping. To manage conflict, one has to recognize and cope with one's own internal experiences, as well as recognize and respond to the behaviors of at least one other person. Conflict resolution involves both dealing with one's inner world of feelings, thoughts. and sensations and one's outer world of other people.

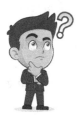 **Questions to ponder 2.1:** Conflicts between clients, between staff and clients, and between staff regularly occur in mental health treatment settings. These conflicts can cripple a program or they can be a source of skill development. Recognizing and working to resolve conflicts can create a healthy skill-based treatment setting. How well does the program you work for handle such conflicts?

Common Conflict Resolution Skills

Like coping skills, conflict resolution or conflict management skills develop as children mature into adulthood and learn to use more complex problem-solving capabilities. For example, preschoolers who are learning to "share," "listen," and "take turns" are using developmentally appropriate conflict resolution skills. Children who "flip a coin" or act out "rock, paper, scissors" to make decisions also are using conflict resolution skills that are typical for their level of developmental. This is the theme of Robert Fulghum's book, *All I really need to know I learned in kindergarten*, quoted in the introduction (Fulghum 2003). Similarly, adults who resolve conflicts by voting are using techniques and strategies that are appropriate for their age and stage of development. Mediators and diplomats working with people and nations at war also use conflict resolution skills and strategies albeit at a far more sophisticated level.

When preparing the people you serve to participate in CBT, you need to be able to recognize, model, teach, and reinforce developmentally simple skills. However, some of the people you serve, and even some staff members, may have difficulty mastering them. The bottom line is that you want to help the people you serve to develop the skills they need in order to solve problems effectively.

Glickman (2009, pp. 230–231) offers these common conflict-solving skills:

- Noticing and naming the conflict, then seeking a peaceful resolution.
- Building and using key foundation communication skills.
- Building and using foundation negotiation skills.

Let's look at each more closely.

Noticing and Naming the Conflict and Seeking Peaceful Ways to Solve it

This includes being able to:

- understand what a conflict is
- notice that a conflict is happening
- realize that the conflict provides an opportunity to use a skill
- identify (name) the conflict
- see the value in solving a conflict peacefully.

The following scenario illustrates this "notice and name it" skill.

Scenario 2.12

Jason and Will are roommates in a residential program. They don't like to go food shopping together because they always argue over what to buy. Both grab food items that they want and put back items the other wants. They argue and sometimes end up pushing and shoving each other. Understandably, staff members don't like to bring Jason and Will shopping together. Finally, the program manager sat the two down and told them that neither of them could go shopping, which they both liked doing, unless they could do it together peacefully. He insisted they make a plan in advance for what they would buy, and, when they disagreed, that they needed to talk about it. They role played this plan several times. The program manager helped them practice saying, "This is a conflict. We can solve it." He then walked them through very basic solutions like flipping a coin, taking turns, and compromising.

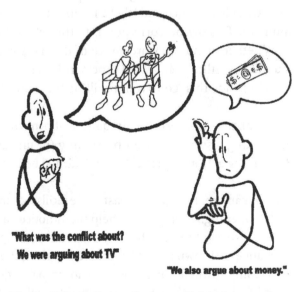

"What was the conflict about?
We were arguing about TV"

"We also argue about money."

Figure 2.8 Noticing that conflict is happening

Foundation Communication Skills

Many people with learning and language challenges have difficulty mastering some common foundation communication skills. They are:

- Using non-verbal communication skills and recognizing them in others.
- The ability to notice and name feelings.
- Listening without interruption.
- Using clean, safe communication.
- Using I-statements.

Let's look at each of these in more detail.

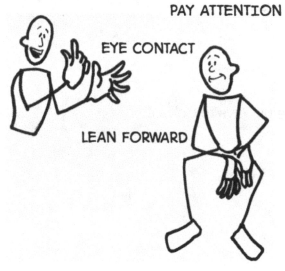

Figure 2.9 Non-verbal attending skills

Using Non-verbal Cues

Recognizing and properly interpreting non-verbal cues is a very powerful communications foundation skill. Very often you will need to begin by helping people understand will what a physical posture of listening looks like. It's easy to contrast this with non-verbal behaviors that show one isn't listening. This posture is easily demonstrated and imitating poor non-verbal attending skills can be a very amusing role-play exercise.

Notice it, Name it

The ability to notice a feeling and then be able to name is an important foundation coping skill that is an essential part of conflict resolution. This skill corresponds to the red light in the traffic signal model you learned about in Lesson 1. It is the profound "stop and notice" moment that makes all skill building possible. You may find yourself spending a great deal of time helping the people you serve to stop reacting and, instead, begin to pay attention so that they are able to notice and label a feeling. You can use a breathing or simple counting exercise to stretch out this moment. This period corresponds to the yellow "calm down" light in the traffic signal.

Whether or not they are aware of it, a person must have had a "stop and notice" moment whenever they handle a conflict well. When a person becomes upset and goes to his room, he probably doesn't realize that hidden inside this "go to room skill" is the more profound moment of:

1. Realizing he's upset and in danger of behaving badly.
2. Taking responsibility for preventing the unwanted behavior.
3. Taking action to prevent the unwanted behavior.

As you can see, there are at least three skills occurring whenever someone takes an action to avoid something bad happening. Your job is to help them notice each of these skills.

You also want to help them notice that by taking these steps, they have already shown *they* can do something to change their own behavior. They are making the change, not you. *They* are showing self-control. That is quite an accomplishment for someone who probably doesn't see themselves as capable of controlling any aspect of their life. Instead, they are accustomed to looking to staff or other authority figures to fix things for them. This may be a momentous step so it is crucial that you help them notice and capture it.

Scenario 2.13 shows how this skill can be seen in everyday situations.

Scenario 2.13

Sol and Terry are roommates who frequently argue with each other. Sol usually starts the argument and often complains about how sloppy Terry is. When Alicia, a staff member, visits the two, she notices that dirty plates have been left on the table and that Sol is about to yell at Terry. To her surprise, Sol picks up the plates, brings them to the sink, and washes them himself. Then, he sits down to watch TV.

Alicia says to Sol:	*"Wow. Something amazing just happened."*
Sol responds:	*"What?"*
Alicia:	*"I saw you do something amazing. Do you know what it was?"*
Sol:	*"No. I just washed the dishes. I do that all the time."*
Alicia:	*"Yeah, that was good, but not amazing. What was amazing was that you were ready to yell at Terry, but you didn't. You stopped yourself. How did you do that?"*
Sol shrugs:	*"I don't want to fight today."*
Alicia:	*"You don't want to fight today? So you noticed you were ready to fight, but you stopped yourself. You decided it wasn't worth it. Then you did something else. You washed the dishes. I'm guessing they were Terry's dishes?"*
Sol:	*"Yeah, he's a slob."*
Alicia:	*"But today you chose not to argue. I wonder if you were using some good 'living with roommate' skills?"*
	Sol smiles.
Alicia nods:	*"I agree. And one more question? Who kept this fight from happening? Was it staff or was it . . .?*
Sol replies proudly:	*"I did."*

Listening without Interrupting

People with learning and language challenges often have difficult listening. It can be difficult for them to pay attention long enough to understand the other person's point of view. In addition, many are impulsive, which makes it difficult to listen well. A good way to improve listening skills is to help the person try to understand what the other person is feeling. A concrete way to develop this skill is to repeat what the other person said but change the wording slightly by either paraphrasing the statement or to use slightly different words or word order. The staff person models this listening skill.

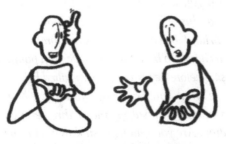

**TRY TO UNDERSTAND
WHAT OTHER PERSON FEELS**

Figure 2.10 Understand the other person's feelings

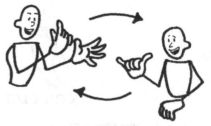

**PAY ATTENTION.
LISTEN.
DON'T INTERRUPT.**

Figure 2.11 Pay attention and don't interrupt

Scenario 2.14 illustrates this technique.

Scenario 2.14

Tim is a patient in a hospital. He's obviously frustrated and unhappy at being there. He says, "I hate this place. I want to get the Hell out of here."

Joseph, a staff member, paraphrases Tim's statement, by saying, "You've had it with this hospital and with us. You just want to be discharged. You want to be out of this damn place."

Clean Communication

The concept of "clean communication" comes from an approach to conflict resolution created by Marshall Rosenberg called non-violent communication (Rosenberg 2003, 2005). The term refers to calmly describing something that happened without threats, criticism, blame, or insults. In other words, describing something "cleanly."

Clean communication occurs when:

- A person says, "I'm mad at you," but doesn't try to bully the person.
- A person says "My watch is missing and I'm concerned that someone took it" instead of "You stole my watch, you jerk!"

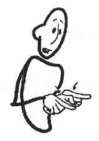

DESCRIBE CALMLY WHAT HAPPENED

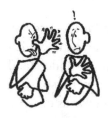 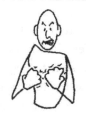

NO INSULTS   **NO THREATS**

NO BLAME   **NO CRITICIZE**

Figure 2.12 Clean communication

Sometimes a primary therapeutic goal can be simply helping a person learn to express his or her feelings safely, without using or exhibiting problem behaviors. For example, you are witnessing "clean communication" when a person says, ""I'm angry" and is willing to talk about that feeling instead of threatening or hitting the other person. Whenever possible, you should point out specific times where a person expresses him or herself safely. These are concrete examples that the person has developed or is developing important foundation skills. Good conversations require many skills. Much of what we want people to develop is evident when we talk to each other effectively.

The following example illustrates the importance of "clean communication."

Scenario 2.15

Pedro was very angry with staff. His typical pattern was to quickly escalate from insults to racial slurs to threats and, finally, physical assaults. On one occasion, he began telling Brian, a staff person, that he was angry. Given Pedro's past history, Brian could anticipate how the situation would escalate. Brian took control of the situation by interrupting Pedro before he had a chance to become aggressive, and pointing out to him a skill he was using before he moved into unskilled behavior.

"Pedro. Do you see what you are doing? You are telling me that you are angry, but you are not insulting me or threatening me. This is great communication. Are you willing to sit down with me and tell me more about what's bothering you, but stay safe? No insults or threats? I really want to hear what you have to say."

The first time Brian tried this, Pedro didn't last long before becoming abusive. When the abusive language started, Brian said, "Pedro, I can't listen to you right now. We'll talk when you are calm." Then, Brian walked away. Pedro approached Brian a few minutes later, and the conversation went better. Pedro was able to stay calm, and try again, thanks to his positive relationship with Brian, Brian's empathetic attitude, and Brian's clear intention to continue talking to Pedro later, under better circumstances.

Bright idea 2.3: Don't let good conversations go by unnoticed! A good conversation is one in which the people you serve use respectful, skillful communication. Many ordinary conversations provide concrete evidence that the people you serve are using the communication, problem-solving, and conflict-solving skills you want to help them strengthen. However, in many cases, the individual isn't aware he or she is using any skills. When we provide specific examples of what a person has already done well, the person will be more inclined to believe they can do it again and, then, repeat the behavior.

Using I-Statements

I- statements are a particularly skillful way of expressing emotions. An I-statement has two parts. It begins when someone describes something specific that has happened, something someone else did, or something another person said. The second part occurs when the person expresses their personal reaction to it. I-statements are always made in a "clean" manner. In other words, without blaming, criticizing, insulting or threatening the other person.

Here are some examples of how I-statements and clean communications go hand in hand:

"When you look at me that way, I feel uncomfortable."
"When you act like a bully, I feel like I don't want to be around you."
"When you express your feelings safely, I want to talk to you more."

A statement like "When you are rude to me, and interrupt me, and disrespect me, I feel really angry at you and I don't want to be with you" is skillful communication. Can you see how less skillful communications, such as the following, can be harmful and potentially dangerous?

"You are a stupid loser."
"You are a jerk."
"This program stinks."

Note that it is not an I-statement just because the pronoun "I" is in it. "I think you are a jerk" is not an I-statement. An I-statement is where you describe your reaction to something. It is a way to communicate how what the other person did affects you. I-statements may communicate painful information (e.g., "When I see you bully people, I don't want to be around you"), but they are much more skillful and helpful than the usual accusations like "You are a bully!"

Skillful I-statements offer you and other staff members a way to give direct, honest, and helpful feedback to persons with challenging behaviors. Done well, they are a constructive way to confront someone about problem behaviors: "When you talk to me that way, I feel like pulling away from you. I want to have a better relationship with you but this isn't helping."

You will often find yourself focusing on the basics of non-verbal attending, listening, clean communication, and I-statements when you are working with people to improve their communication skills. As a staff member, you can teach these skills by modeling them yourself and pointing them out when they occur.

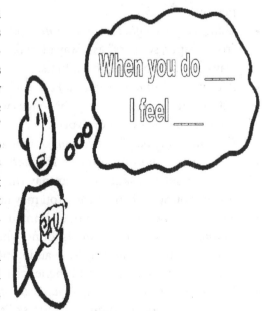

Figure 2.13 I-statements

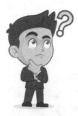

Questions to ponder 2.2: How "clean" are your own communications? When you disagree with someone else, how many of your statements are about what you think they are doing wrong? Do you add in threats or bullying? How often do you use I-statements? Or, do "you" statements dominate your communications with clients, other staff members, and people in your personal life?

Foundation Negotiation Skills

Negotiation begins to come into play when a person realizes that other people are not here just to do what they want; when they recognize that other people have emotions, wishes, and points of view; when they accept that other people have the ability to affect their life. Obviously, people need ways to persuade others. Unskilled communicators try to force their thoughts and wishes on others. Skilled communicators realize they are working with people who want to be treated respectfully, just like they do.

Realizing that other people have similar feelings and desires can be compared to realizing—and accepting—that you have emotions that need managing. Realizing that "this is an opportunity to use a skill" is another key "stop and notice" moment. This profound realization can be easily skipped over because people often take this skill for granted. That's why it's important to point out when you see someone act in a considerate way or take someone else into account. It's also important to help the person "stop and notice" when someone does something constructive as way of dealing with negative emotions. See Scenario 2.16 for an example.

Scenario 2.16

Demetrius, a client in a program, approaches Sandra, a staff person, with a friendly "hello," then asks her how she is feeling. They have worked together for months, and this has never happened before. Sandra, somewhat astounded, seizes the moment.

She replies, "Demetrius. Thank you for saying hello and asking me how I am doing. I really appreciate that. Your friendly smile helps start my day off in a happy mood. How are you?"

Some common foundation negotiation skills include:

- *Discussing a problem with an open mind.* In other words, trying to solve a problem, not defeat another person.
- *Using simple conflict resolution methods.* Flipping a coin, taking turns, sharing, challenging the person to "rock, paper, scissors" as a way of making a decision, voting, and seeking help are all examples of effective ways of resolving simple conflicts.
- *Accepting when one loses or others don't share their opinion.* This can be particularly hard for some people with language and learning challenges who find it hard to understand opinions or accept a solution that is not the one they want or expect.
- *Brainstorming possible solutions* or being able to recognize and consider that other options exist.
- *Weighing the pros and cons of a situation.* Recognizing and weighing pros and cons is so foundational a problem-solving skill that you may think everyone can do it. Don't assume that. Check out whether the people you serve can do this. You may have to spend a lot of time teaching this skill, and if people are very language delayed, it may not be immediately possible for them to learn it.
- *Compromising.* If a solution is found where everyone benefits, it can be presented as "win-win." Again, it's important to use this as a "stop and notice" moment. Be sure to explain how this happened, the skills that the person used and why it is beneficial.
- *Asking for—not demanding—what you want.* Like the concept of "clean communications," this principle is one of the "non-violent communication skills" identified by Marshall Rosenberg (Rosenberg 2003, 2005). Making demands, especially in an effort to stop negative behaviors (e.g., "Stop bothering me!" or "Stop this racist

language!") is not as skillful as requesting specific actions. It is much more effective to ask someone to do something specific than it is to ask someone to stop doing something vague. It is usually more productive too!

Compare the statements in Table 2.1. Which do you think will produce better results? If you are like most people, you responded better to the second of the two statements. These also fit well as I-statements. For example:

"When you act like a bully, I feel angry and I want nothing to do with you."
OR
"When you treat me differently because of my race, it turns me off. In fact, it enrages me, and I just want to fight you."

While this manner of talking can seem phony at first, it quickly becomes natural with practice. When people do this well, they find it is much easier to manage and resolve conflicts. You may want to do an internet search of "non-violent communication" to learn more about this great conflict resolution method.

- *Offer and accept apologies.* The "say sorry" skill is often overlearned. People usually can do it, but it may be superficial and unfelt. Real apologies require more than just saying or signing that you are sorry. Nonetheless, it still counts as a skill, and can be a springboard for learning what more heartfelt apologies are like. Accepting someone's apology is also important to conflict resolution. People in American culture often represent this process by shaking hands. All this represents conflict resolution in a simple form.

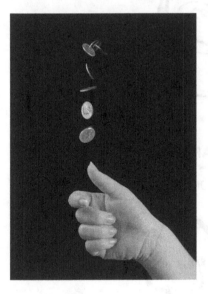

Figure 2.14 Flip a coin skill
©iStock.com/Alexey Stiop

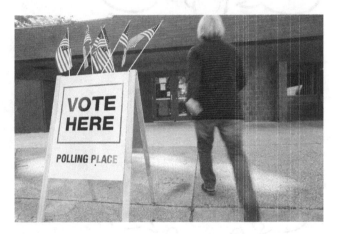

Figure 2.16 Voting is a more advanced conflict resolution skill
©iStock.com/YinYang

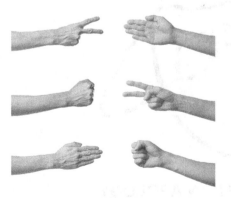

Figure 2.15 Rock, paper, scissors skill
©iStock.com/Evgeny Dubinchuk

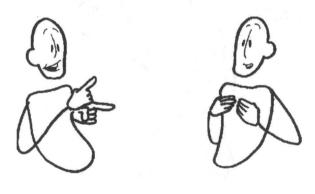

ACCEPT WHEN YOU LOSE

Figure 2.17 Accept when you lose

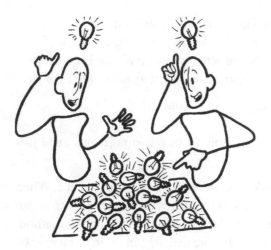

Figure 2.18 Brainstorming

TABLE 2.1 Demands vs. Specific Requests

Stop being a bully!	I would like you to talk to me in a friendly way, without pressuring me to give you money or cigarettes.
We demand that you stop these racist tactics!	We want you to treat everyone the same way, with the same rules and standards, and with respectful language.
Stop oppressing me!	I want you to listen to me and consider my feelings before you make a decision.

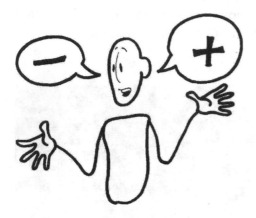

Figure 2.19 Pros and cons

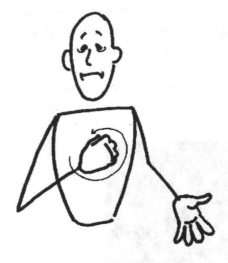

SAY YOU ARE SORRY

Figure 2.21 Offering an apology

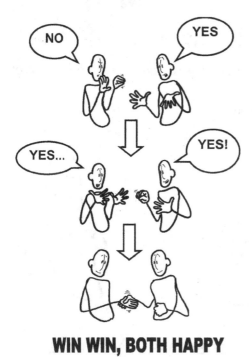

WIN WIN, BOTH HAPPY

Figure 2.20 Win-win, both happy

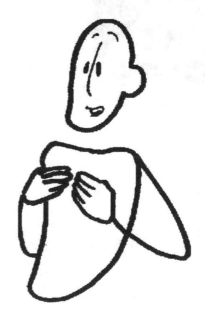

ACCEPT AN APOLOGY

Figure 2.22 Accepting an apology

Scenario 2.17

Matthew and Ida, two program residents, were arguing over who got to sit in the front seat of the car with staff person Armond. With a little help from Armond, they were able to come up with a solution. Matthew would sit in the front on the way to their destination, and Ida would sit in the front on the return. Armond saw the conflict resolution going on and seized the moment to introduce the concept of win-win.

Armond: *"Do you see what you two just did, what skills you used? They were awesome."*
           Matthew looks puzzled. Ida smiles.
Armond: *"You both wanted to sit in the front seat. You talked about it, you negotiated, and you figured out a solution that works for both of you. You both win. Mathew sits in the front seat on the way there, and Ida sits in the front seat on the way back. You both win. We have a name for that skill. We call it win-win skill. You both just did it! I'm really impressed!"*

Note again that most of these skills are very familiar. They normally develop in childhood. As basic as they are, however, adults who are in regular conflict with other people usually are not using them. It is almost always safe to assume that many of the people you are working with have either never learned these skills or, at the least, have not mastered them. This, again, makes your work *developmental*. Because you are not engaged in sophisticated conflict resolution work, these skills can seem so basic that counselors may think they don't—or shouldn't—have to do it. With this clientele, and surprisingly often with people who have stronger language skills, this *is* our work: Helping people develop foundation life skills.

Once you realize that it is essential to work with people to develop such basic skills, it will become easier. When staff look for and name these skills, and engage people with language and learning challenges to develop them further, everyone involved will be more likely to share a language and schema for what "getting better" looks like.

In addition, we should not underestimate how challenging these basic skills can be even for higher functioning adults. Ask yourself, for instance, how often your own communication is "clean" when you are in conflict and how well you use "I-statements."

Bright idea 2.4: Fundamentally, conflict resolution skills are communication skills. The best way to learn to handle conflicts better is to practice these basic, foundational communication skills.

Attitude Is Everything

It's no surprise that attitudes play a key role in effective resolving conflicts. One attitude that is especially helpful to any kind of skill building is willingness. The opposite, of course, is stubbornness. When people are capable of behaving more skillfully, but aren't willing to do so, it can be helpful to ask them outright, "Are you willing?" If you have already established that the opposite of being "willing" is being "stubborn," you might ask, "Are you willing or stubborn?"

It's nearly impossible to solve a conflict peacefully if the people involved aren't willing to participate in the process. You can see this in international conflicts when mediators offer a variety of solutions but neither side is really interested in compromise. The biggest challenge for a mediator often is, "How do I engage all of you in the process?" The process of establishing a willingness to work on problem solving can sometimes be much more difficult

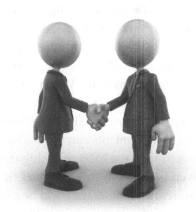

Figure 2.23 Are you willing or stubborn?
©iStock.com/Henrik5000

than actually developing skills once an individual is willing to learn them. The following example highlights the importance of a willing attitude.

Scenario 2.18

Several residents of a group home are arguing with each other about the food in the refrigerator. One accuses a housemate of stealing his food. Another blames him for something unrelated. Another isn't really understanding their complaints but gets involved simply because he's not feeling well. Each in turn goes to Sarah, the staff member on duty, to complain. Sarah wisely chooses not to get involved and, instead, made the housemates responsible for resolving the conflict.

Sarah:	*"I can see you are upset and angry. I'd like to help you talk to each other. I can't fix this for you but I can help you talk to each other. Are you willing to try?"*
	Frank is furious with Sarah. He approaches her and starts yelling at her.
Sarah steps back:	*"Whoa, Frank. I can see you are angry. Do you want to talk about it?"*
	Frank continues to yell at her and assumes a threatening posture.
Sarah continues:	*"Frank, I'm willing to listen to you. But I have to feel safe. Right now, I don't feel safe. Are you willing to calm down and talk to me in a safe way?"*

If Frank's behavior continues to become more aggressive, Sarah has several options for keeping Frank engaged in resolving the conflict with her and the others. She should move away from him and, if needed, call for help. She can approach him at a later time, when he is calmer, and ask him again if he is willing to talk and stay safe. She also may decide to ask someone else to mediate the conflict. She wants to have a good conversation with Frank. By asking "Are you willing to talk to me safely?" Sarah is trying to create an attitude and mindset that will promote a good conversation.

Sarah uses the same approach with all the members of the program. As they continue to complain about each other, Sarah keeps returning to the issue of whether or not they are willing to talk about it.

Scenario 2.18 (continued)

Sarah:	*"I can see you are all angry, but I can't fix this without you. Are you willing to talk about it in a safe and respectful way?"*
	The residents don't answer her question and continue to argue. Sarah repeats, like a broken record, her question about their willingness to fix the situation.
Sarah repeats:	*"Are you willing to talk about this in a safe and respectful way? I can't help you if you aren't willing."*

Sometimes clients are willing to talk through a conflict; at other times, they are not. Sarah doesn't make the mistake of trying to coach skills out of people who haven't indicated a willingness to learn the skills. By way of contrast, she is looking for moments of skillful communication. When she sees them, she points them out. She knows that at those times, if she asks if they are "willing" or "stubborn," that they will say "willing." Then, she can ask a new question: "When you're willing, when you try, does it help?"

Obviously, there are times when staff must step in and fix a situation when conflicts occur in a program. However, whenever possible, it is best to try to engage the clientele to resolve the conflict themselves. Then, any positive developments can be attributed to their own work, their willing attitudes, and their skills.

By getting in the habit of asking the "Are you willing?" question, you can prime people to expect they will be involved in problem solving. Over time, your clients will come to expect that they will be asked to participate in conflict resolution. They will be called on to use their skills.

In Lesson 5, we will explore another important conflict resolution skill: The "ask permission" skill. This skill is used to engage someone in a conversation that is difficult or emotional. For example, you might ask a client, "Is it okay with you if we talk about this?"

This and other attitude questions set the stage for resolving conflicts effectively. By asking, "Are you willing to work on solving this conflict? Are you willing to show the attitudes needed for good conflict resolution?," the individual has the option to say "no" and still remain safe. And, staff has the opportunity to commend the individual on his or her ability to say "no" safely. For example, you might say, "I appreciate you saying 'no' in a safe way. I guess we can't work on this more now. I'll ask you about it again later."

Bright idea 2.5: Before trying to help people solve a conflict, it is often a good idea to ask them if they are willing to try to solve the conflict. They may say "no," but if they say no, it is unlikely you would have been successful by jumping into it. Saying "yes" can create the mind set and attitude needed for conflict resolution. It creates the framework that they are responsible for the outcome. It prepares people for participation and skill practice.

Advanced Conflict Resolution Skills

All of this work is developmental. With some people, we are working on very simple skills. With other people, we are working on more advanced skills. The more that you have a large vocabulary for skills, and the more that you know how conflict resolution skills progress from simple to advanced, the more prepared you will be to recognize and build on skills that are appropriate for the persons you work with. Table 2.2 provides a list of some more advanced conflict resolution skills. It is helpful to be aware of these skills even if you don't get to use them.

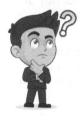

Questions to ponder 2.3: When you review this list of conflict resolution skills, how strong would you say your own skills are? Are you working on foundation skills or more advanced skills? Do you see any kinds of skill that you are not good at? How can you improve them?

Noticing and Labeling Skills That Already Exist

As with coping skills, noticing and labeling skills that already exist is the single most powerful way to engage persons in the process of developing psychosocial skills. To do this, you must have a broad vocabulary for describing skills and the ability to think about skills as a developmental progression. For instance, you must be able to notice and label skills that are evident when a person:

- Has a productive conversation.
- Expresses emotions safely and respectfully.
- Does something that recognizes the personhood, feelings, and perspective of someone else.
- Uses any method at all to resolve a problem to their satisfaction.
- Employs basic skills, such as non-verbal attentiveness.

Wrap-Up

When working with persons with language and learning challenges, it is important to be mindful of whether or not they have a schema for what "getting better" looks like:

- Do they know how you and your program are trying to help them?
- Do they readily understand and agree to a schema that shows them specifically what they can do to advance towards goals?

TABLE 2.2 Advanced Conflict Resolution Skills

Reflective listening	In its simplest form, this means repeating back what the person has said to you. Deeper reflections involve using empathy to infer what the person might be feeling (e.g., "You seem sad").
Being able to distinguish feelings from thoughts and beliefs	You will learn about and practice this skill in Lessons 8 through 10.
Being able to distinguish feelings from wants and from needs	For example, I may *want* to go to the movies right now, but I don't need to. I *need* to eat, breathe, have relationships, and have some fun and recreation in my life, but that doesn't mean I need to go to this movie at this moment.
Being able to distinguish positions from interests	For example, two people are arguing over what television show to watch. The *position* of each is, "I want to control the television." However, the underlying *interest* is in being able to watch shows that are important to them, while keeping harmony in the house. It is easier to help people reconcile their *interests* than to reconcile conflicting *positions* (Fisher & Ury, 1981).
Understanding the concept of *point of view*	It is enormously helpful to be able to recognize and appreciate that the other person has a point of view that makes sense to him or her, even if you disagree.
Understanding varying points of view	Recognizing that there is more than one way to understand a problem is important to coming up with a compromise. Each person involved has an opinion and beliefs about what is happening and what to do. Your way of seeing things might not be correct. Someone else may have a more helpful or accurate viewpoint.
Self-analysis	The ability to understand one's own feelings wishes, beliefs, points of view, needs and goals. Most forms of counseling strive to help people develop this kind of self-awareness. Self-knowledge is also vitally helpful in conflicts.
The ability to understand what two people have in common or both need or want	This requires abstract thinking. For example, "We both want the same thing. We both want to live in a happy house."
Use of more advanced I-statements	These statements go beyond just, "When you do X, I feel Y." They are expanded to "When you do X, I feel y, *because* my need for Z is or is not met." For example, "When you ignore me, I feel angry and hurt because my need to be close with my partner isn't met. That's when I start to look elsewhere for attention."
Paying attention to the feelings, wishes, beliefs, points of view, needs and goals of other people	Not only does self-knowledge help resolve conflicts, but in-depth knowledge of other people also helps. This knowledge skill is usually connected to the skill of empathy.
Feeling empathy	Empathetically placing oneself in the shoes of one's opponent even when you really dislike the person.
WIN-WIN-WIN!	Whenever both sides in a conflict feel they have won something, there is a third win. The relationship wins. For instance, after a new couple works though a few conflicts, they discover they have the ability to weather the ups and downs of being partners. Their relationship wins, and they are a stronger couple. Knowing this can happen, can motivate people to work on conflict resolution.

When the language of a program focuses on skills and this language is consistently reinforced, the people receiving services will eventually start speaking this language. They will start talking about skills and working on skills. They will understand the skills schema. This will also begin to develop the belief that "I can do it."

The first method of doing strength-based work, then, is to notice and label the skills people already have. In Lesson 3, we'll explore three other methods.

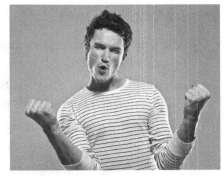

 Practice Exercise 2.4

Figure 2.24 "I did it!"

©iStock.com/Izabela Habur

1. Consider a recent incident in which you were involved in a conflict with another person. Can you identify the specific conflict resolution skills that you or the other person used?

_____

_____

_____

_____

2. Can you identify specific skills that you could have used, but didn't, that would have helped you resolve this conflict? What skills could the other person have used to improve the situation?

_____

_____

_____

_____

3. Consider a time when you sat down with someone you serve to discuss an incident where the person had exhibited really bad behavior. Did the person use skills in the follow-up discussion that he or she wasn't able to use when the problem behavior occurred? What specific skills did you see later, after the conflict was over, that weren't present when the conflict occurred?

_____

_____

_____

_____

Lesson 2 Skill Sheet

- Participant will develop an extensive vocabulary for conflict-solving skills, especially for simpler skills usually learned in childhood.

- Participant will think about skills developmentally, recognizing that they may be looking for the kind of skills that normally develop in childhood.

- Participant will practice noticing and labeling skills that the people they serve already use.

- Participant can help people identify crucial "stop and notice" moments that occur when a person stops him or herself before doing something problematic.

Lesson 2 Quiz

1. Two residents are fighting over which television show to watch. Which of the following conflict resolution skills would you want them to demonstrate? (Check all that apply.)

   a. Taking turns.

   b. Negotiating.

   c. Sharing.

   d. The "around the world" technique.

   e. Expressing feelings safely.

2. You sit with an angry person after she has calmed down to discuss what happened. The person was able to participate well in this discussion and willingly role played ways to handle the stress better next time. Which of the following statements are true? (Check all that apply.)

   a. The person is using some good conflict-solving skills now in this follow-up discussion.

   b. It is a good strategy to help the person recognize the skills she is using at this moment.

   c. It is helpful to practice using skills after they are reviewed.

   d. The person should lose points for blowing up.

   e. She should be punished for her bad behavior, otherwise she will never learn to behave better.

3. Conflict resolution skills vary from simple to complex. Which of the following is an example of a complex skill that is normally learned in adulthood, if it is learned at all?

   a. Sharing.

   b. Taking turns.

   c. Cross-cultural perspective taking.

   d. Expressing feelings safely.

   e. Using I-statements.

4. People from different cultures or subcultures often have cross-cultural conflicts that lead to misunderstandings. This can be true when Deaf and hearing people interact. Which of the following skills are important when resolving Deaf-hearing cross-cultural conflicts? (Check all that apply.)

   a. Listening.

   b. Having respect and empathy for each other.

   c. Clean communication.

d. Perspective taking.

e. Accurately understanding of each other's language.

f. Winning the argument.

5. Three people successfully plan a party together. The staff person observing them notes that they used a number of conflict-solving skills. Which of the following skills did they likely use? (Check all that apply.)

a. Clean communication.

b. Taking turns

c. Problem solving.

d. Planning.

e. Compromising.

f. Win-win.

g. Demanding.

Extra credit: Marshall Rosenberg developed an important approach to conflict resolution that places a lot of emphasis on the development of clean communication. What is the name of this approach?

Lesson 2 Questions for Discussion

1. Do you consciously pay attention to conflict resolution? Are you already working on this in your personal and/or work life?

2. What conflict resolution skills do you feel very confident using? Where do you see weaknesses in your own conflict resolution abilities? How can you develop them further?

3. Consider the colleagues you work with, including supervisors and other staff members. Who seems to have particularly strong conflict resolution skills? What skills in particular do these persons regularly exhibit?

4. Consider the people you serve in your agency. What skills do you see them regularly using? Has anyone helped them to recognize and name the skills they already have? If not, why not?

5. Do you and other members of your team regularly help the people you serve to notice and label the skills they already have?

6. Do you think it is important to establish in your program the idea that you are all working on building skills? Do you think this shared schema will be helpful?

7. You have a good conversation with a person you serve. Can you identify all the skills that each of you likely used that made this a good conversation?

8. Using a developmental framework, identify skills and strengths in a person you serve that you haven't recognized until now.

9. Working with people on conflict resolution requires adopting a framework that applies not just to *them*, but to service providers as well. Everyone, including staff members, has strengths, weakness, and skills that can be improved. Are you willing to have conversations with the people you serve in which you humbly admit that you could have been more skillful? Would you be willing to acknowledge and apologize for times you made mistakes or behaved less skillfully?

10. People in power in organizations sometimes resist work on conflict resolution because they don't want to have to make decisions without input. Indeed, the more power you hold, the less likely the idea of

conflict resolution may appeal to you. Why work on conflict resolution when you can just tell people what to do?

Who in your organization is likely to be receptive to this model and who is likely to be resistant? Will the people with more power be more resistant?

Lesson 2 Quiz Answers

1. Answers *a*, *b*, *c*, and *e* are all types of conflict resolution skill. To my knowledge, there is no such thing as the "around the world technique."

2. Answers *a*, *b*, and *c* are strength-based approaches that will be discussed more in Lesson 3. The pre-therapy approach presented here does not involve either a level or point system or punishment. Both of these approaches go against our emphasis on engaging people in skill development.

3. The correct answer is *c*, cross-cultural perspective taking. This advanced skill requires the ability to appreciate another person's perspective, as well as the ability to appreciate another culture's frame of reference. Cross-cultural perspective taking also may require the ability to appreciate that some of your own deeply held beliefs are, in fact, historical and cultural. These beliefs are often acquired because you lived or were raised in a specific social and historical context. If you had lived in another time and place, you'd probably think very differently. Response *e*, "I-statements," also refers to a skill that is advanced for many people.

4. Answers *a* through *d* are important skills for resolving cross-cultural conflicts. While *e* is helpful, it is not required. People who don't share a language can work out conflicts with each other, although interpreters and cross-cultural mediators and educators will likely be needed. Winning an argument (*f*), without the other person feeling they have won also, will likely result in a damaged relationship.

5. The group is likely using all of the skills, with the exception of *g*.

Extra credit: Marshall Rosenberg's approach to conflict resolution is called "non-violent communication." It emphasizes communication skills and is the basis of much of the information presented in this lesson.

Note

1. This example is taken from *Deaf mental health care*, p. 61. Multiple other examples of Deaf/hearing cross-cultural conflicts can be found in that book.

References

Fisher, R., & Ury, W. (1981). *Getting to yes*. New York: Penguin.

Fulghum, R. (2003). *All I really need to know I learned in kindergarten*. New York: Ballantine.

Glickman, N. (2009). *Cognitive behavioral therapy for deaf and hearing persons with language and learning challenges*. New York: Routledge.

Rosenberg, M. (2003). *Nonviolent communication: A language of life*. Encinitas, CA: Puddle Dancer Press.

Rosenberg, M. B. (2005). *Speak peace in a world of conflict*. Encinitas, CA: Puddle Dancer Press.

Introduction

In Lessons 1 and 2, you were introduced to this program's emphasis on noticing and labeling skills people already have. We used a developmental framework so that we can see developmentally simple skills, or skills that are just emerging, and bring these to the attention of the people we serve. In Lesson 3, we will expand on this strength-based approach. We will discuss three new ways to look for skills. We will contrast problem-based and strength-based interventions, and provide examples of what the latter look like. We will also learn about asking questions that help people discover their skills and strengths.

Scenario 3.1

Becky and Irene are two roommates in an apartment. An outreach worker, Ben, works with them. Becky and Irene have horrible arguments with each other, especially over the television remote. They have each become insulting and threatening, and Ben is very worried about their ability to live together safely.

One day, Ben goes out to a restaurant with them and the three of them share a nice meal together. At the end of the meal, Ben comments on how pleasant it was. They talked about how they joked around, listened to each other, agreed on what food to order, and how they were all nice to the waitress. After this discussion, Ben asks them, "Could you use some of these same social skills at home?" He wonders out loud, "How would your home life be different if you used these skills at home the way you used them here in the restaurant." Becky and Irene say they will try.

Of course, they quickly resume fighting at home. But now, Ben has a reference point for positive skills. "Remember the great restaurant skills you used when we went out together? Are you using them now?"

Working in a strength-based way is possibly the single most powerful way to engage people in mental health treatment. In a strength-based approach, staff members recognize, talk about, and build on skills that people already have. They talk to people about what they do well and invite them to consider ways they could do things differently or better. For many programs, this means shifting their thinking 180 degrees, from focusing on a person's skill deficits to focus on their individual strengths. In practical terms, staff members who are working in a strength-based way are not saying, "Stop that." Instead, they are saying, "Do more of that!"

Changing Expectations

Strength-based work is especially important when you are working with people who function poorly and have challenging behaviors. They typically receive a lot of criticism from people in authority, including staff members in mental health programs who are often very focused on what the individual does wrong or doesn't do at all. Individuals with problem behaviors commonly encounter staff members who try to control or influence them by telling them what they need to do or improve.

Sometimes, staff members simply say, "Use your coping skills," as though this advice is enough. Staff members often complain that "she won't use her coping skills" when a person isn't able to meet staff expectations. They've forgotten that the art and skill of pre-therapy work is about *engagement*, about creating people's *willingness* and *ability* to develop and use these skills. Focusing exclusively on an individual's problems inevitably creates resistance. This should not come as a surprise. After all, who wants to take on the hard work of changing behaviors when no one recognizes their progress? At some point, most people would say, "Why should I work with you when you only want to talk about what I do wrong?" or "Why should I do that? You know that I can't."

Usually, the people you are serving have been referred to your program because they have very severe problems—either they are functioning at what society considers very low levels or they are hurting themselves or other people. For example, they may be failing in school, can't take care of their basic needs, or are physically aggressive. Some may show all of these behaviors. When people are in treatment because of such overwhelming life challenges, it can be difficult for staff members to focus on strengths and skills because they are not readily apparent. Cultivating the ability to see the skills and strengths people have usually takes intention and effort. It's a vitally important skill for staff to master.

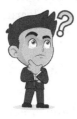

Questions to ponder 3.1: Most programs today give some attention to client strengths. Sometimes strengths can be observed but often staff doesn't really know how to build on these strengths in their treatment efforts. How are client strengths attended to and built on in your setting?

Four Key Strategies

Identifying skills is at the heart of strength-based work. There are four key strategies that you can use to identify coping and conflict resolution skills in the people you are serving. You can find them in Bright idea text box 3.1. In this lesson, we will elaborate on each.

Bright idea 3.1: Four methods of doing strength-based work

1. Find skills that are developmentally simple.
2. Find skills when the problem behavior is absent.
3. Find skills when the problem behavior is improved.
4. Find skills when the person is engaged in recovery from problem behaviors, including when they offer any repair to damaged relationships.

Let's look at each strategy more closely.

Finding Skills by Thinking Developmentally

The first strategy was discussed in Lessons 1 and 2. As you'll recall, these lessons focused on basic coping and conflict resolution skills. Identifying these skills can be called "thinking developmentally." Remember, skills develop from simple to complex. You need to look for simple skills. You are thinking developmentally when you recognize that a person is using coping skills by rocking in a chair, doing headstands, listening to music, or laughing. You are thinking developmentally when you recognize that a person is using conflict resolution skills when he or she takes turns, flips a coin, shares food, or expresses themselves safely. These skills are simple ones that are usually first shown in childhood.

While it sounds easy to think developmentally, it is actually a complex skill. It can become harder to remember and recognize simple skills as your own skills advance. Even seasoned professionals find this difficult, as shown in Scenario 3.2.

Scenario 3.2

Staff members on a hospital psychiatric unit were working with an adolescent who became aggressive very easily. The adolescent received a weekend pass to visit her residential school. On Monday, the hospital social worker called the school counselor and asked how the weekend had gone.

School counselor: *"Fine, but she didn't use her coping skills."*
The hospital social worker was puzzled.
Social worker: *"What do you mean?"*
School counselor: *"Well, she didn't blow up at all, but she just stayed in her room a lot, watching TV."*
Social worker: *"Oh. What else did she do?"*
School counselor: *"Just the usual stuff. She talked to some of her friends and used the PlayStation. I think she did some drawing."*

The hospital social worker explained that she thought the young woman must have been using her coping skills because she was safe and in control. She said, "Well, to me her behavior shows that she did use her coping skills. She used 'stay in her room skill,' 'talk with friends skill,' 'PlayStation skill' and 'drawing skill.' And I bet, if you look more closely, you'll find she used other skills as well. When you say she didn't use her coping skills, what were you expecting?"
The school counselor couldn't really answer that question.

Perhaps the counselor thought that coping skills had to be something more sophisticated. While it would have been wonderful if the adolescent had chosen to meditate, practice yoga, write in her journal, or draw pictures to express herself, those were more sophisticated skills than she had. Her skills were developmentally simpler. But, the important thing is that she used them.

Problem-based vs. Strength-based Responses

Consider how a problem-based response would differ from a strength-based response in the situation we have just discussed above.

In a *problem-based response*, staff pay attention to problem behaviors, including the inability or unwillingness to use an agreed on treatment strategy. For example, following an outburst, a staff member might say: "You didn't use your plan to come to staff when you are upset to talk things out. What kept you from using this plan? How can we help you do better?"

In a *strength-based response*, staff members search for any skills the person did use, no matter how simple. They then seek to build on them. For example: "I noticed that you used a number of skills this weekend. You kept yourself safe. What did you do? We noticed that you stayed in your room a lot. That seemed to help. How did it help? We also noticed that you talked with your friends, used the PlayStation, and did some drawing. All of these are good skills. What else did you notice?"

Again, the goal is to help this student to do better than she did. Of course, you intend to build on this beginning but, for now, you want to engage her. Which of these two approaches do you think will engage her more successfully?

Think back to the scene from the Temple Grandin movie that we discussed in Lesson 1. As you'll recall, Temple's overwhelming anxiety was triggered by a series of what most people would consider to be very small irritations, such as a piece of paper out of place, the metallic sound of the fan turning, the shapes of the curtains rusting in the wind. She responded by running outside to put herself in the squeezing machine used to calm cattle. This behavior was initially puzzling to her aunt who didn't understand the very clever coping skill that Temple was using. Temple had discovered that a sensory-based skill used to soothe cattle—applying pressure to both sides of the body—also soothed her. Most people use some sensory- or movement-based coping skills (think about exercise, for example), but when people have language and learning challenges, their sensory-movement strategies may be their primary coping skills. In Temple's case, she developed a highly effective, sensory-based approach to helping children with autism deal with meltdowns.

In the following example, staff members at a group home help residents recognize both obvious and easily overlooked skills (Scenario 3.3).

Scenario 3.3

Joan, a staff person, is having a house meeting with Frank, Bob, and José, three deaf residents of the program. The focus of the meeting is a discussion about skills. Frank and Bob are very talkative, but José is quiet. However, when Frank makes a comment about a skill that he uses that he calls the "bubble skill," José asks what that is. Then José is quiet again. While Frank talks about the bubble skill, José sits uncomfortably in his chair and interrupts three times to ask, "When is the group over?" Frank continues telling his story. He describes how he was walking down the street when a person bicycled around him. As the person passed him, Frank noticed that he looked angry. Then, he gave Frank "the finger." Frank realized that the person had probably been telling him to get out of the way but Frank hadn't heard him. Frank said he normally would have responded by returning the gesture. But, this time, he just kept walking. Frank said he imagined that he was in a bubble where nothing bad could happen to him. Then, José started talking about a time when someone gave him an angry face and he used his "shield."

Before the group meeting ended, Joan made a point of noting that, even though José had been quiet and seemed uncomfortable, he had used several skills. Their discussion went something like this.

Joan:	"José, I'm really impressed with some of the skills you used in the meeting today. Do you mind if I point them out?"
José looks puzzled:	"OK."
Joan:	"I'm happy to do that, but first I wonder if you *noticed* the skills. For example, could you tell me, on a scale of 0 to 10, how comfortable you felt during the meeting? I'm guessing you didn't feel very comfortable. Am I right? What number would you give it?"
José:	"I was bored."
Joan:	"Oh, you were bored. So, on a scale of 0 to 10, how bored were you?"
José:	"Ten."

Joan:	"Ten, wow. So here's what is so impressive. You were so bored that you gave it a 10 on the scale, but you still asked questions. . . You still stayed in the group . . . You still told your own story about how you used your shield. All of these are skills you used to handle the boredom and anything else you might have been feeling."
José:	"Oh."
Joan:	"Here's a harder question. How did you manage to use these skills when you were so bored?"
José:	"I don't know."
Joan:	"Well, I don't know either. I just know you did it, and I appreciated that you stayed in the group. See, it is really easy to use skills when you are interested and comfortable, but when you use skills when you are bored or uncomfortable, that's really when you show coping skills!"
Joan (to everyone):	"Not only did you all talk about skills. You were also using all these great skills, like sharing stories, expressing yourself clearly, listening, and supporting each other. Great job everyone. I really enjoyed this meeting!"

As this scenario shows, recognizing and pointing out developmentally simple skills is a great way to help the people you serve discover skills they already have.

Finding Skills when the Problem Behavior is Absent

Another strategy for doing strength-based work with people with language and learning challenges is to find coping and conflict resolution skills when a problem behavior is absent.

No matter how much we talk about strength-based work, the reality is that most of us use a problem-based approach most of the time. This is partly because mental health training is very concerned with helping people address specific problems. It's also because problems are more obvious and, as a result, easier to notice. You can't help but notice when someone becomes angry and throws a chair. You may not notice, however, when a person with a history of chair throwing *doesn't throw the chair* and instead

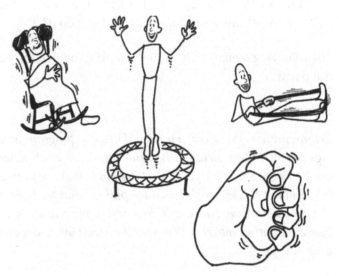

Figure 3.1 Sensory-based coping skills

chooses to go outside for a break or just pushes the chair slightly and walks away. You also may not make the connection that the person is demonstrating important skills when he participates in a very good conversation the next day about throwing the chair and how he might do better.

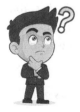

Questions to ponder 3.2: How often do you comment on the coping and conflict resolution skills that people you are working with are using?

No one shows problem behaviors all the time. Even if the person you are working with is the most aggressive or self-harming person you've ever encountered, he or she is not aggressive or self-harming every moment of every day. It's physically impossible. Everyone has times when problem behaviors are not evident. These in-between moments often offer insights into the person's coping skills.

For instance:

- A person who tends to "blow up" leaves a situation to calm down.
- A person who normally makes insulting, racist comments acts in a socially respectful way with a person of color.
- A person doesn't drink or use substances even though he craves them.
- A person who is usually assaultive or self-harming every day goes a week without any problem behaviors.

When problem behaviors are absent, attend to what the person *is* doing. It pays to be curious. Ask the person how he or she managed to avoid the problem behavior at those times. What did he or she do differently?

Before you start asking questions, however, you want to make it clear that your intention is to ask questions about what the person is doing well. Remember, the person may be so used to being criticized or asked problem-based questions that he or she becomes defensive whenever staff ask anything. The person is expecting criticism. Signaling that you are going to ask about something positive can lessen the person's defensiveness. For instance:

"I'm so impressed with something good you just did. Can I ask you about it?"

"Wow. Did you notice how well you just handled that situation? It seemed like Joe was picking on you. How did you feel? Angry? But you didn't hit him, like you often do. Awesome. How did you manage that?"

"I noticed you chose not to drink this time. I think that's awesome. Do you? I know it's been so hard for you to resist those cravings. How did you do it?"

The following scenario illustrates how to recognize and reinforce the skills used when a problem behavior does not occur.

Scenario 3.4

Brianna receives services at a partial hospital program in a building that also houses program offices where meetings are often held. Brianna is easily bored and tends to leave her program and go into the offices while meetings are in progress. She barges in and demands that the people in the meeting talk to her. Staff members have spoken to her about this many times and explained that the behavior disruptive and disrespectful. But she keeps doing it.

One day, however, she didn't do it. She went up to a conference room, looked in and, for some reason, walked away. However, staff members noticed that she hadn't interrupted them. After the meeting, the senior staff person approached Brianna.

Staff member: *"Wow. I'm so impressed and so appreciative. Did you notice what awesome skill you used today?"*
          Brianna shrugs.

Staff member: *"You did something really good, really helpful and really skillful. Do you know what it was?"*
          Brianna looks interested but still says nothing.

Staff member: *"When you came up to the room, we thought you were going to come in and disrupt the meeting, but you didn't. You saw that we were having a meeting. You stayed respectful. You were willing to wait to talk to us until later. That was so awesome! How did you do it?"*

Brianna: *"I was looking for Joanna."*

The staff member continues, determined to frame this as a skill.

Staff member: *"You were looking for Joanna, and she wasn't in the room. But you didn't come in and ask where Joanna was. You didn't come in and talk about something else. You used your skills of being polite and respectful and waiting. We all just thought it was so good."*

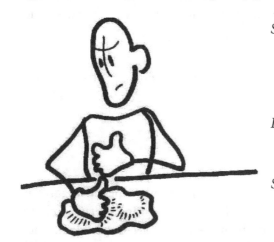

Figure 3.2 Pounding clay as a coping skill

Brianna stops and thinks, then says: "Uh-huh."

It often takes some creativity to discover and name the skills used when a person isn't showing problem behaviors. As you read Scenario 3.5, try to identify the skills that Angelo is using.

Scenario 3.5

Angelo is a 16-year-old boy who lives at a residential school. He has an artificial leg that can be detached. When Angelo is angry, he sometimes takes off his leg and throws it at another person. It's not surprising that this action invariably elicits strong reactions and has become a real problem in the program. However, because it takes some time to detach his leg, sometimes Angelo doesn't bother. One of his teachers has taken to praising him each time he expresses anger without detaching and throwing his leg. She praises him for his "leg-keeping skills."

She asks: "Why were you able to be angry yet still keep your leg on?"

She shows genuine interest in his success and also offers a personal I-statement response.

She says: "When you talk about your feelings like you are doing now, and don't throw your leg around, I like being with you much more."

If you are looking for evidence of coping skills, try to spot times when the person doesn't show aggressive or self-harming behaviors in situations in which they normally would have. If you are looking for evidence of conflict resolution or other social skills, look for instances when people who often argue or fight get along instead.

In Scenario 3.6, a counselor helps a couple begin to recognize skills that they have and are using to avoid the conflicts that characterize their relationship.

Scenario 3.6

Bruce and Tricia are a couple that argue over very simple matters. Neither listens to the other particularly well and neither appreciates that the other has their own needs, wishes, and ideas. They finally agree to see a counselor.

When they are in the counselor's office, they can't identify any specific problems even though they have been arguing all week. In their minds, they have no problems because they are not arguing at that exact moment. Each says everything is fine. This isn't denial or an unwillingness to open up to the counselor. They are genuinely unable to identify conflicts or reflect on behaviors that, in their minds, are over. They may not like the other person's actions, but neither has the abstract thinking skills needed to see how their failure to develop and use a set of skills to manage their feelings and behaviors makes new conflicts highly likely. They certainly aren't able to recognize patterns in their conflicts. In their minds, when they aren't fighting, everything is fine.

The counselor's job is to help them establish the schema for skills. Once that is done, the counselor will be able to help them see how not using skills can lead to conflicts. Since they aren't identifying conflicts on their own, the counselor asks them to talk about what they like in each other and what is going well.

In one session, Bruce talked about how Tricia agreed to play basketball with him and they played together for an hour. From this example, the counselor helped them identify the skills they used when they were not arguing such as:

- *Identifying what I like to do.*
- *Asking my partner to do what I like to do.*
- *Negotiating a time and place.*
- *Arranging to get to the basketball court.*
- *Playing together for an hour.*

- *Having fun together.*
- *Accepting when one person wins and the other lost.*
- *Thanking the person for doing what you asked them to do.*

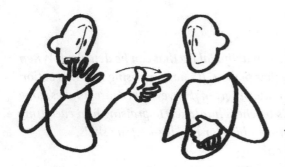

ONE PERSON TALKS, THEN THE OTHER.

Figure 3.3 Turn taking in conflict resolution

Similar discussions occurred numerous times before Bruce and Tricia were able to talk about skills on their own. It was much easier for them to notice the skills they used when things went well—that is, when the problem conflicts weren't present—then to recognize the skills they needed when they fought. However, once the idea of using skills was established, and once a set of useful skills were named, discussed, and practiced, it became much more possible for the counselor to have Bruce and Tricia practice using these skills in situations where they actually needed them. In particular, they practiced the skills of talking to each other without interrupting, taking turns, showing respect, and trying to understand what the other person wanted.

 Bright idea 3.2: Sometimes people who have many problems talk to you but they aren't able to identify any problems. It may be that they don't recognize a problem because it isn't happening at that particular moment. You may be able to open up a skills discussion by shifting the conversation to ask, "What is going well now? What are you doing to help things go well?"

 Bright idea 3.3: What we call a skill is somewhat arbitrary. You may not feel, for instance, that playing videogames is a skill. The point is that it is useful to frame it as a skill in your conversations because it creates a schema that skills are important. You may also discover that playing videogames actually does require a number of distinct skills, such as patience and taking turns, not to mention a variety of cognitive skills.

 Practice Exercise 3.1

1. Think of a person you serve in a program who exhibits very problematic behaviors.
2. Consider moments when these behaviors are not present.
3. Think about the following questions and write down your answers in the space below:
   - Why didn't the problem behaviors happen?
   - What did the person do instead?
   - What was different?
   - Is there any way you can give the person credit for using skills that kept him or her safe?

_____

_____

4. If possible, pose these same questions to the person you have chosen as the subject of this exercise. Write down the person's responses in the space below.

_____

_____

Finding Skills When a Problem Behavior is Less Obvious or Intense

You also may be able to spot skills when a problem behavior is less intense, an episode is shorter, or the recovery from an episode is quicker. Scenario 3.7 illustrates this opportunity.

Scenario 3.7

Charlotte is a hearing adolescent in an inpatient program. She had a horrible meltdown that lasted well over an hour. During that time, she tore apart her room, physically attacked several people, and shouted insulting, racist comments. Staff members were unable to stop her. Staff eventually resorted to restraining her after she threw her body against the wall and was in danger of seriously injuring herself. It was a miserable experience for everyone. When it was over, staff struggled to find anything about the episode that they could put a positive spin on.

A few days later, Charlotte was again upset. For about 10 minutes, she knocked over the furniture in her room, threw her clothing on the floor, and screamed. Then, she sat on her mattress, covered herself with blankets, and cried until she calmed down. After a few minutes of crying, she was willing to talk with a staff person who had sat down beside her. The incident ended without any restraints being used.

In this situation, staff members can choose to use a problem-based or strength-based approach. Let's examine how each might look:

Problem-based staff response:
   Staff member: "I'm concerned that you are still having these meltdowns where you try to destroy furniture and hurt people. How do we help you keep from destroying your room when you get upset? Why didn't you use your coping skills?"

Strength-based staff response:
   Staff member: "You seemed to handle this stressor better this week. Do you notice the difference?"
   Staff member waits to see if Charlotte can tell her. When Charlotte doesn't respond, the staff person continues.
   Staff member: "Last week, you were aggressive and self-destructive for over an hour and didn't stop until we restrained you. Do you remember how you assaulted three people, called people racist names, and hurled your body against the wall so powerfully that we were afraid you would hurt yourself?
   Staff member again waits to see if Charlotte recalls her behavior. Charlotte is listening but says nothing.
   Staff member: Today, you were still upset, but what did you do differently? Did you notice that you didn't assault anyone? Did you notice you made no racist comments this time? Did you notice you used a sensory strategy of calming yourself with blankets? Did you notice that you allowed yourself to feel your feelings and cry and that you were then willing to talk with staff? My question is, how were you able to cope so much better this time? Why did you do so well today compared with last week?"
   After some discussion, the staff member continues: "What do the skills you used this time, the fact that you did so much better, say about what you are capable of?"

   Which approach do you think is likely to be more helpful to Charlotte?
   The same principle applies to finding conflict resolution skills when conflict behaviors are less intense. Scenario 3.8 illustrates this principle.

Scenario 3.8

Bruce and Tricia have had some really serious conflicts that resulted in physically aggressive behaviors, like pushing and hitting each other. However, more recently, they have not been getting physical with each other, just yelling. Their counselor could focus on their continuing problem of mistreating each other. The counselor could ask something like: "What can you do instead of yelling at each other?" The counselor could also note the improvement and ask questions to help them recognize some of the skills they were using to improve their interactions. For example:

Counselor: "Remember how you used to hit each other and push each other? You haven't done that in, I think, three or four months, right? It seems as though you are learning some skills that help you stay safe with each other. What skills do you think you are using?"

The first time the counselor asked Bruce and Tricia these questions, they were puzzled and didn't know how to answer. They were not used to thinking about their behaviors as skills, and they didn't think they were doing anything well. However, after they became used to talking about skills, they were better able to answer the question. They agreed that they followed the "no hitting rule." The counselor expanded on this "rule" and framed it as a "skill."

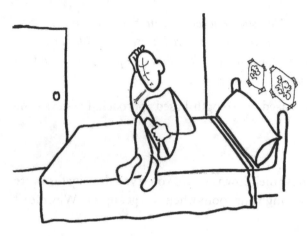

Counselor: "So you both learned that a good rule for relationships was no hitting, and you are using the skill of following the 'no hitting rule.' When you follow that rule, do you feel better? Do you like the other person more?"

After exploring how this was true, the counselor helped them see that they had just used another skill.

Counselor: "Notice that you are talking about what you do and how you feel? When you are safe with each other, when you don't hit, you feel happier and you like each other more. It seems that you are learning some skills about controlling your behavior. You are doing this right now. How are you doing it? How are you staying safe?"

This conversation led to a discussion about "time-out skills," which they also have used on a few occasions.

Figure 3.4 Time out skill

Bright idea 3.4: If a person graduates from physical assault to verbal assault, the verbal assault is not a skill. Whatever the person did to *improve* their behavior is the skill. The point is not to focus on the "less bad" behavior but on the reasons *why* it is less bad. Of course, you want to discuss what even more skillful behavior would look like. Recognizing and validating skill improvement is designed to be the start of a conversation, not the end.

Bright idea 3.5: When asking why or how improvement occurred, be attentive to signs of self-talk. It's very likely that the person engaged in some helpful self-talk, but isn't aware of it. It may have been something like, "I don't want to get in trouble again," or "I'll just ignore this jerk." The skill is *thinking*—in particular *thinking about consequences*. Finding evidence of this kind of helpful self-talk allows you to help the person develop this skill further.

Practice Exercise 3.2

1. Read Scenario 3.9.
2. Think about what a *problem-based conversation* between Jeremiah and staff might look like. Write it down in the space provided.
3. Think about what a *strength-based conversation* between Jeremiah and staff might look like. Write it down in the space provided.

Scenario 3.9

Jeremiah has a history of self-harm, including head banging, cutting, swallowing objects like batteries, paper clips and pens, and other dangerous behaviors. He is being treated in a psychiatric hospital. Staff members notice that for the past month Jeremiah's self-harming behavior has lessened considerably to some fairly minor cutting. However, he still cuts himself whenever he gets hold of something sharp.

Problem-based conversation:

_____

_____

_____

_____

Strength-based conversation:

_____

_____

_____

_____

Finding Skills at a Later Time, in the Recovery or Relationship Repair Process

You might be concerned that this style of work reinforces bad behaviors by calling them skills. Can you think of any situations in which you can say that a behavior was unskillful, unhealthy, and/or bad in every respect? Should even the worst behaviors be framed positively as skills in order to do strength-based work? What about times when people have the skills to behave better but choose not to?

The intention of strength-based work is not to sugarcoat destructive behaviors. Rather, it is to engage people in the process of self-development. We are opening a conversation about how to do better by getting the topic of skills on the table.

It is usually a good treatment idea to help people see what they do well. However, it's vital to do this with people who don't think of themselves as having any positive skills and qualities because it gives the person a language for "doing better" and a belief that they have the capacity to do better. People get better by using skills. Once people are engaged in a conversation about skills, you can start asking them to evaluate whether their skills are adequate, whether these skills are helping them to reach their goals, or whether they think they need stronger, better skills. We'll move to the topic of promoting this self-questioning in the next four lessons.

For now, however, let's focus on situations in which no skills can be observed when an individual is in the midst of a problem behavior. In this type of situation, referring to something that is obviously destructive as a skill is unconvincing at best and, at worst, runs the risk of reinforcing a problem behavior. This might include times when an individual has skills but chooses not to use them and behaves badly. How can you find strengths then? Even if you can't find strengths at the time that the problem behavior is happening, you can often find strengths in the recovery process after the problem behavior has passed. You may be able to identify skills in the way people calm themselves down, get back on track, or attempt to "repair" relationships that they have damaged. Often, you can find important skills in the conversations the person engages in to explain why and how the problem happened and what they might do better in the future.

In Scenarios 3.10 and 3.11, you will see how the recovery from destructive behaviors can be used to recognize, reinforce, and build skills.

Scenario 3.10

Brady became really aggressive with staff when a trip he wanted to go on was postponed. He spat, kicked, punched, and hurt two staff people. There was simply no way that anyone could see that Brady used any skills in this incident.

The next day, Brady was willing to talk about what happened with a counselor. He could identify what he was upset about, what he felt, and even a little bit about what he was thinking. He said he felt that "It's not fair! I never get what I want! Staff lied to me!" He talked about the situation for about 20 minutes. Throughout that time, he remained calm and was able to identify what he could have done differently. After 20 minutes, he said he wanted to stop talking.

Before they finished the conversation, the counselor asked Brady whether he noticed all the skills he had just used. Brady didn't initially see them, so she helped him out. The counselor pointed out:

- *"You were willing to talk. You showed a willing attitude and an open mind."*
- *"You stayed calm and expressed yourself safely. You didn't threaten me or insult me. You used what we call 'clean communication' to talk about what happened."*
- *"You were able to say what bothered you, what triggered your anger."*
- *""You were able to identify how you felt."*
- *"You even used a really difficult skill—identifying how you* think*. You said you thought that postponing the trip wasn't fair, that you never get what you want and that staff lied to you. You showed a lot of self-awareness skills."*
- *"You listened and we had a good back and forth discussion. The conversation felt respectful to me. Did it feel respectful to you?"*

- *"You were able to identify two things you could have done differently. You said you could have gone to your room or you could have talked to staff."*
- *"You were able to say when you had enough and to end the conversation in a skillful way."*

The counselor recognized that Brady isn't ready to practice any of these skills yet, so she doesn't propose it. But, she does finish with a question that will pave the way for future discussions,

Counselor: "Look at all these skills you just used with me. What do you think this says about what you are capable of doing if you decide you want to?"

Brady shrugs.

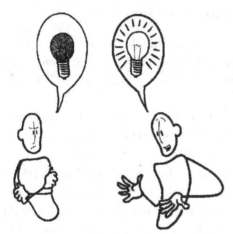

"It won't work!"
"Impossible!"

"We will find a way"
"We can solve this!"

DISCUSS WITH OPEN MIND THINK HOW SOLVE PROBLEMS

Figure 3.5 An open mind is a skill

By posing this last question, the counselor has planted a seed. The counselor is setting the stage for work she wants to do in the future when Brady is ready. She hopes to eventually invite him to work on developing more and stronger skills. However, he's not ready for that quite yet. Staff will have to continue to search for evidence of skills that he already has, however developmentally simple they are. Then, staff will need to help Brady discover them as well.

Scenario 3.11

Yesterday, Samuel, a Deaf signing resident of a program, became agitated while in a conversation with a staff member and punched him. Today, Samuel has expressed some regret and is willing to explore what happened. He talks calmly about how angry he felt when the staff person said "no" to him, how he just couldn't control himself, and that he is sorry now. Dax, the staff person who is helping Samuel to explore the incident, helps Samuel notice some of the skills that he has just used, like EXPRESS FEELING SAFE SKILL (express feelings safely skill). Dax invites him to role play the conversation that had ended so badly the day before, then walks Samuel through the RED, YELLOW, GREEN LIGHT coping skill.

Samuel apologizes to the person he assaulted and is willing to role play the conversation they had yesterday, only to do it in a better, safer way. Of course, it is easier for Samuel today because he isn't feeling the same emotions as he felt yesterday. Even so, he is using a variety of skills. The whole conversation engages him in doing better next time.

At the end of the conversation, Dax helps Samuel to name the skills he just used in their conversation.

Dax: "This was a great conversation. Do you see how this conversation was different than yesterday? What did you do differently today, in this meeting?"

Samuel: "Stayed safe."

Dax: "Yes, exactly! You didn't hit me, you didn't yell at me, you didn't make racist insults, and you didn't break anything. You stayed safe. How'd you do it?"

Samuel: "I used my coping skills."

Dax: "What skills did you use?"

Samuel: "Uh, red, yellow, green."

Dax recognizes that Samuel is saying what he thinks Dax wants to hear. Dax seizes the opportunity.

Dax: "Yeah, I think you did you use that. When we role played, you noticed the moment you were mad. You used the 'red light, stop and notice' skill. Then you used the 'yellow, calm down' skill when you did some slow, deep breaths. Then you used the 'green light, think then act' skill when you talked calmly. You also used great conflict-solving skills. What were they again?"

Samuel: "Talk safe."

Dax: "Yes, talk safe. What else?"

Samuel: "I don't know."

Dax: "Did you listen? Did you take turns talking? Did you apologize?"

Samuel: "Yes."

Dax: "Are these skills too?"

Samuel: "Yeah."

Dax: "Awesome job!"

 Bright idea 3.6: If you can help someone see how current behaviors are more skillful than previous ones, it may help them acknowledge that the previous behaviors were problematic. You are providing evidence of how they can do better. This reduces any shame that may be attached to acknowledging the previous "bad" behaviors.

Strength-based work comes down to this: Staff *notice, label, comment on,* and *invite discussion of skills* that people already show.

As a staff person, you can develop this ability by thinking developmentally and having a very large vocabulary for the kind of behaviors that could be considered skills. In ASL, you can sign the idea of "turning your head around" to convey the idea that you are seeing the world in a new and different way. Instead of seeing problems, you see what people do well. Instead of just seeing when problems occur, you also recognize when they *don't* occur, are less intense, or end sooner. Then, you can ask, "Why the improvement?"

Finally, you can find skills by watching what the person does to calm down, feel better, or repair any damage after a problem behavior has occurred. This is one way to understand "recovery." Recovery might occur in conversations or may be seen in actions that suggest the person is trying to reconnect with someone who was hurt by his or her actions or words.

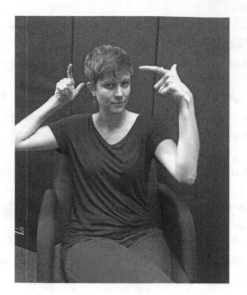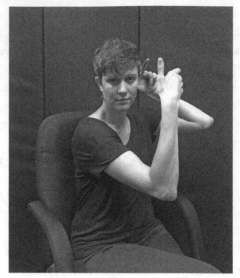

Figure 3.6 ASL sign for TURN YOUR HEAD AROUND
Used with permission

In some cases, the improvement may have something to do with a change in the environment (e.g., the person wasn't triggered as much) or with medication. Regardless of the circumstances, it is important to find a way to attribute the improvement to a skill that the person used. For example, you can say: "Yes, people didn't bother you, so you found it easier to use your skills." Or, "Yes, the medicine helped you stay calm enough to use your coping skills." People will do better if they attribute their own improvement to something they did, not circumstances or medication.

Of course, common sense must play a role when you are helping a person find strengths. Framing a behavior as a skill must be reasonable to the person you are talking to. If you don't believe this yourself, you are not likely to be convincing.

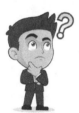 **Questions to ponder 3.3:** Why would we want someone to attribute their positive behaviors to their own skills and not to circumstances or medication? Does it make sense to do this even when medicine or the environment clearly played a positive role?

 Bright idea 3.7: Never let someone's successful use of skills go unnoticed. Always point it out. This is an easy way to reinforce positive coping and social skills.

 Practice Exercise 3.3

1. Consider the last conversation you had with someone you serve that felt productive and positive. How many skills can you identify that were used by either of you in this conversation? Write them down in the space below.

_____

_____

_____

2. Go back to the person and explore together what each of you did right. List them in the space below.

_____

_____

_____

3. Identify the skills that were used. Give the skills names. Write them in the space below.

_____

_____

_____

Asking Strength-based Questions

Throughout our daily work with the people we serve, we have countless opportunities to choose between telling people something (usually what to do or not to do) or asking them questions to help them figure something out on their own. For example:

1. "You can't do that right now," or "Can you do that right now or can you wait? If you insist on doing it right now, what will happen?"
2. "You did terrific work on that," or "Did you see how terrific your work on that was? I can tell you what you did that was terrific but I'm wondering if you already know. Can you tell me?"
3. "We need to talk about this," or "Can we talk about this?"
4. "I think you have a problem," or "I'm worried about something. Can I talk to you about it? I'm wondering if you already know what I'm worried about?"

Generally speaking, it is better to ask questions than to give answers. When you ask good questions, you encourage the people you are working with to figure things out on their own. Asking questions engages people and fosters skill development. The best questions help people discover their skills and strengths. For example, these questions are variations on the same theme:

"What did you do that worked?"
"How did you succeed in doing that?"
"What skills did you use?"
"How did you manage to stay in control or handle that situation?"
"You did that really well. What do you think that says about how you are changing and growing?"

Staff members can find skills by asking questions that help people discover what they do, no matter how simple, that helps them to function better. You can find skills by asking why and how a problem behavior did not recur or how and why a behavior improved. You can ask questions that help people see what they are doing to recover and repair relationships that might have been damaged by problem behaviors. See Table 3.1 for some common questions that you can consider asking in specific situations.

It's also important to notice that asking questions, especially questions about what people do well, is a more respectful approach than acting as an authority and *telling* people what they do well. When done properly, the process of asking questions empowers the person receiving services and establishes him or her as the authority and the person with the answers. It also fosters better relationships. We will explore relationship-building skills, such as empathy, in the next two lessons.

TABLE 3.1 Strength-based Questions that Help People Discover Skills

When	Consider asking
A person does something that he or she doesn't realize is a skill	"Did you notice how you calmed yourself down? Did you notice how you felt after you went to your room and watched television? I wonder what skill you were using."
A person's behavior is better than it was previously	"Did you notice how you handled this trigger today?" "How was this different than yesterday?"
A person didn't show a problem behavior	"Today I noticed you used some awesome skills. Did you notice? What were they?"
A problem behavior is less intense	"Did you notice you seem to be showing a different attitude today than yesterday? What's the difference? Do you see a difference in how people are responding to you today?"
A person's attitude or mood has improved	"Wow. That was awesome. Did you notice whether you used 'open mind' or 'closed mind' skill? What do you think?"
A person recovers more quickly from a problem period	"Last time you drank, it took you a week to get back on track. Did you notice that you seemed to recover more quickly this time? What did you do differently this time?"
A person does a good job of "repairing" a relationship after a problem behavior	"Did you notice how well you discussed the problem this time? How does that compare with the way you handled it yesterday? What did you do differently today?"

Practice Exercise 3.4: Practice asking strength-based questions

In this lesson, you learned four strategies for finding skills. They were:

1. Thinking developmentally.
2. Noticing when a problem behavior is absent.
3. Noticing when a problem behavior is improved.
4. Noticing when the person is recovering from problem behaviors, including when they are interested in or offering to *repair* damaged relationships.

Using these four strategies:

1. Create some strength-based questions that you could ask in the following situations.
2. Write them in the space provided.

Situation 1: Samuel is struggling with a strong caffeine addiction. He drinks several huge cups of coffee or caffeinated soda each day. As a result, he becomes very confused and is unable to form clear sentences. He twitches, makes jerky movements, and sometimes becomes aggressive. Staff members have been working to encourage him to cut down on his caffeine intake. This morning, he limited himself to two cups of coffee when he would normally drink four.

What are some skills that Samuel might have used?

_____

_____

_____

What questions could staff ask to help Samuel recognize these skills?

_____

_____

_____

Situation 2: Julia has a problem picking at her skin. She can't seem to stop herself and will pick to the point that she creates an open wound. She has been willing to use anti-itch creams. A few times, when she felt overwhelming urges to pick, she was willing to wear gloves. A staff member notices that Julia is putting anti-itch cream and Band-Aids on the area she often picks at.

What are some skills that Julia might have used?

_____

_____

_____

What questions could staff ask to help Julia recognize these skills?

_____

_____

_____

Situation 3: Sebastian lives in his own apartment. Outreach staff visit him and help with shopping. He looks forward to these shopping trips with staff. However, recently Sebastian's apartment was so filthy that when the staff person arrived, she said they had to focus on cleaning and would not have time for shopping. Sebastian was very upset about this. But, the next time she came, the apartment was much cleaner. Sebastian said that he didn't want to waste their time cleaning. He wanted to go to the mall.

What are some skills that Sebastian might have used?

_____

_____

_____

What questions could staff ask that will help Sebastian recognize these skills?

_____

_____

_____

Bright idea 3.8: Staff are at their most skillful when they ask questions that guide people to discover their own abilities. A person is more likely to own positive feedback and use it if staff are able to draw it out of the person by asking good questions.

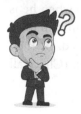

Questions to ponder 3.4: How comfortable are you asking questions of the people you work with? Do you think you are being less skillful when you are asking questions than you are when offering answers?

- Participants are expanding their skills vocabulary by understanding how a large number of everyday behaviors can be considered skills.

- Participants notice when problem behaviors don't happen and ask why. They ask what enabled the person to *not* show a problem behavior.

- Participants identify the skills used by name when a problem behavior is less severe than before. They ask, "Why are you doing better?" They look for skills to help explain this progress.

- Participants identify the skills used by name when a person they are serving tries to *recover* from a problem behavior and offers some *repair* of damaged relationships.

- When things go well, participants make an effort to give the people they serve credit for the improvement by connecting the positive outcomes to the skills they used.

- Participants help the people they serve to discover skills they already have by asking strength-based questions.

Lesson 3 Quiz

1. Patty is angry because she expected a trip home but her family had to postpone it. In the past, when she has not gotten something she wanted, she has become aggressive with other people and destroyed property. Today, she screamed and then went outside for a long walk. Which responses are most likely to engage her in learning skills? (Check all that apply.)

    a. "You have to learn to stop screaming. You're scaring other people."

    b. "You should not go outside without telling staff."

    c. "You seemed upset when your parents said they had to postpone the visit. How did you feel?

    d. "Last time you got bad news, you hit the staff person. This time you just screamed and went out for a walk. It seems like you used more skills this time. Did you notice that?"

    e. "You got bad news. How did you handle it? What skills did you use?"

    f. "Could you use even more skills?"

2. Which of the following are strategies for strength-based work? (Check all that apply.)

    a. Understanding how simple skills develop into complex skills.

    b. Mindfully pay attention to what people are doing well.

    c. When a person has a good day, ask why and seek to give them the credit for whatever positive developments happened.

    d. Pay attention to the way people calm down after they have lost control.

    e. Notice efforts that people make to reconnect with someone they have hurt.

    f. No matter what happens, look for the skill.

3. Ahmed is a 22-year-old male who has a problem with head banging. In the past, he has banged his head against the wall hard enough to cause a head injury. Staff recognized that he bangs his head when he is anxious, frustrated, or angry. They have helped him to explore other sensory strategies to help him cope with these feelings. One day, Ahmed became upset and started to bang his head and then stopped. He then rolled on the floor until he calmed down. Which of the following are strength-based responses? (Check all that apply.)

a. Ask Ahmed why he didn't use his coping skills.

b. Praise Ahmed for using "roll on the floor skills."

c. Notice that Ahmed stopped himself from banging his head.

d. Notice that Ahmed only banged his head a little before rolling on the floor.

e. Take away five points because Ahmed is still banging his head.

4. Which of the follow represent opportunities to find skills in a person's recovery from an incident of problem behavior? (Check all that apply.)

a. The person calmed down much more quickly this time.

b. Sam hit his roommate, but then he went to staff asking for help.

c. Josephine stopped herself from drinking after two beers.

d. Asa slammed the door to her room, then stayed inside for two hours.

e. After pushing someone, Arthur gives a quick, insincere apology, but won't discuss it further.

5. John had a bad blow-up yesterday and ended up punching another person. Today you sit down with him and are able to have a good conversation about what happened. Which of the following are skills he might be using today? (Check all that apply.)

a. Listening.

b. Taking turns.

c. Expressing himself safely.

d. Practicing new skills.

e. Saying he was sorry.

f. Making excuses and blaming other people.

6. Turn the following strength-based observations into questions that could be used to guide people to discover strengths on their own.

a. "I noticed you used your 'going to your room to chill out skill' today."

b. "Usually when I tell you 'no,' you start screaming at me, but today you didn't."

c. "Last time it took you a full hour to calm down after a meltdown. Today you calmed down in only 10 minutes. It seemed like rocking back and forth was a skill that helped you calm down."

d. "Today you are talking to me in a very skillful way. You're listening. You are not screaming at me, but instead you're expressing yourself calmly, saying how you feel."

Lesson 3 Questions for Discussion

1. In your work setting, when you observe staff interacting with clientele, what percentage of the time would you estimate that staff members are focused on problems they see? What percentage of the time are staff members focused on skills or strengths they see?

2. Consider your coworkers. What skills and strengths do you think other staff members are *not* seeing in the persons they serve? Why do you think they are not recognizing these skills and strengths?

3. Think of a situation where a problem behavior did *not* occur. What skill could the person have been using to avoid the problem behavior?

4. Think of a situation in your work in which a problem behavior occurred but less badly than previously. In this case, did staff focus on how the problem behavior was continuing or how the problem behavior was improving?

5. People often attribute their progress to medication or to someone else helping them. Why is it important for people to attribute their progress to their own skills, not to medicine or another person?

6. Can you think of a situation where a person showed very few skills in a problem situation but did a very skillful job of processing the situation later?

7. How could a "processing session," where you talk about what happened, be turned into an opportunity to rehearse using skills better?

8. This lesson is based on the assumption that most of the "bad" behaviors we see in our programs are due to a lack of psychosocial skills like coping, communication, and conflict resolution skills. Is this always true? What if the person has the skills but chooses not to use them? What if the problem is a lack of motivation, not a lack of skills? What if the problem is that the person has different values, or is motivated to commit crimes? Is there any benefit to identifying positive skills even in those situations?

9. Are there times when it is more helpful to focus on increasing motivation than on teaching skills?

10. Bright idea 3.7 was "Never let someone's successful use of skills go unnoticed. Always point it out. This is an easy way to reinforce positive coping and social skills." Do you do that now? If you did more of that, what do you think would happen?

Lesson 3 Quiz Answers

1. Response *d* is the most strength based and the most likely to engage her. Response *c* shows some empathy and asks questions. Both are good responses. Response *a* is setting a limit. Could questions have been used to help Patty see the impact of her screaming on other people? The least helpful response is *b*. It just sets a limit and tells the person what they did wrong. *E* and *f* are good questions to ask later in the process.

2. Answers *a* through *e* are all examples of strength-based work. *F* goes too far. If someone does something really bad, look to see if there are skills in the recovery or the repair, but don't minimize the impact of really bad behavior. One of the better ways to respond to bad behaviors (depending, of course, on what they are) is with I-statements. For example, when you threaten or hit me, I feel afraid, angry, and I lose motivation to work with you.

3. Answers *b*, *c*, and *d* are strength based. You can find skills in the moment Ahmed noticed his problem behavior and did something else, in the fact that the problem behavior wasn't as bad and in choosing the alternative less harmful behavior of rolling on the floor.

4. With a bit of digging, it's possible to find skills in answers *a* through *d*. Answer *e* is trickier. Arthur says he is sorry, but the way in which he does it indicates it is just his way of not dealing with the consequences of his aggressive behaviors. Perhaps you could find a tiny bit of skill in this behavior—he recognizes the need for apology—but it might be more useful to continue looking deeper. For example, does Arthur's behavior change, even for a short time, after his aggressive behavior? Does he do anything differently, like act friendlier, after the aggression that might suggest that he is trying to repair the relationship? If staff can find more evidence of skills in the recovery than a weak "sorry," this approach will be more effective.

5. Answers *a* through *e* are skills that might be happening in that conversation. Response *f* would not be skillful in recovery or repair.

6. The statements and questions could be framed as strengths in the following ways:

   a. "How did you calm down? What did you do?"

   b. "Did you notice how much better you coped today when I had to say 'no' to you? What did you do differently today?"

c. "Last time it took you a full hour to calm down after you lost at cards. Today you calmed down in only 10 minutes. What did you do that helped you calm down so much more quickly today?"

d. "How do you think this conversation today went? Did you see all the skills you were using? What were they?"

References

There are many sources for this approach to strength-based work. One can find it in the solution-oriented brief therapies developed by William H. O'Hanlon and Michele Weiner-Davis as well as that developed by Steve de Shazer. One can find it in the narrative therapy approach developed by Michael White. One can also find it in the works of Donald Meichenbaum, especially in his later constructivist narrative CBT and his works on resilience.

I like the book by Matthew D. Selekman, which summarizes and extends these solution-oriented and narrative approaches and a recent work by Meichenbaum on finding resilience in military, trauma victims, and their families.

Meichenbaum, D. (2012). *Roadmap to resilience: A guide for military, trauma victims, and their families*. Clearwater, FL: Institute Press.
Selekman, M. D. (1993). *Pathways to change: Brief therapy solutions with difficult adolescents*. New York: Guilford Press.

Introduction

In Lesson 4, you will learn about empathy and the important role it plays in developing strong therapeutic relationships. You will learn that pushing people to learn skills often fails if you have not also developed a strong therapeutic relationship based in your ability to communicate an empathic understanding of your client's inner world. In Lesson 4, you will also learn about the importance of asking for and using feedback to improve our abilities to show empathy.

Acceptance and Change

Scenario 4.1

Joe is a direct care worker in a group home for Deaf people living with mental illness. He understands the importance of helping people learn skills and that the best way to get a conversation going about skills is to notice and discuss the skills a person is already using. However, when he tries to talk about skills to the people he is working with, they aren't always interested.

Sharon is a young resident at the group home who often cuts herself. Sometimes she makes vague threats about wanting to harm herself or others but when staff members want to talk about it, she refuses. Staff members find this behavior alarming and don't know what to do. They've been told that they should talk to her about skills, but Sharon doesn't always want to.

One day Sharon got some bad news. She wasn't offered a job that she really wanted. At the house, she seemed both angry and depressed. She started scratching herself, eventually causing her arm to bleed. She came to Joe to show him her bleeding arm.

Sharon: *"I cut myself. I can't stop."*
Joe: *"What about your coping skills? What coping skills can you use?"*
  Sharon became angry with Joe, screamed at him in sign language, and then went up to her room where she proceeded to do even more serious cutting.

  Did Joe do something wrong?

The Role of Empathy

Dr. Marsha Linehan identified an important problem with standard cognitive behavior therapy, particularly as it applies to many persons who have experienced a great deal of abuse and neglect and have been diagnosed with "borderline personality disorder" (Linehan 1993).

Dr. Linehan recognized that the success of any form of counseling and therapy depend on the counselor's ability to demonstrate empathy. Empathy and acceptance are the foundation of dialectical behavior therapy, or DBT, a successful therapeutic approach she developed in the late 1980s. DBT combines empathy and acceptance with the skill building techniques that are at the heart of traditional CBT.

Dr. Linehan pointed out that many people are unwilling to accept help from someone if they feel that person doesn't "get" them in a deep and meaningful way. This is a widespread problem in all forms of counseling and therapy. She noted that CBT is primarily an approach to help people learn skills that they can use to change themselves and achieve their goals. Problems arise, Dr. Linehan said, when too much emphasis is placed on change. If you push people too hard to change, they may feel that:

- They aren't accepted.
- They aren't receiving the support they need.
- They aren't being heard.
- Their needs and challenges aren't being validated
- They aren't receiving the respect they deserve.

The result may be that they push back and refuse to change. They may begin to view your efforts to help them to change as criticism. Your relationship with the person suffers and they pull away from the work you've been doing with them.

When too much emphasis is put on a specific therapeutic technique, such as skill building, it's easy to overlook the critical step of building an empathetic connection with the person. Without empathy, the other techniques often fail.

Invalidation

Consider, for instance, the idea of "invalidation." You invalidate someone when:

- You do *not* recognize what the person feels and thinks.
- You tell the person that their feelings and thoughts don't make sense.
- You tell them that they should *not* think and feel as they do.

For instance, when Jason feels angry, his father responds by telling him that he has no good reason to feel angry and that he should feel happy. This invalidates Jason's feeling and most likely makes him feel frustrated and even angrier. His father also likely feels frustrated.

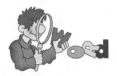

Emotional invalidation

Definition 4.1: Emotional invalidation: Emotional invalidation occurs when a person's thoughts, feelings, or experiences are criticized, ignored, or rejected.

Example of emotional invalidation: When her abusive father dies, Miriam has mixed feelings. She feels sad but she also feels angry and relieved. She tells her mother that part of her is happy that he is gone. Her mother tells her it is a sin to feel happy when your parent dies and that Miriam should be ashamed of herself for feeling that way.

Borderline personality disorder is a set of emotional, behavioral and identity problems that are the result of an extensive history of abuse. Dr. Linehan theorizes that borderline personality disorder develops, in part, when a person receives an enormous amount of invalidation from parents and other key persons during childhood. Emotional, sexual, and physical abuse all involve emotional invalidation. When children are victims of abuse, they learn not to know or trust their feelings. As children, they learn unhealthy coping strategies, such as self-harm, and do not learn how to form healthy attachments or relationships. As a result, they often find themselves forming other unhealthy relationships as adults.

A classic example is a person who was sexually abused as a child who later seeks out adult relationships with abusive people. Why would a person do that? The people trying to help the individual may feel the urge to shake him or her and shout: "Don't you see that you are getting involved in the same type of abusive relationship again and again? Why don't you work on finding someone who will treat you well?"

Oh, if only helping was that easy!

The Purpose of Unhealthy Behaviors

People who have unhealthy or challenging behaviors found them to be helpful, at least initially. At one time, it made sense to harm themselves, use alcohol and drugs to avoid feeling pain or behave with other people the way that people had behaved with them. These behaviors are usually very hard to change. People can't be expected to just turn off a behavior simply because a counselor tells them to "wake up" or use skills. However destructive they may be, these unhealthy behaviors and coping strategies are what people know. They become a kind of comfort zone. It is often easier for people to stay in this zone, to repeat destructive behaviors, than it is to risk change.

Counselors who don't understand this, who push too hard for change without striving to understand the person's experience at a deep level, will usually find that the person resists change. Instead of feeling safe, the person receiving services may just feel criticized or blamed. He or she may continue engaging in—or return to—the unhealthy behaviors that helped them cope with negative feelings in the past.

To make matters worse, a lot of CBT is focused on helping people change how they think. This is the "C," or cognitive, part of CBT. We'll discuss it in depth in Lessons 8 through 10. However, recognizing the impact of the way a person thinks is critical to being empathetic. Because CBT often focuses on how people think in incorrect or unhelpful ways, there is a risk of further invalidating the person. The person gets the message that they "think wrong" and that they should change. Chances are, the person has heard this his or her entire life. Hearing it now, from a counselor this time, doesn't feel helpful and may re-traumatize the person.

Balancing Change and Acceptance

Dr. Linehan's brilliant insight was that a therapeutic focus on change had to be *balanced with a therapeutic focus on acceptance*.

Most people will not try to change if they don't feel accepted. Dr. Linehan designed a form of therapy that brought together techniques designed to help people change with techniques that help people feel validated and accepted. She drew from the world of CBT to find change strategies; she looked to the world of Buddhism for acceptance strategies. This movement back and forth is called a *dialectic*. Hence, the name of her treatment approach: Dialectical behavior therapy, or DBT.

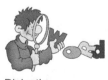

Dialectic

Definition 4.2: Dialectic: A method of examining, discussing and using opposing ideas in order to find a higher truth.

Example of dialectic: Arnold is a staff member working in a group home. His job is to coach clients to learn skills and he understands they can change by learning skills. He learns that sometimes he should not push clients to change by learning skills. Instead, he should empathize, to offer them support for how they feel. This means that instead of pushing them to change, he is helping them accept themselves as they are.

The idea of sometimes helping clients change and other times helping them stay the same is confusing to Arnold at first, but after a while he realizes there is something very smart in this idea.

Linehan uses the term "dialectic" to refer to two seemingly opposing ideas that are essential for mental health care: Acceptance and change. Depending on the individual's situation and needs at the time, you may work on helping the person accept themselves as they are. At other times, you may work on helping the person change behaviors that are unhealthy. This movement between acceptance and change is like a dance, a *dialectical* dance. All good mental health care moves back and forth, like a slinky or a pendulum, between acceptance and change strategies. In other word, all good mental health work is *dialectical*.

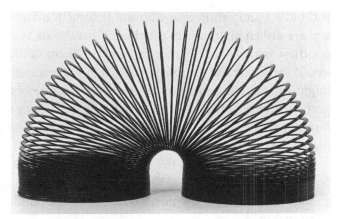

Figure 4.1 "Dialectic" is like a slinky. Movement between opposing ideas: Accept people as they are and help them change

©iStock.com/cass greene

Let's get back to Joe from Scenario 4.1. Joe did a good job of remembering that an important part of his job is helping the people he serves to use coping skills. Unfortunately, he didn't realize that *you can't just jump into skill work*. If you immediately encourage someone who is in pain or distress to use skills, they usually will feel unsupported. Or, they may think that you are criticizing them. What people usually want first is emotional support. How do you think Sharon would have reacted if Joe had responded like this?

Scenario 4.1 (continued)

Sharon: *"I cut myself. I can't stop."*
Joe: *"I see. Do you want to talk about it?"*
Sharon: *"I have to cut myself."*
Joe: *"You feel like you have to cut yourself. Are you willing to tell me more?"*
Sharon: *"I didn't get the job."*
Joe: *"Oh. You must be really disappointed."*
              Sharon nods.
Joe: *"You really wanted that job."*
              Sharon nods and starts to cry.

The Power of Relationships

There is wide agreement in the mental health world that a good therapeutic relationship trumps every other therapeutic tool. In a therapeutic relationship, counselors use their powers of empathy to convey understanding of and support for clients' experiences and feelings. It is more important to develop a good relationship with someone than to do any other therapeutic intervention, including focusing on skills. Nothing happens in counseling outside of a therapeutic relationship.

Any treatment approach can be implemented badly. Empathic and nurturing relationships are critical to successful treatment. If you apply a specific technique as if you were a machine, it will probably fail because you have forgotten to be a warm, caring person. The technique isn't at fault—the fault lies in the way you performed it.

CBT offers many techniques that can be put into a treatment manual or completed on a computer. If the person is ready and able to use these CBT manualized or computerized techniques, they may benefit, even without a therapist. People who use treatment manuals on their own readily understand these approaches and are driven internally to use them. Chances are very good that because these people understand and seek out these manualized approaches, and use them skillfully on their own, they will benefit. Research on them would show that the approach works, but the research might draw the wrong conclusion as to the reason. It might conclude that the person got better because of the specific techniques they used, whereas they might get better because they are enthusiastically following a self-help method that they find personally meaningful. It might be the personal meaning they find in the approach, and not the specific techniques themselves, that makes the difference.

In any case, this is not the clientele this workbook seeks to help. We have no way to bypass the human connection that is essential to recovery for most people and certainly for our clientele. We've been talking about skills, but now we must be sure any skill building occurs in the context of an empathic therapeutic relationship.

The human connection is particularly important at the early stages of treatment work, such as when you are trying to engage people initially. Since this pre-therapy workbook is focused on giving you ways to engage people in CBT, it is critical that you pay close attention to your relationships and your ability to empathize.

You focus on skills to give people a language and practical strategies for "getting better." You demonstrate empathy to move people to want to work with you.

As the example from Scenario 4.1 shows, Joe means well. He's trying to use what he learned. But, he isn't truly attending to how Sharon is feeling. He also isn't focusing on their relationship. At the moment, Sharon isn't ready to talk about coping skills.

The example in Scenario 4.2 illustrates how CBT techniques can actually push someone away if they are used improperly.

Scenario 4.2

A staff person is frustrated with a client and doesn't want to spend time with her. She says to the person in a scolding manner, "Go use your coping skills." The client interprets this attitude as a rejection and responds by becoming more aggressive. The staff person then complains that CBT isn't working.

Some people who receive mental health services may tell you that they are sick of talking about skills. In this situation, the person has likely worked with someone who has practiced CBT or DBT techniques badly. Clinicians or staff may have criticized the person for "not using skills." They may have forgotten to use empathy. They may have over-emphasized the CBT techniques while not attending sufficiently to the therapeutic relationship.

Think about the situation described in Scenario 4.2. Can you think of a more skillful response? A more effective—and respectful—response would be to stop and attend to her feelings. For example:

"You seem upset. Would you like to talk? I wonder if you can wait 10 minutes. I have to finish this task, and then I can sit with you. Is that okay? I really want to hear what you have to say."

Contrast this with the staff member's earlier abrupt response. In the second example, the staff person shows empathy, caring, and respect. She also is negotiating around both of their needs if she can't, as often happens, be available immediately. (If the person does accept this negotiated plan, she will have also demonstrated negotiating skills, something the staff person can point out to her later.)

In pre-therapy work, the goal is to create a model of care that is simple, clear and engaging. This involves using skill-building strategies for helping people change. It also means *switching to relationship building* and *backing away from skill building* when the person isn't ready.

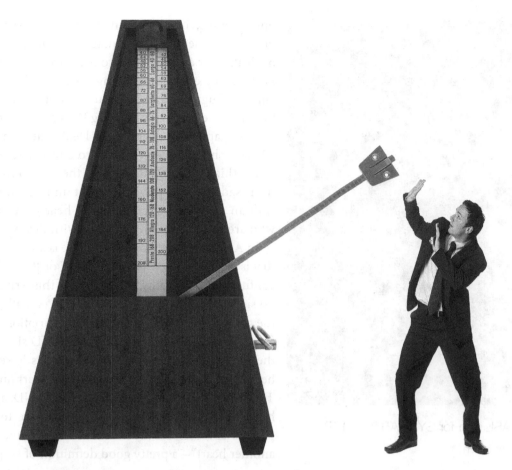

Figure 4.2 Person not ready to work on change? Then work on acceptance!
©iStock.com/kkgas

Bright idea 4.1: In mental health care, you must balance two strategies that can seem opposing—helping people accept themselves while also helping them to change. You need to have a toolbox for each of these strategies, and learn how to skillfully choose between them.

Bright idea 4.2: The most important tool in the therapist or staff counselor's toolbox is *empathy*.

Skill with Empathy

Empathy and skills are the two guiding concepts in this CBT pre-therapy program. Counselors showing empathy help people feel accepted and safe enough to consider change-oriented strategies like developing skills. People become more willing to learn new skills when they believe that the people working with them can put themselves in their shoes and appreciate just how tough this work is.

Empathy is the ability to understand how another person feels and thinks. It is often confused with sympathy or pity. Sympathy is feeling badly for someone else because you imagine or assume they are suffering.

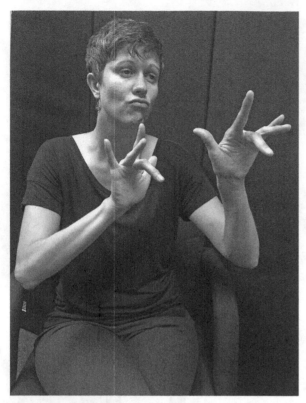

Figure 4.3 ASL sign for SYMPATHY or PITY
Used with permission

For example, many hearing people feel sympathy for deaf people because they imagine it must be terrible to be deaf. They are surprised to learn that, in reality, many deaf people experience being Deaf in relation to their culture, language, and community, not as the absence of hearing. They experience being Deaf as a benefit, a "gain" and are happy and proud to be Deaf (Bauman & Murray 2014) As hearing people learn to empathize rather than sympathize with Deaf people, their emotions change from sadness and pity to respect and admiration. This shift in attitude better prepares hearing professionals who are in helping roles to work with deaf people.

In American Sign Language, there is a well-known sign that is usually glossed as SYMPATHY or PITY and is often confused with empathy. At the time of this writing, there is no single universally accepted sign for empathy. One way the concept is conveyed is by using a variation of the sign for UNDERSTAND. The UNDERSTAND sign is made at the forehead. For EMPATHY, the sign is lowered to the heart level, conveying the idea that the heart understands. Then the second hand signs UNDERSTAND, again at the heart level, but closer in the signing space to the other person. This conveys the idea of "one heart understanding another heart"—a pretty good definition of empathy!

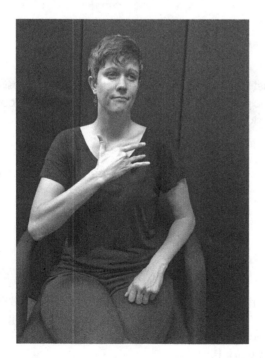
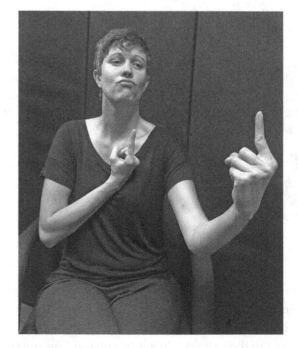

Figure 4.4 ASL sign for EMPATHY (HEART UNDERSTAND)
Used with permission

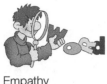

Empathy

Definition 4.3: Empathy: The ability to sense what another person is feeling and thinking and communicate that to the other person.

Example of empathy: Betsy is telling her friend Joseph how she felt when a strange man followed her home. Joseph listens carefully and makes comments like, "Wow, that must have been terrifying!" He is aware of past bad experiences that Betsy has had with men. He gently asks, "Did this bring back all those memories of what happened before?"

Anyone who wants to become an effective counselor must develop strong abilities to empathize. You can develop your empathy skills over time by learning to listen well. It can't be taught or learned in one simple lesson, but it can become a focus of mindful attention and practice. People can learn about this skill, and begin the daily practice of empathy that must continue throughout their careers.

Most people learn empathy in childhood when the adults in their lives exhibit empathy in their interactions with them. People also develop greater empathy when they find themselves in a position where they need help from others. For instance, it is commonly believed that Franklin Delano Roosevelt's capacity for empathy with the poor was enhanced when he became sick with polio. For the first time in his privileged life, Roosevelt found himself needing help from other people.

Empathy has four characteristics (Wiseman 1996):

1. The ability to understand another person's feelings.
2. The ability to understand another person's thinking or point of view.
3. The ability to respond to another person without judgment.
4. The ability to communicate one's understanding of another person.

A good way to start any intervention with a person you want to help, therefore, is to ask yourself:

"Have I been able to *accurately understand* how this person feels and thinks and to *accurately communicate* this understanding to the person without judgment?" If you answer "no" or "I'm not sure" to this question, there's a good chance that, at this moment, you may not be as effective in helping the person develop skills as you hope to be.

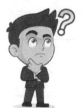

Questions to ponder 4.1: How well developed is your own ability to feel empathy for other people? How skilled are you at accurately perceiving and understanding how other people feel and think? How good are you at conveying this understanding in a non-judgmental way?

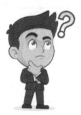

Questions to ponder 4.2: When you are working with someone to change their behavior, how often do you stop and ask yourself whether you really understand how that person feels, thinks and sees the world? Do you see the world from their point of view? It's important to answer these questions honestly before you begin therapeutic work.

Practice Exercise 4.1

Part 1

Examine the photograph in Figure 4.5.

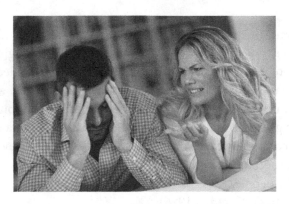

Figure 4.5
©iStock.com/laflor

1. Create a scenario that you think describes what might be happening in the picture.

    _____

    _____

2. Try to imagine what each person might be *feeling*.

    Man: _____

    Woman: _____

3. Try to imagine what they might be *thinking*.

    Man: _____

    Woman: _____

4. Can you distinguish the difference between what is being felt and what is being thought?
5. What would you say to *accurately* and *without judgment* communicate your understanding of the way each person feels and thinks?

    _____

    _____

Part 2

Examine the photograph in Figure 4.6.

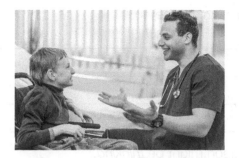

Figure 4.6

©iStock.com/Christopher Futcher

1. Create a scenario that you think describes what you might be happening in the picture.

_____

2. Try to imagine what each person might be *feeling*.

Staff person: _____

Child: _____

3. Try to imagine what each person might be *thinking*.

Staff person: _____

Child: _____

4. Can you distinguish the difference between what is being felt and what is being thought?

5. What would you say to *accurately* and *without judgment* communicate your understanding of how each person feels and thinks?

_____

_____

Part 3

Examine the photograph in Figure 4.7.

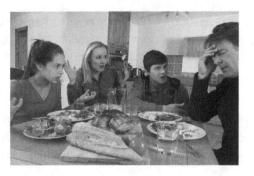

Figure 4.7

©iStock.com/monkeybusinessimages

1. Create a scenario that you think describes what you might be happening in the picture.

_____

2. Try to imagine what each person might be *feeling*.

   Man: _____

   Woman: _____

   Boy: _____

   Girl: _____

3. Now try to imagine what each person might be *thinking*.

   Man: _____

   Woman: _____

   Boy: _____

   Girl: _____

4. Can you distinguish the difference between what is being felt and what is being thought?
5. What would you say to *accurately* and *without judgment* communicate your understanding of how each person feels and thinks?

   _____

   _____

Part 4

It's more effective, of course, to practice empathy in real-life situations:

1. Think of a time when someone else was able to convey to you that he or she really understood how *you* feel. What did the person do to show you how well he or she understood you?
2. Write your thoughts in the space provided.

   _____

   _____

   _____

 Bright idea 4.3: Whenever you don't know how to help another person, try to empathize more deeply. It is easy to get stuck looking for ways to fix a problem. Stop trying to fix anything. Work on understanding and on communicating non-judgmentally this understanding instead.

Human service workers frequently find that people they serve are angry at them. Many of us go into this field with a desire to help other people and a related expectation that people will appreciate us for helping them. Working with people who are not only unappreciative but openly hostile to us is very challenging. Perhaps nothing is more challenging in our work than finding a way to empathize with people who are hostile to us.

Scenario 4.3

Glen is working with Tyler, a 25-year-old male who is struggling in the early stages of recovery from substance abuse. Glen tries to help Tyler but finds that Tyler is often hostile to him. Tyler criticizes Glen for just about everything; he insults Glen and has made vague verbal threats like, "You better watch out." Glen finds Tyler really unpleasant to work with and asks his supervisor, Susan, if he can be assigned to work with someone else.

Susan encourages Glen to try to get inside Tyler's head. Why might Tyler be angry and hostile? What has Tyler had to face in his life that may have shaped the person he is now? She asks Glen to consider what it must feel like to be in the early stages of recovery from a serious addiction. Susan asks Glen how he thinks the key people in Tyler's life may have treated him.

Glen argues that no matter what Tyler has gone through, he has no right to treat Glen this way. After all, Glen says, he's only trying to help Tyler. Susan agrees and says they will figure out a way to confront Tyler about his abusive behavior. She also says she'll consider Glen's request for reassignment but they can't proceed with that until they understand Tyler better. Glen and Susan then review what they know about Tyler's life and try to imagine what it is like to be him. They also consider some ways in which Glen's responses to Tyler might actually be provoking Tyler's anger.

The best way to develop empathy skills is through focused, intentional practice. Use the following practice exercises to help you build your skills.

Practice Exercise 4.2: Listening practice

1. Pair up with a person you don't well.
2. Ask the other person to tell a personal story about something that triggered an emotional response.
3. Repeat the entire story or at least the story's highlights:
   a. Ask: "Did I get that right?"
   b. Try to determine what the person was feeling. Say something like, "In that situation, I think you were feeling . . ."
   c. Ask, "Is that right?"
4. Repeat back to the person what you think the person was *thinking*:
   a. Say something like, "You seem to be thinking that . . ."
   b. Ask: "Is that right?" Try to clearly separate the *emotional* (feeling) response from the *cognitive* (thinking) response.
5. Reverse positions. The storyteller should now be the listener and the listener should share a story.
6. Repeat the process.

Practice Exercise 4.3: Developing empathy at work

1. Pair up with a coworker you don't know well.
2. Think about and answer the following questions about your work:
   Question 1: What inspires and engages you in the work that you do?
   Question 2: What do you dislike about your work? What discourages you about your work?
3. Share your answers with your partner.
4. Take turns repeating back what you heard the other person say. Try to:
   a. Identify the person's feelings.
   b. Identify the person's thoughts.
   c. Check in to determine whether or not you picked up on the person's feelings and thoughts correctly.

Practice Exercise 4.4: Common situations in therapeutic settings

In this exercise, you will read about a situation in which a person receiving services behaves in a way that is challenging for the staff person. After you read about the situation, set up a role play involving three persons. One person role plays the staff person who is reacting to the challenging behavior from the client. Most likely the staff person feels frustrated or angry. He or she may also feel unprepared to deal with this challenge. Perhaps they feel embarrassed. The staff person may express strong emotions about the way they feel they are being treated. A second person role plays the supervisor offering empathic support. He or she practices skillful listening and communicating, but *not* problem solving. That person should say back what he or she heard and check in about whether they got the feelings right. The third person is there to coach the supervisor to communicate empathy is a non-judgmental way.

   Note that in each situation, the staff person and supervisor will likely feel a strong urge to do some problem solving, to decide how the staff person should respond. Try, for this exercise, to resist the urge to solve the problem. The supervisor should focus instead on helping the staff person express his feelings and thoughts, communicating empathically, without judgment.

Example scenario

Tim works at a residential program and is the staff person on-call. Camilla, a person in the program, calls him at 3:00 in the morning to say she is thinking of killing herself. When Tim asks her what is going on, Camilla replies, "Never mind. I don't want to talk about it." Then, she hangs up. Tim is awake the rest of the night.

Example role play

One person role plays Tim. He shares his experience with Wes, a coworker. Tim: "I'm feeling really frustrated with Camilla. She has no consideration for staff. She calls in the middle of the night, wakes us up and then isn't even willing to talk. Really, I'm pissed off at her!"

   Wes (practicing being empathic with Tim): "You are feeling angry at Camilla. You are thinking that she doesn't respect staff. But you know, Camilla is doing the best she can. You shouldn't be upset with her."

   Amir is the third person helping Wes communicate empathy. He comments to Wes: "I think you heard what Tim was saying, but then you started to correct him and you became judgmental. You started defending Camilla. Can you get Tim to express more about how he feels without cutting him off?"

Practice scenario 1

Levi used most of his Social Security check to buy lottery tickets, even though he was supposed to use it to pay for rent, heat, and food. Levi's service plan, which he agreed to, says that Levi is supposed to be working with staff on budgeting skills. When Gideon, his staff member, asks to sit with him while he makes a budget, Levi lashes out angrily and accuses Gideon of treating him like a baby. Now, having wasted his check, Levi calls Gideon's supervisor to complain that he is hungry and that Gideon is letting him starve. He tells the supervisor he may get kicked out of his apartment because Gideon isn't helping him stick to a budget.

Practice role play 2

One person role plays Gideon. A second person role plays his supervisor showing empathy to Gideon. A third person offers the supervisor support to stay empathic, not making judgments or telling Gideon what he should do.

Practice scenario 2

Emiliano says all the time that he wants to be "independent." Staff member George agrees with this goal and proposes to work with him on specific skills to improve his independence, like using public transportation. However, Emiliano would rather get a free ride from George than use his money to pay for a bus or train.

Practice role play 2

One person role plays George. A second person role plays George's supervisor offering empathy to George. A third person offers the supervisor support to stay empathic, not making judges or telling George what he should do.

Practice scenario 3

Elena has a serious cocaine and crack addiction and has been prostituting herself in order to get money to feed her drug habit. She just found out she has been diagnosed with HIV and Hepatitis C. She lashes out at her staff person Byron for not providing enough help, saying this is all his fault.

Practice role play 3

One person role plays Byron. A second person role plays his supervisor offering him empathy. A third person coaches the supervisor on showing empathy without judgment.

The Importance of Gathering Feedback

If you did the exercises, you may have discovered that developing and communicating empathy is not as easy as people sometimes think it should be.

You are in good company if you have trouble perceiving what other people feel and think and communicating this to them without judgment. It turns out that many highly trained and experienced therapists are not nearly as empathetic as they believe they are. Counselors and therapists are sometimes poor judges of whether or not their clients see them as empathetic and often think they are more empathic than they are (Bachelor & Horvath 1999). Many counseling and psychotherapy professionals need more training in what is, without question, the foundation of successful therapeutic work: Tuning in to other people with empathy.

It also turns out that one of the best way to improve one's empathy skills is to ask for feedback from both the people you service and your coworkers. It is important to ask them to evaluate your skills, particularly in two areas:

1. Empathy (how well understood they feel).
2. How helpful you are.

David Burns is a psychiatrist and one of the primary developers of CBT (see the website www.feelinggood.com). In recent years, he has increasingly focused on the importance of developing clinicians' ability to empathize. Burns strongly encourages counselors to check in with the people they serve about how empathetic they are and helpful their work is. His workbooks and conference materials provide tools that professionals can use to measure counselor empathy and helpfulness.

Resistance to Gathering—and Accepting—Feedback

Unfortunately, most counselors do not want to ask for feedback from the people they serve. We especially do not want to ask for feedback from people who might regard us with anger or hostility. Why do you think professionals tend to be so resistant to asking for feedback?

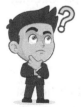

Questions to ponder 4.3: How do you feel about asking for feedback about how empathetic you are and how helpful your work is? Are you reluctant? If so, why? Are you worried that you'll receive negative or unfair feedback? Are you worried that your agency or supervisor will use this feedback against you in some way?

While every person has their own reservations, there are three common reasons that mental health professionals are reluctant to solicit feedback:

1. *Fear.* People are afraid to ask for feedback because they don't want to hear something negative. After all, who wants to hear that they aren't doing good work? They also may believe that the people they work with may not respond fairly, honestly, or reasonably. This can certainly be true at times.

2. *Lack of confidence.* Sometimes people are just not confident enough in their own abilities to be open to considering potentially critical feedback. With greater experience and confidence, there is often a greater ease with hearing critical feedback.

3. *Unsafe work environment.* Professionals may be reluctant to ask for feedback because they don't trust their supervisors or don't believe their agencies will support them if an evaluation is negative. It is also important for supervisors to recognize that the person asking for feedback is placing him or herself in a vulnerable position and needs to be supported for doing this. Supervisors can make this easier by modeling an openness to feedback about their own abilities at empathy with their supervisees.

If you are willing to ask for feedback on a regular basis, you are likely to be advancing your empathy skills much more rapidly than those who don't ask for feedback. (Duncan, Miller, Wampold, & Hubble 2010) It may help you to remember that virtually everyone gets bad ratings at some points. This is partially because *all of us fail at empathy at times.* These bad ratings offer important opportunities for learning and developing relationships. *Always ask for more information about a bad rating*: What did I miss? What didn't I understand? How could I be more helpful? Responding openly to bad ratings can significantly improve the sense of safety and trust of the people who work with us have.

Empathy can be measured. A number of formal instruments are available to measure empathy. I'd recommend, in particular, checking out the set of instruments included in the *Therapist toolkit* developed by Dr. Burns. Unfortunately, all of these instruments depend on strong reading abilities, something you can't assume when you are working with people with language and learning challenges. For our purposes, a simple check in with the people you serve may be enough.

Ask a question, such as "Do you think I understand how you feel?" Then ask the person to use a scale to rate your performance. A rating scale can be as simple as these:

- "Thumbs up, middle, and down."
- 0 to 5 rating scale.
- Facial expressions—happy face to sad face.
- Other rating that participants are familiar with or that are relevant to their situation.

Figure 4.8

What Should You Ask?

While evaluation formats and processes may vary, the basic questions you ask are all variations on the following:

a. Do you think I pay attention and listen when you are talking?
b. Do you think I understand how you feel? *(Note: This question may be too abstract for some people and may have to be "unpacked" for clarity.)*
c. Do you feel that I support you?
d. Am I helpful? What do I do that helps you? What do I do that isn't helpful?

Always thank the person for their input, regardless of the rating that you receive. Thank them for their honesty and their willingness to help you improve your skills. Consider asking the person if he or she is willing to give you more detailed feedback on what you do well, not so well, and how you could be more helpful.

 Bright idea 4.4: Counselors who regularly ask for feedback, especially about empathy and helpfulness, are likely to continuously deepen their therapeutic abilities.

Practice Exercise 4.5: Asking for One-to-One Feedback

1. Choose one person that you serve, a peer, a supervisor or other colleague.
2. Explain that you are trying to improve your ability to understand other people and that you would like some honest feedback.
3. Ask the person questions like:
    "When we talk, do you think I listen well?"
    "Do I seem to understand how you feel?"
    "Am I easy to talk to?"
    "What could I do better to listen to you more skillfully?"
    "Do you feel I help you?"
4. Write down their answers in the space provided.
5. Thank the person, regardless of the feedback you receive.
6. Review the feedback. Are there any areas for improvement? If so, what will you do differently?
7. Write your thoughts in the space provided.

_____

_____

 Practice Exercise 4.6: Asking for feedback from a group

If you work in a setting such as a hospital, day program, or group home where group work is done, consider inviting some of the people you serve to provide feedback to the staff on a regular basis, such as during a community meeting. Use this also as a teaching opportunity for offering constructive feedback.

1. Discuss some ground rules for giving feedback. These ground rules should reflect the skills of "clean communication" and the use of "I–statements," as discussed in Lesson 2. Feedback sessions also can be opportunities to work on these communication skills. That is, when people give you feedback skillfully, you have an opportunity to stop and notice, label, and comment on the communication skills they are using.
2. Ask the group questions like these:
    a. What is one thing staff did well this week?
    b. What is one thing staff could do better?
3. Document the results and look for opportunities to improve your own work or the work of the group.
4. If people used skillful communication in offering feedback, be sure to tell them what they did skillfully and to thank them.

Responding to Negative Feedback

The next time someone criticizes you, try not to respond defensively. This can be difficult, especially if the person's criticism seems completely off-base and you passionately disagree with their perspective. Focus on listening and hearing what they have to say.

If the person uses abusive language, help the person to express his or her feelings with "clean communication" and "I-statements." Tell the person you can hear them better if they use these positive communication skills.

Take, for example, this exchange between Jack, a program participant, and a staff member:

Jack: "You're a jerk."
Staff member: "I think you are saying you are angry at me. Can you tell me what I did wrong and how you're feeling without insulting me? Just say what I did and then what you feel. That will help me to listen better."

Wrap-Up

In this lesson, you learned about the important role that empathy plays in building relationships with the people you serve. Remember, empathy is not the same as sympathy or pity. Empathy needs to be learned and practiced regularly. One of the best ways to improve your empathetic skills is to ask for, accept and use feedback from the people you serve and your coworkers.

In Lesson 5, you will learn about working "one-down," another way to build therapeutic relationships.

Lesson 4 Skill Sheet

- Participant demonstrates empathetic responses to other people involving:

  a. Understanding how the other person feels.

  b. Understanding how the other person thinks.

  c. Communicating this understanding skillfully and without judgment.

- Participant ask for feedback from a person they work with, either in informal conversations or using a rating scale.

- Participants considers the feedback they receive, especially if it is negative, and consider non-defensively if they can learn something from it.

- Participant understands that offering and receiving constructive feedback are both valuable skills to develop in the people they serve and in themselves.

Lesson 4 Quiz

1. A staff person asks Mary to clean her room before going on the trip. Mary delays and doesn't do it. As the time for the trip gets closer, Mary gets more anxious and angry. Finally, she screams at staff and runs out of the house. Which of the following show an empathetic response to Mary?

   a. "You need to clean your room before we can go."

   b. "Stop screaming. Use your coping skills."

   c. "You seem very upset. Are you worried about something? Is something bothering you?"

   d. "I thought you wanted to go on this trip."

2. Which of the following skills could Mary be missing or need to develop? (Check all that apply.)

   a. Difficulty organizing space.

   b. Difficulty handling anxiety.

   c. Poor language skills.

   d. Poor planning skills.

   e. Poor ability to read non-verbal social cues.

3. Look at the photograph in Figure 4.6 again. What are some of the things that the adult appears to be doing to develop a relationship with the child? What cues are you using to make these assumptions? Write your ideas in the space provided:

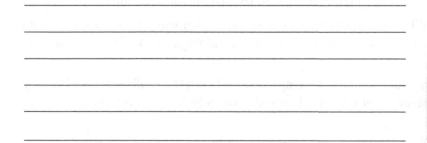

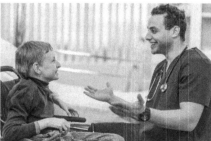

©iStock.com/Christopher Futcher

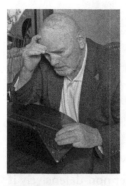

Figure 4.9

©iStock.com/Ana
Abejon

4. Look at the picture in Figure 4.9. What do you think this person is feeling? What cues are you using to make these assumptions? Can you imagine a few different things he might be thinking? Write your responses in the space provided.

_____

_____

_____

_____

_____

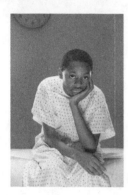

Figure 4.10

©iStock.com/FangXiaNuo

5. Make up a brief story to go with the photograph in Figure 4.10. What happened? How is the boy feeling? What might he be thinking? What cues are you using to make these assumptions? Write your responses in the space provided.

_____

_____

_____

_____

_____

Lesson 4 Questions for Discussion

1. Do you ever feel confused and overwhelmed by the challenges of your work? How do you tend to behave when you feel confused and overwhelmed?

2. How hard do you work on developing relationships with the people you serve? What are some of the techniques that you can use to develop these relationships?

3. Do you ever feel that your job is to give advice?

4. Do you sometimes feel uncomfortable when the people you serve express strong emotions? How do you typically respond at those times? How would you evaluate the effectiveness of your response?

5. Do you ever feel angry towards the people you serve? How do you handle this emotion?

6. Consider the people you serve. Who do you feel the strongest connection with? Who do you struggle to connect with? What do you think might be getting in the way of developing a good relationship with some clients?

7. Do you feel that your supervisors and administrators empathize well with the challenges you face in your job? Do they have a good understanding of what it is like to do your job? What things do you want them to know?

8. Have you ever found yourself telling someone you're working with to use their "coping skills" as a way of getting the person to leave you alone?

9. How do you feel about asking clients for feedback regarding your empathy and helpfulness? Are you reluctant to do that? If so, why?

10. Do you feel your workplace is a safe place to ask for feedback on your work performance from the people you serve? Do you feel that you can trust your supervisor and administrators to use this information to enhance your professional growth and overall agency performance? Do you fear that it will be used negatively (e.g., as the basis for disciplining staff members, etc.)? If you are a supervisor, would your team feel safe knowing that you have that kind of feedback about them?

Lesson 4 Quiz Answers

1. Answer *c* is the most empathic response. Answers *a* and *b* are limit-setting responses. The response in *d* seems to be sarcastic.

2. This question brings us back to the issue of skills and skill deficits that were discussed in Lessons 1 and 2. When you appreciate Mary's skill deficits, you will be able to empathize more with her situation. All of the responses are possible skill deficits. If you see her as lacking some basic skills, perhaps you can appreciate that she is doing her best. Perhaps you also can begin to appreciate that she might feel frustrated, embarrassed, inadequate, anxious and/or depressed.

3. The adult's open body posture and broad smile appear to reflect a warm, emotionally open approach to the boy. The man's open arms, strong eye contact, and smile seem to say, "I care about you."

4 and 5.   There are no *right* answers to these questions. They are presented for you to consider and come up with your own conclusions. You can get clues from observing body posture and facial expressions as well as context. (The boy appears to be in a medical setting and the clock behind him suggests time is passing.)

References

Bachelor, A., & Horvath, A. (1999). The therapeutic relationship. In M. A. Hubble, B. L. Duncan, & S. D. Miller (Eds.), *The heart and soul of change: What works in therapy*. Washington, DC: American Psychological Association.

Bauman, H.-D. L., & Murray, J. J. (Eds.). (2014). *Deaf gain: Raising the stakes for human diversity*. Minneapolis, MN: University of Minnesota Press.

Duncan, B. L., Miller, S. D., Wampold, B. E., & Hubble, M. (Eds.). (2010). *The heart and soul of change: Delivering what works in therapy* (2nd ed.). Washington, DC: American Psychological Association.

Linehan, M. (1993). *Cognitive behavioral treatment of borderline personality disorder*. New York: Guilford Press.

Wiseman, T. (1996). A concept analysis of empathy. *Journal of Advanced Nursing, 23,* 1162–1167.

Additional resources

These two YouTube clips are especially useful in trainings about empathy:

*   http://www.onbeing.org/blog/an-empathy-video-that-asks-you-to-stand-in-someone-elses-shoes/5063
*   http://www.youtube.com/watch?v=1Evwgu369Jw

As mentioned, many of the tools developed by David Burns are focused on improving therapist empathy abilities (see http://www.feelinggood.com).

The Power of Working "One-Down"

Introduction

In Lesson 4, you learned about the important role that empathy plays in your work. You also learned why it is critical to establish an empathetic connection with the people you serve before you begin to encourage them to learn and use skills. In this lesson, you will explore another crucial pre-therapy tool: How to invite—not

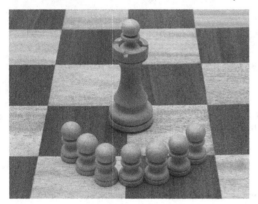

force—the people you serve to participate in taking control of their development or recovery. The overall name we give to the process of inviting, not compelling, people to engage in recovery is working "one-down."

Using Power and Authority in a One-Up Stance

In cognitive behavioral therapy, we help people explore connections between their emotions, thoughts and behaviors and we help them develop and use important life skills. If people are ready and willing to do this, there isn't much need for pre-therapy. If they aren't, and if the obstacles have to do with language and learning challenges, we are in the world of pre-therapy. Our pre-therapy work includes:

Figure 5.1 Authority

©iStock.com/Luis Francisco Cordero

- Creating a shared understanding (schema) that *skill building is what we do here.*
- Creating a positive mindset that says: *"I can do this. Staff doesn't need to do this for me."*
- Using empathy to convey that we understand how difficult it can be to learn new skills.
- Becoming skillful at *inviting* people to participate in this difficult process.
- Helping participants to develop foundational problem solving abilities.

The stance you take towards the people you serve will play a key role in how effective you are in achieving these goals. A *stance* literally means the way a person stands, their posture. In this workbook, however, the word "stance" refers to the attitude you assume toward the people you serve, especially with regard to the way that you use your power and authority. Of course, at times, a person's attitude may literally show up in the way you stand and move.

You are in a position of authority over the people served in your program. Take a minute to consider your stance toward the people you serve and how you use the power that comes with your position:

- Do you act like you are their boss?
- Are you very concerned with whether or not the people you serve listen to you and respect you?
- Do you spend a lot of time telling people how they should behave?
- Do you tell people what they should feel or think?
- Do you think your job is to manage and control people?
- Do you see it as your job to rescue people if they make bad choices?

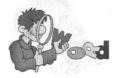

Stance

Definition 5.1: Stance: The attitude a person assumes, especially with regard to how much power they believe they have over another person.

Example of stance: Betty assumes a stance of authority. She tells the people she serves how they should behave. Melissa assumes a more humble stance. She is endlessly curious about why people behave as they do and asks them lots of questions. She assumes they understand themselves better than she does.

Most people in human services act from a one-up stance unless they have been specifically trained to work in another way. That is, many of us use our power to try to directly influence people we serve. This is especially true of staff who work in programs that serve people who are thought to be very impaired. In various ways, we tell them what they should do.

Look at Table 5.1 and Figure 5.2 to see what is involved in a *one-up stance.*

TABLE 5.1 Examples of One-Up Stances

Stance	Description	Example
Directing	Telling people what to do or giving them advice about what you think they *should* do	• "You should just ignore him" • "You need to take a time out right now" • "You need to use your coping skills now"
Informing	Telling people what is right or wrong, appropriate or inappropriate, healthy or unhealthy Informing includes giving both praise and criticism	• "That behavior is inappropriate" • "You are not respecting my boundaries" • "You are being manipulative" • "This is what you need to do now"
Controlling	The person's overall intent is to control the way others behave. Within this framework, clients are typically described as either "cooperative" or "resistant" based on whether or not they accept staff control. If the person responds by attempting to control staff in return, the individual is often labeled "manipulative".	• Staff work on "fixing" a behavior without the person's knowledge, participation or consent. This can include creating a behavior plan designed to reinforce certain behaviors • A program is based on rules. Staff's job is to get program participants clients to cooperate and follow the rules

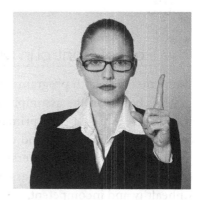

Figure 5.2 "I'm the boss!"

©iStock.com/Ostill

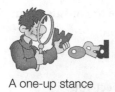

A one-up stance

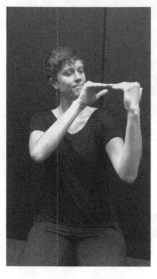
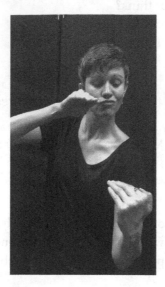

Figure 5.3 ASL sign for ONE-UP

Used with permission

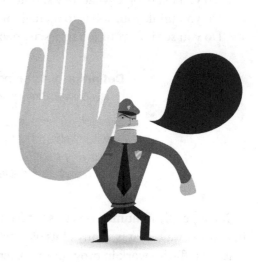

Figure 5.4 Are program staff members substitutes for the police?

©iStock.com/alashi

One-up treatment environments focus on rules. Staff members view their work as primarily to make sure everyone in a program follows the rules. They are authority figures; they are in charge. As a result, staff members sometimes behave like police. Even if staff members have good intentions, they spend the majority of their time telling people what to do. This work style is extremely common.

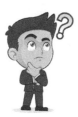

Questions to ponder 5.1: How many of your interventions with clients take the form of directing, informing or controlling? If you haven't thought about your stance toward the people you serve until now, chances are that most of your interactions are done with a one-up stance, meaning you are directive and controlling.

The Role of Control in Mental Health Programs

Many mental health programs are preoccupied with staff having control over the people they serve. If a program is based on the assumption that the people being served are "impaired," then staff members are more likely to believe that their primary job is to fix or correct problems. For staff members working in these programs, fixing, correcting and controlling are all viewed as forms of helping. This often leads to the unstated assumption that staff members, themselves, are *not* impaired because they are being paid to do the helping. In other words, staff members assume they are healthy and competent while assuming the people they serve are unhealthy and incompetent.

Many staff members work in these programs because they want to help people. However, many never examine how easy it is to cross the line that separates helping from controlling. They may believe that helping means to correct, fix, guide, shape, protect or control *for the person's own good.*

Recently, however, many people who receive services have begun to challenge this model. They are speaking out, saying things like: *Stop treating us like children! Respect our ability to make decisions and, yes, to make mistakes.* They are talking about the "dignity of risk," meaning that, like everyone else, they have the right to make mistakes and deserve to have this right respected by the professionals who support them.

Many programs are based on a medical model which assumes that the people served in the program are *patients* who are *sick*. In this model, medical professionals, with their expert knowledge and skills, are trained to try to fix patients' problems, to help them "get better." This is the traditional way the medical field has worked. This stance or attitude often promotes a passive model of recovery—the patient follows the doctor's orders, takes medication as prescribed. The doctor knows best.

Fortunately, this stance is changing as more of today's medical professionals recognize that medication is not enough and begin to understand that patients get better through learning to manage their illness, and more broadly, their own lives. People receiving services don't simply follow a doctor's orders. Rather, they *partner* with the professionals that support them on mutually agreed upon goals.

The process of becoming an active *agent* in your own recovery or development is at the heart of modern thinking about health care. People get better when they start to take some control over their recovery process. They learn to manage their sleep, diet, exercise, attitudes, stress and relationships with the help and support of others. They develop a deeper understanding of the problems they face and they learn strategies to manage those problems. In other words, they learn to manage their illness, *as well as their wellness.* This is just as important for people with language and learning challenges as it is for people with better language and thinking abilities. The best mental health programs today promote this teamwork between clients and providers. Often this involves teaching people who receive services how to assume a more active role in their treatment and recovery.

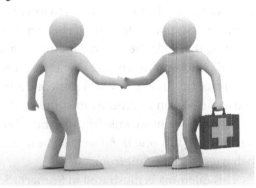

Figure 5.5 Partnering in health care
©iStock.com/Sergey Ilin

To work actively with a counselor or doctor, to participate actively as a partner in the process, one needs a sense of "personal agency." Personal agency is a person's belief that:

"I can make a difference in my own life."
"I'm responsible for my health."
"I can take steps to make my life better."
"It's not the pill that makes me better."
"I make myself better, and the pill, the surgery, the support from others, are resources I can draw upon."

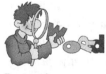

Personal agency

Definition 5.3: Personal agency: The belief in your ability to make and carry out decisions that impact yourself and the world.

Example of personal agency: After being diagnosed with cancer, Beth decided to radically change her lifestyle. She changed her diet, began a regular exercise routine, and cut down her work hours. She believed she could extend how long she lived and how well she lived by taking more control over her day-to-day life.

Personal agency is especially important when you are working with someone with emotional problems that don't have a clear biological cause. Indeed, many people with language and learning challenges or other disabilities don't consider themselves capable of directing their own lives. They may not have sufficient language and thinking skills to consider such an abstract concept. They have always been dependent upon other people and don't know any other way to live.

Yet, many people with language and learning skills struggle, often unskillfully, to exert more control over their fate. They may not know how to control their lives because nobody has tried or been able to teach them essential foundational life skills. If they have never developed good social skills, they may treat people the way they have been treated. They may bully, threaten, and try to force their will on other people. They may assert themselves in unskillful, hurtful ways through alcohol and drug abuse or other destructive behaviors.

How do you engage people who don't see themselves as having the power or capabilities to shape their own lives in the process of developing important skills? An important first step is recognizing that you can't help a person begin to control his or her life if you continue to control every aspect of it yourself. You won't achieve this goal unless the person begins to make decisions, including risky decisions, and experiences the consequences.

In most programs that are attentive to this, it can be very hard to decide what to do when someone is engaged in very risky behaviors, especially when they endanger other people. There is no one simple answer, but it is very hard for mental health programs to force people to accept supervision, follow rules or behave safely. If we work with the assumption that unsafe behaviors are due to skill deficits, then we must find a way to engage people in learning the skills they need. One-up authority stances usually don't do this.

Staff who want to engage clients in learning skills, and who don't want to take controlling, one-up stances, often face this dilemma when someone is behaving in a very dangerous way. If they set greater limits, they may cause the person to rebel against them. Their therapeutic relationship may suffer, and the person may decide to behave even more unsafely. On the other hand, staff and program leadership are very uncomfortable about backing off. It is one thing to talk about empowerment, but empowering people who have not learned skillful behaviors can be dangerous.

This dilemma is illustrated in Scenario 5.1.

Scenario 5.1

Cliff is a 25-year-old deaf male who was language deprived and delayed and lacks social skills to find female sexual partners. He also struggles to communicate clearly, and literally lacks the language to negotiate a complex interaction like a decision to have sex.

Staff in Cliff's program attempt to help him by teaching him how to approach woman, start a conversation, and assess whether or not the woman wants more contact with him. They strive to help him appreciate the woman's feelings, but Cliff's skills at empathy are very undeveloped. Negotiating sex is very hard for Cliff, even if the other person signs, and usually women don't want more contact with him. In his desperation and despair, he pressures them, and this pressure has escalated to sexual assault.

Cliff lives in a group home where staff attempt to supervise his interactions in the community; but Cliff hates it when staff hover around him, always, from his perspective, telling him he can't do something. The program staff struggle because they want to support his desire for independence but they recognize the danger he poses to women in the community. When Cliff has been arrested in the past, he has never been charged with anything, because police, court and even the women he assaulted felt bad for him. Consequently, he hasn't faced legal consequences. He's only experienced the program staff becoming upset with him and limiting his freedom. Practically speaking, Cliff lives in an open, unlocked setting; and staff have no way to force him to accept supervision, especially when no court or police holds him accountable.

The agency leadership has many discussions about how to handle this problem. They have responsibility to the community (as they've assured worried neighbors), but they have no legal backing for any attempt to control Cliff; and they also know that he rebels against these attempts to control him. Staff realize that Cliff is less dangerous when he is engaged with them, when he sees them as allies and supports, not as bosses telling him what to do, but they are worried about giving him too much independence and freedom.

Ultimately, the agency decides on a two-sided strategy. First, they urge the legitimate social authorities, the police, courts and probation, to hold Cliff responsible to the same standards for safe behavior as everyone else. They have police talk to Cliff, and they urge the police to use their full authority, and tell him the rules and consequences for hurting someone. When there was an incident, they urged the police to arrest him. After he was arrested, they pressed hard that he be tried and assigned a probation officer who would meet with him regularly and, if necessary, threaten him with jail if he doesn't follow the rules. Staff fought against the tendency of the police to treat his anti-social acts as mental health problems, bringing him to a psychiatric emergency room rather than arresting him. They said he needs the police and courts to insist on rules; and then the program can help him comply with the rules.

Secondly, they strove to collaborate with Cliff to help him avoid legal trouble he did not want. They strove to teach him skills and also to provide him with social opportunities to meet peers of the opposite sex. They continued the work of helping him consider what each woman feels and wants, and how to cope if she says no.

Staff understood that the more they could get the legal system to act like the agents of authority they are supposed to be, the easier it would be for mental health practitioners to ally with Cliff, to support him in his desire for independence and relationships while assisting him in learning the skills he needs to be safe. For the program to help Cliff, they need to worry with him about how the police might arrest him, and discuss with him what they can do to keep this from happening. They can't do this if they also must act as police themselves.

Staff, then, strove for a collaboration with police and courts, urging them to stay one-up with Cliff, so staff could engage him one-down.

Behavior Modification and Other Rationales for Behaving One-Up with Clients

Placing doctors, nurses and other professionals in charge of someone else's recovery often interferes with that recovery. The same can be true with some behavior modification models.

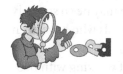

Behavior modification

Definition 5.4: Behavior modification: An educational and treatment approach designed to create motivation by using a program of rewards and punishments.

Example of behavior modification: Every hour that Andrew gets through without hitting himself or another person, staff award him 10 points. At the end of the week, he can exchange the points he has earned for items in the program's reward store.

In behavior modification, staff members use rewards, and sometimes punishments, to motivate people to behave differently. These are called "reinforcers." Staff members in programs that use behavior modification almost always assume a one-up stance because these programs are designed around trying to control people's behaviors by controlling their environments. Usually, the focus in these programs is on rewarding positive behaviors. Staff decide what the positive behaviors are and when they are being used, and staff decide when to give or withhold a reinforcement. The responsibility for the clients' behavior, then, remains with the staff.

Behavior modification is very common in programs that serve people with developmental disabilities. It is also found in many mental health programs, especially those where people show extremely challenging behaviors.

Behavior modification has some significant drawbacks as a treatment approach. To begin with, implementing behavioral modification plans successfully requires a great deal of consistency in staff. Everyone needs to know and follow the plan. This is difficult to achieve in programs that are staffed seven days a week, 24 hours a day. This well-known problem is voiced when staff complain that *other* staff aren't following the plan.

An even bigger problem, however, is that behavior modification gives too much power to staff. Behavior modification programs are designed to turn staff into control agents who are responsible for creating environments that shape other people. If a staff member has any tendencies at all towards abuse of power (and most humans do), behavior modification principles can make these tendencies more pronounced. The result can be an unnecessarily controlling environment in which staff members' abusive behaviors surface over time. Another result is that this kind of treatment setting can actually create resistance and negative behaviors from the very people the program is designed to serve.

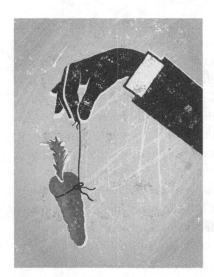

Figure 5.6 One form of behavior modification

©iStock.com/Meriel Jane Weissman

Risk management is another force that encourages staff to exert control. This isn't surprising, given that many programs work with people who engage in dangerous, high-risk behaviors. They hurt themselves and other people or are unable to take care of themselves. Some people with language and learning challenges, like Cliff, have not learned how to establish healthy social and sexual relationships. This lack of skill can be compounded by communication problems. As a result, they may force themselves on other people, engaging in bullying behaviors. If they engage in sexual bullying, or sexual assault, staff will feel even more compelled to try to control them. Treatment programs are under mandates to keep clients and community safe. The *pull* on staff to do this through overt control is enormous.

Funding sources often worry about negative publicity and the fall-out if bad things happen. They too have good reason to be concerned. For example, it is not uncommon for agencies and personnel to be sued if a person participating in a state-run program injures or kills someone. Outside observers often assume that mental illness is to blame whenever someone commits a violent crime. People ask, "Why didn't the mental health system [or other programs] prevent this? They should be sued."

Agencies that serve people with developmental disabilities are especially notorious for being controlling and risk averse. They know that when a client does something bad, the agency will be blamed so the safest path is to create treatment settings that seek to control people *for their own good*. These controlling environments also are designed to protect other people and agencies from bad publicity and potential lawsuits.

Finally, the reality is that many of the people you serve have been referred to your program because they *aren't* yet capable of living safely. Many have very poor judgment and impulse control. Some may be so severely impaired that it is unlikely that they will ever live independently. Furthermore, some individuals who have been charged with criminal behavior might not be considered competent to stand trial.

Obviously, serving this population is complicated. The fact is that you are in the business of working with people with very significant impairments, many with unsafe and dangerous behaviors. These individuals need help. And, in some cases, society needs to be protected. The problem is that mental health agencies are expected to substitute for police and courts. This places staff in a police-like role which can interfere with mental health treatment.

All of these forces push staff to be controlling, to act from a one-up stance. In some situations, this may be necessary. However, staff may begin to think this is the only way to behave and may never realize that a humbler stance could work better, even with people who engage in high-risk behaviors.

Drawbacks to a One-Up Stance

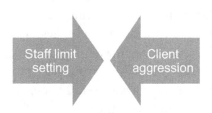

Figure 5.7 A common struggle in treatment programs

You will find programs and staff working from a one-up stance throughout the human services field. You also will see resistance among the people being served in these programs. In many cases, one-up behaviors may actually *trigger* strong reactions, including aggressive behaviors. Indeed, the more violently a client acts, the more likely staff will be to respond with strong directives. This can create a vicious cycle where staff and the people they serve become increasingly aggressive with one another. In effect, they trigger one another.

A Common Struggle in Treatment Programs

Working from a one-up stance has other potentially negative consequences. First, expertise in a particular treatment approach is not the same as wisdom and kindness. Staff members are human. They may make mistakes and implement treatment badly, regardless of their training or credentials. Staff members have their own skills and skill deficits. Some may even experience the same psychological challenges as the people they serve. For instance, staff members in your program may:

- Have experienced or are experiencing significant trauma.
- Struggle with anxiety, depression, anger, and other emotions.
- Abuse substances.
- Struggle with other addictive behaviors.
- Have poor coping and conflict management skills.

One-up treatment environments often bring out staff members' least skillful behaviors. They can allow, even subtly encourage, staff to become petty tyrants, bossing their clientele around.

Second, even the most benevolent environments are often more controlling than necessary. When a program is based on the assumption that program staff knows best, staff members are set up to act as authorities, and, almost inevitably, they make mistakes. Staff often do not know how to respond well to the people they serve. They may just set up arbitrary rules, or tell people to do things, and not even think about how they could be more collaborative. Direct care staff are supposed to be well supervised, but in busy, understaffed programs, supervisors are not always available; and when they are available they aren't always helpful.

Third, one-up stances tend to push people away. Efforts to control people often backfire because people get angry and resist staff efforts when they feel that they are being bossed around. This is the very opposite of what you are trying to achieve when you are trying to engage people in self-development.

Fourth, this type of intervention is designed to control behavior, not teach skills. As a result, participants may behave one way in the programs, but quite differently when they are on their own. They've learned to follow the rules of a setting, not how to use skills they need in all realms of their lives. Because they have been very dependent on staff, they continue to have a weak sense of personal agency. They were never helped to discover and learn how they can solve problems on their own.

Consider how you typically respond when someone tells you to do something. Now, imagine you are participating in a program where just about everyone is telling you to do something. Would you begin to feel frustrated and angry? Would you have any reason or incentive to comply?

Scenario 5.2 provides an example of staff using a one-up stance.

Scenario 5.2

Joe is a 32-year-old deaf male with a developmental disability who lives in a group home and attends a day treatment program. Joe has poor independent living skills such as cooking, self-care, money, and medication management. He also lacks general problem-solving skills. However, he constantly talks about wanting to be "independent." From Joe's perspective, this seems to mean being in a situation in which staff does not tell him what to do.

Joe's parents live nearby and oversee his care. They strongly resist his efforts to become more independent and are happy with his living situation. They directly ask staff to supervise him closely and "keep him out of trouble." They are strongly allied with a case manager from the state's Department of Developmental Disabilities who also expects staff to tightly manage Joe's day-to-day life.

Program staff believes that their job is to supervise Joe and make sure he is "good." However, Joe challenges staff's authority multiple times a day. He goes out into the community without asking anyone; he refuses to do his chores; he won't take his medication. Sometimes he threatens others and at times becomes physically aggressive and pushes and hits people. He has destroyed several pieces of furniture and punched holes in the wall. Some staff members are afraid of him. They all feel caught in an unhappy dance in which staff feels obligated to control a dangerous person and Joe feels staff won't let him be independent. It doesn't help that staff turnover is high.

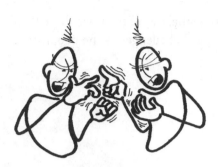

Figure 5.8 Conflict

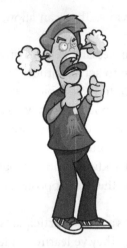

Figure 5.9 A familiar problem

©iStock.com/Dan Bailey

Does the staff dilemma with Joe sound familiar to you?

A serious communication barrier often exists when deaf people are served in hearing treatment settings. Consider all of the interventions that depend on a shared language. If a shared language is lacking, staff naturally begins to rely more on other tools, such as medication and behavior modification. Without an effective means of communication, staff usually becomes more directive and controlling. The lack of communication alone can be triggering for the deaf person who likely feels isolated, frustrated, and anxious. Poor care and bad outcomes are almost guaranteed when you couple staff's inherent tendency to be controlling and bossy with the assumption that staff members are expected to enforce the rules.

The people served in mental health programs all have unique personalities and challenges. Some are passive and dependent. Others are just the opposite and may be bossy and demanding, even bullying. They may be accustomed to using threats or aggression to get what they want. In fact, it's very common for staff to be afraid of some of the people they work with. A major concern for many staff members may be their own safety at work.

In the following scenario, a very socially unskilled person uses bullying to get his way. Staff have no idea how to engage this person, who seems to have too much power, in the process of becoming more socially skillful.

Scenario 5.3

Simon is a 20-year-old deaf male who was referred to a Deaf services group home after being expelled from a Deaf residential school. He is physically large and very strong. He has assaulted peers and staff in his schools and in the community. However, he has never been arrested because of his perceived mental illness and deafness. Each time that police intervened, Simon was brought to a hospital and eventually discharged to return to whatever program he was in at the time. As a result, Simon has never really faced legal consequences for hurting other people, although in most instances he was kicked out of the program and referred to another. He always blames others when this happens.

In the group home, Simon makes constant demands on staff. He demands to be taken to visit people, some of whom live hours away. He doesn't care whether there is enough staff to do this. He demands that the program buy electronic devices and special movies for him. If a staff member isn't immediately available, he sometimes "blows up" and ends up pushing or hitting staff and peers or destroying property. Most staff members are afraid of him.

Initially, it doesn't appear that Simon is a person who thinks he has no power in the world. On the contrary, Simon seems to be someone with too much *power. The fact that he can harm people and never be arrested adds to his power. However, a deeper look reveals that Simon's only power lies in his ability to threaten to harm others. He doesn't know how to get what he wants by using his own skills. Indeed, he has no concept of skills such as negotiation and problem solving. He knows how to intimidate other people, but doesn't know any other ways to get his needs met.*

There is no question that Simon is hard to serve in a program. Some staff may respond by setting firm limits, which provoke confrontations. Others may just give in, reinforcing his bullying behaviors. Both are currently happening and likely have been happening for years. This means that Simon has learned that bullying often works.

How would you engage Simon in the process of learning coping, conflict resolution and other skills? Why should Simon even try to learn new skills when bullying often works quite well? What would motivate him to change his behavior?

There is a saying that "if the only tool you have is a hammer, every problem looks like a nail." If the only tool that a program has to help someone is medication, staff will tend to assume that people have an illness and need medication. If the only tools staff members have to help people are rewards and punishments, staff will begin to assume that clients are only motivated to behave well if they get the right rewards and punishments. If the only approach one knows is to direct people, you will tend to assume that everyone served in a program needs direction.

In Simon's case, staff members have few tools. They can set limits or give in. They can try to make him take medication. At times, they may have used a behavioral incentive plan with rewards for good behaviors, but it's very hard to get everyone in a program to follow the plan. In addition, his family and case manager may not follow the plan.

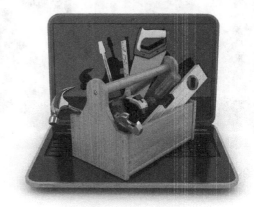

If the staff can't sign with enough skill to communicate with Simon, or if interpreters are not available enough, it will be impossible to teach him much. However, even when staff are Deaf themselves and sign well, they may have no idea how to work with Simon. Staff burnout is an enormous problem, especially in programs with challenging persons like Cliff, Simon, and Joe. Program administrators are usually desperate to find qualified staff. It is particularly difficult to find staff with the necessary communication skills. Constant staff turnover means that the people served in a program are continuously making and losing relationships with staff, making it harder for them to trust new people.

Figure 5.10 What's in your work tool box?
©iStock/com/Bet_Noire

There's got to be a better way.

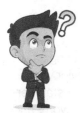 **Questions to ponder 5.2:** The subject of power is rarely addressed in mental health settings but it's one of the most important considerations in effective treatment. Who has the power and how do they use it? What kind of power do the people receiving services have? What role does the way staff uses power play in the challenging behaviors exhibited by people receiving services?

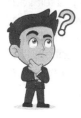 **Questions to ponder 5.3:** What forces encourage you to act with authority (one-up) to control people? Were you taught to act this way? Do your supervisors act this way? Does your program's treatment approach encourage it? Are you worried about preventing bad outcomes? Do you need to act like "the boss" in order to feel satisfied? Are you aware of other ways to interact more positively with the people you serve?

The Awesome Power of Working "One-Down"

The more tools you have, the less likely you will be to make the wrong assumptions about people and the less likely you will be to behave in ways that make matters worse. With more tools, you have more options. Learning how to work one-down will significantly expand your toolbox even in situations in which you must maintain high levels of control.

When working with deaf individuals, your ability to communicate with them in the way they prefer opens up a host of tools that flow from good communication. But, sharing a language does not *guarantee* good care. Bad treatment can occur in Deaf treatment programs where staff members sign well. A common language, whether spoken or signed, does not prevent anyone from approaching people in a bossy, controlling manner

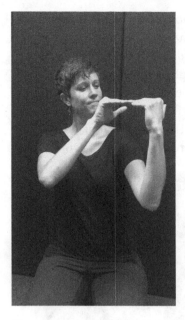
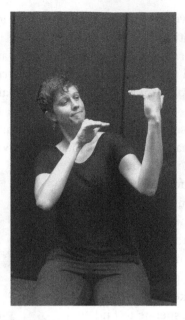

Figure 5.11 ASL sign for ONE-DOWN

Used with permission

and offers no guarantee that the people you serve will be treated with respect.

Working with a one-down stance means strategically lowering your own authority and power so as to better engage people, to bring them to the table of treatment. Instead of relying on the authority of your role, you attempt to cast the people you work with in the role of expert. A one-down stance also refers to attitudes and behaviors that reflect a sense of humility and deep respect for the capacity of other people, including those with great disadvantages, to become capable experts in their own lives.

When you learn to respond to people from a one-down stance, you will discover a wealth of new options for how to intervene in difficult situations. By *inviting* the people you serve to participate in the process, many professionals discover that client aggression drops and meaningful treatment becomes possible for persons who have been labeled "treatment resistant."

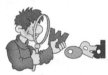

One-down stance

Definition 5.5: One-down stance: The attitude and behavior where one deliberately avoids using power and authority and, instead, shifts the power, authority and role of expert onto the person receiving services.

Example of one-down stance: Joel, a program resident, just had a meltdown during which he destroyed the couch in the living room and punched a roommate. His behavior was so aggressive that staff had to restrain him (one-up). Later, when Joel was calm, a staff person approached him and asked if they could talk. The staff person expressed worry and concern. He asked, "Can you help me understand how you got so angry that you felt you had to punch your roommate and destroy the couch? I'm really worried about you now. I'm worried what will happen if you keep behaving so aggressively. We need your help to figure out a better plan. Can you help us?" Although the restraint was a one-up intervention, the staff member's use of inviting, curiosity, worrying, and asking for help were all examples of one-down interventions.

When you assume a one-down stance, you deliberately adopt the attitude that you don't know the answers and you need the people you serve to help you find them. This may seem like an odd way for a staff person to behave, but the practice of working one-down is well established in the mental health field. However, it may go by other names. For instance, in family therapy, especially among practitioners of "solution-focused practice" (Anderson & Goolishian 1992), this stance is sometimes referred to as "not knowing." That is, counselors strategically downplay their own expertise in order to encourage the people they work with to pull out their own expertise.

As mentioned in the Introduction, most of the ideas in this pre-therapy program are based on the work of Donald Meichenbaum, an originator of CBT. He often describes copying the interviewing style of Columbo, a television police detective who pretended not to know something so that people would feel comfortable sharing their secrets. Working one-down is essentially a "Columbo" technique but, as that television show recedes into history, fewer people recognize this marvelous character or his clever method.

The transition to a one-down style of work must be gradual when you are working with people who are very disempowered, who aren't used to solving problems, or who don't see themselves as able to influence their own fate; that is, people that have no sense of personal agency. It can be jarring and upsetting for people receiving services to suddenly find staff members expecting more of them when they are accustomed to depending on authorities for direction. As much as they may resent being told what to do, it is what they know. They may resent being dependent on others but know no other way to function.

Participating in the decision-making and problem-solving process brings these individuals into an unfamiliar and scary world. Becoming empowered *doesn't* make a person capable. For many individuals with language and learning challenges, such empowerment may bring them face to face with the fact that they lack crucial skills and really do need help.

Becoming empowered, then, may be terrifying and cause an individual to want to retreat to the safe territory where staff make all the decisions.

This is one reason why it is so important for staff to recognize and name the skills that an individual *does* have, no matter how simple. Assuming a one-down stance works better in strength-based programs where staff are continually helping people discover that they do have abilities.

A one-down stance also flows naturally from a feeling of empathy. It's a way of saying: "I want to be there with you for this, to help you find the best path forward, but only with your permission. I don't have the answers but I have some ideas and strategies that have worked for other people. I have hope. I know this work is difficult. I know that we staff may not always understand all you've had to deal with in your life, all the obstacles you have faced. But I've seen other people, just like you, set and reach goals, recover, get better, move closer to the life they want. I've seen people just like you learn more and more of the skills they need to have the lives they want to have. I can't know what works best for you, but I believe that nothing will work if it doesn't come from you. I'm willing to share the tools I have with you and find out together what helps. Are you willing to try them out?"

A *one-down stance* may take forms as can be seen in Table 5.2.

TABLE 5.2 Examples of One-Down Stances

One-down form	Example	
Inviting	"Would you be willing to discuss this now?" "Can we work on a plan to help you with this?"	 Figure 5.12 One-down: Inviting ©iStock.com/jonya
Curiosity	"I am curious about why you do/feel/ think this." "I'd like to understand you better. I'm curious what happened to you that lead you to behave this way."	 Figure 5.13 One-down: Curiosity ©iStock.com/Soubrette

(Continued)

TABLE 5.2 (Continued)

One-down form	Example
Wondering	"I wonder what you think is the best plan right now?" "I wonder what will help. What could we try?"

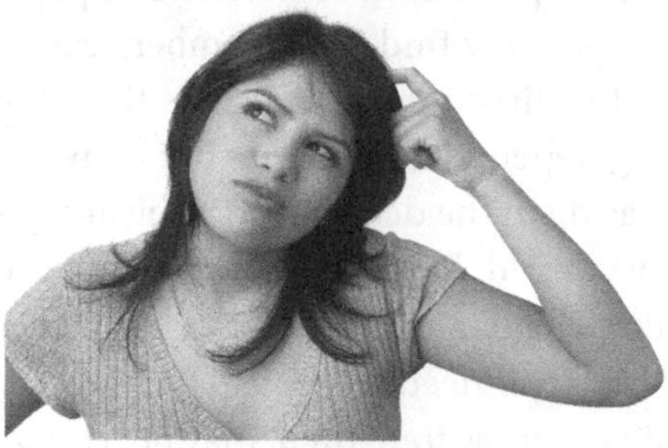

Figure 5.14 One-down: Wondering

©iStock.com/Aldo Murillo

Worry	"I am worried about what will happen to you if you continue to drink." "When you behave that way, it makes other people avoid you. Even staff want to avoid you. I'm worried you are pushing away the people you need in your life."

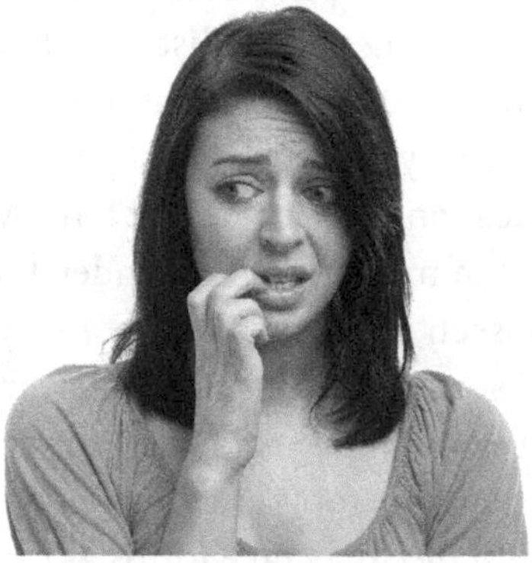

Figure 5.15 One-down: Worrying

©iStock.com/DRB images, LLC

Asking for help	"We really need to figure out a better plan. I need your help on this. Would you be willing to help me?"

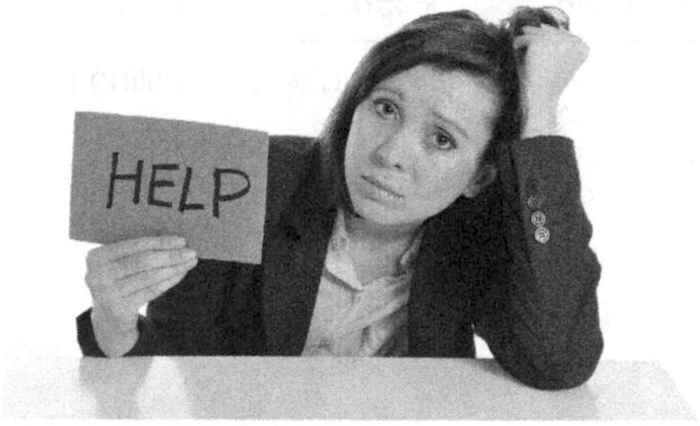

Figure 5.16 One-down: Asking for help

©iStock.com/OcusFocus

One-Down: Humility in Action

In essence, a one-down stance boils down to humility. For mental health workers, humility means:

- Realizing and accepting that you can't make anyone do anything they aren't willing to do.
- No longer trying to force people to change.
- No longer trying to "fix" someone against their will.
- Inviting the people you serve to work with you.
- Accepting that your real power stems from empathy and relationship, and that you are effective in your role to the extent you are able to engage people to collaborate with you on their own development and recovery.

Humility also means accepting that your task as a mental health worker is to help the people you serve develop a sense of personal agency (the belief in their ability to change their own lives). Once a person becomes engaged in the process, you will be in a position to offer tools that the person may find helpful in their growth, recovery, and development.

There is a saying that "the more you know about something, the more you know you don't know." People who study a topic deeply often come to realize just how much they don't know. This spurs them to continue to explore their topic at ever deeper levels. It takes a great deal of knowledge and wisdom for people to appreciate the limitations of what they know. It can also take a great deal of clinical skill to assume the stance of someone who doesn't know, and who invites help.

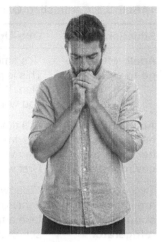

Figure 5.17 Humility
©iStock.com/PeopleImages

Benefits to Providers

Providers also benefit from taking a one-down stance. Mental health work is very difficult. Burnout is common. Staff turnover rates are high in most mental health programs serving people with challenging behaviors. Burnout is more likely if a program is based on unrealistic expectations concerning staff members' ability to change the people they serve. Acting like an expert, and striving to fix people who don't do what you ask them to do, is stressful and exhausting.

For example, if you think, "Why isn't this person getting better?" and then blame yourself, you are likely to feel discouraged and give up. If, by way of contrast, you work with the understanding that you are there to *partner* with other people, not to control them, you are likely to last longer and enjoy greater success. In other words, you will be more successful when you work with a profound sense of humility.

When working with deaf people, there is such a strong need for staff who can communicate effectively that people may imagine, and say, that all you need is good communication to do this work. If that were true, there would never be difficulties in programs where everyone uses the same language. Programs that serve deaf individuals often hire a "deafness expert" who faces great pressure to be all things to all deaf people. That person is often expected to work well with all deaf people, regardless of their communication abilities, age, clinical problems, or the other resources available to help the person. The "deafness expert" often works alone, and the pressures on this person to assume a one-up expert stance are immense. After all, isn't that why the agency hired the person?

This is a set up for burnout. Communicating well with all deaf people is much more complicated than it seems because so many deaf people have been language deprived and therefore aren't good language users in either spoken or signed languages. Many need resources that go well beyond individual counseling. They need a team with multiple kinds of services. Signing counselors last longer if they don't feel responsible to single-handedly fix the world for every deaf person they serve. For such persons, humility can be a key to their own survival in the field.

Regardless of the quality of your education or the number of degrees you have, you are powerless to change people *unless they decide to work with you* and agree with you on a method for "getting better." With practice, you can get really good at partnering with people and helping them discover how change is possible. You can develop skill at what Professor Edgar Schein refers in his book title as *Humble inquiry: The gentle art of asking instead of telling* (Schein 2013).

Common Examples of One-Up and One-Down Stances

Let's compare how one-up and one-down stances might appear in some common situations that occur in mental health settings. As you read through these scenarios, note that statements and directives flow naturally out of a one-up stance, while questions and invitations to partner flow naturally from a one-down stance. An important part of mastering the art of working one-down involves learning to make fewer statements and directives in favor of asking more questions.

Using a one-up or one-down stance when working with adults is examined in Table 5.3.

TABLE 5.3 Contrasting One-Up and One-Down Stances

Situation	One-Up Stance	One-Down Stance
Adult refuses to go to work	"It's time for you to go to work. This is part of your treatment plan. If you don't go to work, you will lose your job."	"I'm worried about what might happen if you don't go to work today. Remember, you decided that working for a year was a goal. What do you think will happen if you don't show up?"
Adult refuses to clean his or her room or environment	"It's time to clean the apartment. If everyone cleans, then we can go to the mall. First we clean, then we go out."	"Can you help us clean up? Everyone wants to go out to the mall, but this place is a mess. My boss told me that the apartment must be cleaned today. I know you want to go out. What can we do?"
Two people are in conflict about food in the refrigerator	"The two of you need to stop fighting. I want each of you to take a time out. Go chill out. I'll set up the dinner."	"Obviously, we have a problem here and I need your help solving it. But, first, you have to be calm enough to talk. Remember the 'red, yellow, green light' skill we discussed? What's the red light? What's the yellow light? Before we get to the green light, what has to happen? Can you come back in five or 10 minutes and we'll try to figure this out together?"
After becoming physically aggressive, a person is willing to discuss the matter	"Remember the plan we discussed? When you hit people, you don't earn any points for the day. We also don't go out that day."	"Can we talk about what happened? What did you do? How did it happen? When you hit people, how do you think they feel? How do they react to you? I'm really worried now. Do you know why I'm worried? Can I tell you? I'm worried that you are losing friends. I'm also worried that staff won't want to work with you. Can we figure out a better plan? What would it be?"
Person has harmed himself	"We are going to continue one-to-one supervision because you are not safe."	"We are really worried about you. Would you be willing to help me understand why you hurt yourself? If I understood it better, then maybe the two of us could come up with the best plan to help you. What do you think?"
Person continues to drink alcohol	"You need to get to a (Twelve Step) meeting today."	"Can I help you get to a meeting today? Many people find that getting to a meeting is the most important thing for them to do after relapsing. Are you willing to go?"

Using a one-up or one-down stance when working with children is examined in Table 5.4.

TABLE 5.4 Contrasting One-Up and One-Down Stances with Students

Situation	One-Up Stance	One-Down Stance
Student doesn't complete a class assignment	"You didn't do the homework so I gave you an F."	"What got in the way of doing your homework? I know you don't want to fail. When you don't finish an assignment, what grade do you think you should get? Can you help me understand what makes this hard for you?"
You are meeting with a student a few hours after he assaulted a peer	"This behavior has to stop. I'm suspending you from school for a week. If you do it again, I will expel you."	"I am really worried about you. The school has a zero tolerance policy for violence. You hit Frank. That means I have to suspend you for a week. If we don't figure out a better plan, I will have to expel you from school permanently. I'm scared about this. Are you?"
Student can't handle unstructured time and starts bothering a peer	"You need to keep your hands to yourself. Here are some things you should do."	"What's going on? Are you bored? Let's see if we can figure out something else you can do."
Student is disappointed and angry that a visit was cancelled	"I understand that you're upset, but you have to control yourself."	"This must be a big disappointment. Do you want to talk about it? Can you stay safe while we discuss it?"
Student wants to stay in bed in the dorm	"You have to get up now. There's no staff to stay here with you. It's time for school."	"It seems really hard for you to get out of bed. I'm worried about your missing school. I'm also concerned because I can't leave you here alone in the dorm. I need you to help me now. Can you do it?"

The "Ask Permission" Skill

A particularly important one-down skill is the "ask permission" skill. This skill can be especially effective when working with people who are very aggressive or don't easily tolerate discussions about problems. The premise is simple: Before trying to address the problem, the staff member asks the individual's permission to proceed.

For example:

"Is it okay with you if we talk about x?""
"Can I ask you a really hard question?"
"Is this a good time to talk to you about this?"

In cases where a conversation is likely to be very difficult, it often helps to lead with a positive comment, such as: *"I noticed you did something good yesterday. Do you know what it was? Can I talk to you about that?"* After the person agrees, the staff person can then proceed with the discussion by saying something such as: *"I'd also like to talk to you about how you handled the stress today. Can we talk about that?"*

If the person says "no," the staff person should end the conversation. Don't feel bad—it is unlikely that the conversation would be productive when the person begins with this negative attitude. The staff person can say something like: *"I appreciate that you were able to say no and stay safe. Nice job. I will ask you to talk about this another time."*

Note that the staff person is asking for permission to help the individual evaluate their skills and response. You can accomplish this by:

1. Expressing a concern.
2. Asking permission to proceed.
3. Asking a series of questions.

These questions are designed to help the person to analyze and solve the problem, as well as evaluate their own behavior and abilities.

A staff person who is using a one-down approach *would not* say, "You didn't use your coping skills yesterday." Rather, the staff person would say something like:

"I'm curious about what happened. Did you use your coping skills like we planned?"
"Did you notice the skills you used? Do you think you could have done better? What would that have looked like?"

Socratic Questioning

The Greek philosopher Socrates asked good questions to guide his students to find their own answers. The method of teaching that is based on asking questions that lead students to discover important truths is called "Socratic questioning." This is a very useful one-down strategy. Even though the teacher has a good sense of the answer she is looking for, she invites and guides the student to discover it. She plays down her own power and authority to help students discover how they are capable of finding answers themselves.

You'll learn more about asking good questions in the next lesson.

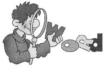

Socratic questions

Definition 5.6: Socratic questioning: The process of asking questions to help guide another person to clarify their thinking or solve problems.

Example of Socratic questioning: "You say you are stupid. What makes you say that? I saw you do several things today that showed me that you are smart. What did you do that showed you are smart?"

Scenario 5.4: Socratic Questioning

Jim is a 22-year-old deaf client with a severe personality disorder who has very poor problem-solving, coping, and social skills. When he wants something, he has difficulty waiting. He hates being told "no," and often becomes aggressive when he has to wait or can't have something. He has learned a bullying style that often intimidates people. He has threatened or assaulted staff on numerous occasions.

Although Jim has been hospitalized for aggressive and self-harming behaviors many times, he is currently being served in his own apartment using a staff outreach model. Staff members meet him in his apartment and assist him with shopping, medicine, budgeting, and socialization.

Over the years, Jim's negative behaviors have improved. Medication has been part of the solution but years of learning about and practicing coping and social skills have also played an important part. Jim understands the concepts and can discuss his own skills. He also uses them often. Over the years, staff members have learned to recognize when he uses his skills and celebrate with him.

Nonetheless, Jim resorts to very threatening postures and words from time to time. Jim doesn't need staff to tell him that these behaviors are bad. He knows it, and will say this himself if staff approach him in a one-down way. In a recent incident, he threatened Joel, a staff person who was driving him in a car. While the car was in traffic, Jim got out, leaving the door open, then gave Joel the finger while he walked away. Joel was understandably upset and frightened. He had to drive the car with an open door through a busy intersection. The next day, Peter, the program director, approached Jim about the incident.

Peter: "Jim, I'm really worried about what happened yesterday. Is it okay if we talk about it?"
Jim: "I don't want to."
Peter: "I know, but we have a problem. I need your help to solve it."
Jim: "What do you mean?"
Peter: "Well, can you tell me what happened yesterday?"
Jim: "Joel was being an asshole. I got mad at him."
Peter: "Yeah, you did. I appreciate that you admit it. Is it okay if we talk about it?"
           Jim shrugs.
Peter: "Actually, I don't really want to talk about it either. This isn't fun for me. But I'm really worried. Do you know what I'm worried about?"
Jim: "You are worried that I might blow up. I won't do it again."
Peter: "I am worried about that, but I'm also very worried about something else. Can you guess what that is?"
           Jim has had versions of this conversation before.
Jim: "Staff?"
Peter: "Exactly! I think you understand a lot. How do you think Joel is feeling about working with you now?"
Jim: "Joel is an asshole. I don't want to work with him."
Peter: "Yeah, and how do you think he's feeling about working with you now?"
Jim: "I don't care."
Peter: "So here's the problem. You don't care how staff feels. How am I going to find someone to work with you?"
Jim: "Sarah is okay. Tell her to come."
Peter: "How do you think Sarah is feeling about working with you?"
Jim: "I didn't do anything to her."
Peter: "Can you take a moment now and think? This is a hard question. Do you think Sarah might be scared? Why might Sarah be scared?"
Jim: "I won't blow up at her."
Peter: "Do you remember saying that to Joel?"
Jim: "I don't want to talk about this."
Peter: "Do you want a break?"
Jim: "OK."

Peter:	"Great. Is 10 minutes okay?"
	They meet again in 10 minutes to continue the discussion.
Peter:	"Thank you for coming back to talk more. Did you notice the skill you just used?"
Jim:	"What?"
Peter:	"It seemed you were getting stressed. This conversation is hard. What did we do? What did you agree to?"
Jim:	"Take a break."
Peter:	"Exactly. You recognized you needed a break and we agreed to a break. That's a really important skill. Did it help?"
Jim:	"I think so."
Peter:	"Hmm. I wonder where else you could use that skill?"
	Jim thinks, then says: "When I get mad?"
Peter:	"Yes! Good thinking. Now can I share the problem we have?"
Jim:	"What?"
Peter:	"How do you think Sarah feels about coming to your apartment? In fact, how do you think all of the staff feel about coming out to see you?"
Jim:	"Scared. But I never hit Sarah."
Peter:	"You're right. But Sarah and other staff feel uncomfortable or afraid. You haven't hit Sarah but you've hit other people, and they're afraid you might hit them. And I don't know how to fix it without your help."
Jim:	"What do you mean?"
Peter:	"Joel, Sarah, me, other staff, we're all on your team. We're the people who try to help you with shopping, money, medicine, having fun, right? But everyone on this team is just like you. Everyone has feelings. Everyone has the right to feel safe. And I can't make other staff members feel safe. I can't make them feel comfortable working with you, without your help. Are you willing to help?"

Peter, the program manager, is not dropping expectations about safety. Rather, he is using a one-down style of questioning to try to make safety a shared problem. He's also sharing a real problem with Jim—program staff members don't want to work with him. Peter's statement about "not knowing" what to do reflects a genuine concern; he really *can't* fix the situation without Jim's help.

This style of one-down work is close to an approach called "collaborative decision making" developed by Ross Greene (Greene & Ablon 2006). An excellent book, *Opening our arms* (Regan 2006), describes the process of changing the culture on a pediatric psychiatric inpatient unit as staff struggles to learn new ways of working that are less dependent on rules and authority and more oriented towards engaging children in skillful problem solving.

It takes much more skill to use a one-down stance than a one-up stance. Asking good questions is more difficult than telling people what to do. It takes a great deal of skill to guide someone through the decision-making process without providing the answer. Keeping one's one ego in check and acknowledging "I can't fix this without you" requires a more mature psychological development. The most talented staff members are able to do one-down work effectively. Less talented staff members usually focus on setting limits and rules.

You will become *more* skillful at your job as you develop the ability to work in a one-down way.

 Bright idea 5.1: Staff who are able to approach the people they serve with humility, using various one-down stances, tend to be most effective at engaging people in their recovery and treatment efforts.

More Examples

Compare the one-up and one-down stances you might take in the situations examined in Tables 5.5, 5.6, and 5.7.

TABLE 5.5 How are These Stances Different?

Situation 1

You are the night staff person in a residence. Joe has been staying up much too late and as a result he is very difficult to wake up in the morning. Morning staff has asked you to "get him to go to bed early." You approach Joe:

One-up stance:	One-down stance:
"You need to go to bed early so you can get up in the morning. You should go to bed by 9:00."	"Can I talk to you about something? It seems like you have trouble getting up in the morning. Is that true? Why do you think that is? I wonder what will happen if you oversleep again. Do you want that to happen? What do you think you should do?"
	Staff used: Curiosity, wondering, Socratic questioning, asking permission, asking for help

---

TABLE 5.6 How are These Stances Different?

Situation 2

You are a staff person in a residential program. One resident, Mark, has gone into the garage and borrowed the bicycle of housemate Luis, without his permission. Luis is furious and ready to hit Mark. Mark has done this many times before and usually admits it when confronted. But, he always says it was a mistake. You need to:

- Keep Luis from hitting Mark.
- Get Mark to apologize to Luis and agree to not borrowing his bicycle in the future.

How would you respond to *each* of them?

To Luis:

One-up stance:	One-down stance:
"I know you're mad, but you can't hit Mark. You need to stay safe and in control."	"I can't believe Mark borrowed you bicycle again without asking you. That must be so frustrating. Are you angry? I would be too. But what what's the smart thing to do now?"
	Staff used: Empathy, questioning, inviting the person to participate in problem solving

To Mark:

One-up stance:	One-down stance:
"You have to stop taking things that belong to other people. We're going to keep the bicycle locked up so you can't get it."	"When you take Luis' bicycle, how do you think he feels? How would you feel if he took your bicycle or something else you have, like your iPhone? If he is angry, what might happen? I'm worried he will hit you again. Do you want him to hit you? What should you do now?"
	Staff used: Worrying, Socratic questioning, inviting the person to problem solve

---

TABLE 5.7 How are These Stances Different?

Situation 3

You're a mental health worker and part of the nursing department staff in a psychiatric inpatient unit. At morning rounds, the treatment team decides which patients have off-the-unit "privileges." The team decides that Sara isn't safe to be off the unit because she has been hiding sharp objects and using them to cut herself. Your supervisor asks you to tell Sara that she does not have off-unit privileges. In the past, Sara has responded to this kind of bad news by screaming, making insulting comments, and banging her head on the wall. You approach Sara:

One-up stance:	One-down stance:
"I'm sorry Sara, but you haven't been safe. You keep cutting yourself. The team doesn't think you are safe enough to be off the unit without staff."	"Sara, you hid some sharp objects and cut yourself again. I'm wondering what happened. Are you willing to talk about it?"
	"We've got a problem. Do you know what it is? You ask for off-unit privileges, but you keep hurting yourself whenever we don't watch you. Can you guess how the team members feel about supporting your off-unit privileges? How can you help us feel more confident that you are safe enough for us to back off supervising you so closely?"
	Staff used: Wondering, asking permission, sharing the dilemma, Socratic questions and asking for help

Practice Exercise 5.1: Asking permission

In this exercise, you will practice the ""asking permission" skill:

1. Identify a person you are anxious to talk with and arrange a time to talk.
2. Before starting the difficult conversation, ask some version of "is it okay if we talk now? I'd like to ask you a few questions."
   Note: This often goes better if you make it clear that you want to comment first on something positive. For example, "First, I'd like to tell you about something really good that you did. I wonder if you know what it was. Can we discuss that first?" If the person says no, thank them for saying "no" in a safe and respectful way, and say you'll ask them again at another time.
3. Document what happened when you asked permission to talk.

_____

_____

_____

Practice Exercise 5.2: One-down vs. one-up

In the following situations, come up with contrasting one-up and one-down responses. You can find sample answers at the end of the chapter. Remember one-down stances usually take one of these forms:

- Inviting.
- Wondering.
- Curiosity.
- Worrying.
- Asking permission.
- Asking for help.

A one-down stance also involves asking more questions, giving fewer directives and, and "sharing the dilemma" you are facing so it is open to joint problem solving:

1. Choose one of the following situations:
   a. Client is threatening to cut himself.
   a. Client pushes another person.
   b. Client refuses to go to work.
   c. Client won't help clean her apartment.
   d. Client refuses to pay her rent, a requirement for living in the residence.
2. Write down a one-up response:

_____

_____

3. Write down a one-down response:

_____

_____

_____

4. Choose another situation from the list in Step 1 or a situation that is not listed but commonly occurs in your program.
5. Write down a one-up response:

_____

_____

6. Write down a one-down response:

_____

_____

_____

Practice Exercise 5.3: Practicing a one-down response

In this exercise, you will intentionally practice using a one-down style:

1. Ask someone else to observe you and comment on how well you use a one-down approach.
2. Pick a situation from the list in exercise 5.2 or use one you have encountered in your work.
3. Practice using one or more of the one-down intervention styles (i.e., asking permission, inviting, wondering, curiosity, worrying, asking for help).
4. Observe how the person reacts while you are talking.
5. Discuss it with the person involved and the observer.

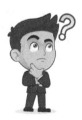

Questions to ponder 5.4: How skillful are you at adopting a one-down stance with the people you serve? How easily does this style of work come to you?

Lesson 5 Skill Sheet

- Participants show skill using these one-down types of one-down intervention:

  a. Inviting (Example: "Would you be willing to discuss this now?")

  b. Curiosity (Example: "I am curious. What do you think about this?")

  c. Wondering (Example: "I am wondering what you think is the best plan right now?")

  d. Worrying (Example: "I am worried what will happen to you if you continue to drink.")

  e. Asking for help (Example: "We really need to figure out a better plan. I need your help on this. Would you be willing to help me?")

  f. Asking permission (Example: "Is it okay if we talk about this now?")

- Participants observe the impact that using a one-up and one-down stance have on participants' willingness to work on developing different kinds of skill.

- Participants observe the impact that these different styles of work have on the level of aggression observed in the people they are working with.

- Participants consider whether a one-up or one-down stance is more likely to be effective in particular situations.

Lesson 5 Quiz

A staff person asks Mary to clean her room before going on a trip. Mary delays and doesn't do it. As the time for the trip approached, Mary gets more anxious and angry. Finally, she screams at staff and runs out of the dorm:

1. Which of the following shows a one-up staff response to Mary? (Check all that apply.)

   a. If you clean your room, you will get 10 points.

   b. First clean your room, then we will go on the trip.

   c. If you blow up, I will drop your level.

   d. Do you need help cleaning your room?

   e. It's OK if you don't clean your room right now. Safety is our priority.

2. Which of the following is one-down response to Mary? (Check all that apply.)

   a. If you clean your room, you will get 10 points.

   b. First clean your room, then we will go on the trip.

   c. If you blow up, I will drop your level.

   d. We have a problem. The house must be clean before we can leave. What should we do about your room? Do you need help?

   e. It's OK if you don't clean your room right now. Safety is our priority.

3. When would it make sense for staff to use a one-up response to Mary? (Check all that apply.)

   a. Mary is refusing to talk about cleaning and a decision must be made about staying home or going on the trip.

   b. Mary is about to hit someone.

c. Mary insists on watching TV

d. Mary's language and thinking skills are so poorly developed, or her anxiety is so great, that she can't participate in decision making regarding the trip right now.

4. A one-down stance is shown in which of the following responses. (Check all that apply.)

a. Curiosity.

b. Worrying.

c. Humility.

d. Asking for help.

e. Inviting.

f. Offering a reward.

5. Why are staff members sometimes reluctant to work in a one-down way? (Check all that apply.)

a. No one has ever showed them how to do this.

b. Staff members were not exposed to this way of working when they were children.

c. Staff think it means they are not skilled.

d. Staff members don't want to have less power within the organization.

e. Staff feel disrespected as workers. Using one-down strategies feels like they are agreeing to accept even less respect in the workplace than they receive now.

Lesson 5 Questions for Discussion

1. Observe the interactions between staff and the people they serve in a particular setting. Do you see staff working primarily from a one-up stance or a one-down one?

2. In the same informal survey, observe how people receiving services react to the one-up vs. one-down stances taken by staff. Do you see any patterns?

3. Do you think that a one-down style of work promotes engagement with the people you serve?

4. What, if any, would be the appropriate times to use a one-up, authority-oriented style with people receiving services?

5. Staff members working in programs that serve people with severe emotional or behavioral problems are often expected to prevent them from doing harmful or destructive behaviors. At times, police, courts, state agency personnel, and the general public expect the program staff to control the behaviors of the people they serve. Do you think there are times that staff working in treatment programs should be responsible for the behavior of the people they serve? When would that make sense?

6. What role is appropriate for the police and the legal system in addressing the anti-social or criminal behaviors exhibited by individuals served in treatment programs?

7. What is your program's policy about calling the police when people who receive services from you act in dangerous or anti-social ways? How do you feel about calling the police?

8. Do you have any fears or concerns about working intentionally in a one-down manner with the individuals receiving services in your program?

9. Are there ways to set limits with people while using a one-down style? For instance, suppose a person acts aggressively and, as a result, staff members feel uncomfortable traveling with the person in a car. Can you confront the person about the impact of their behavior while still using one-down techniques such as invitation, curiosity, wondering, worrying, or asking for help?

10. Do you agree that many of the people served in mental health programs have no real sense of personal agency? That is, do the individuals you serve believe that they can do something to impact their own lives? Do you think a sense of personal agency is central to their recovery, improvement or growth? Do you think it is the job of program staff to help participants develop this sense of personal agency?

11. What is the connection between helping people notice and identify skills they already have and the development of a sense of personal agency?

12. Do you agree with the statement made in this lesson that it takes a great deal of wisdom to recognize your ignorance? Does that make sense to you?

Lesson 5 Quiz Answers

1. Answer *d* is the only one-down stance listed because it focuses on asking Mary what she needs and seeks to problem solve with her, not for her. Answers *a*, *b*, and *c* are all one-up stances because they involve the use of authority and consequences. Answer *e* is also one-up because staff is making the decision. A more skillful response is to empathize, negotiate and then give her credit for negotiation skills.

2. Answer *d* is the one-down response because it involves asking Mary to help you. It also involves sharing the dilemma, not solving it for her. You might think that *e* is a one-down response. People sometimes confuse one-down with backing away from expectations. It isn't that. Rather, one-down work still raises expectations, but decision making is left to the client. One-down work attempts to foster decision making, problem solving, conflict resolution, etc., by engaging the person in the process and developing these skills.

3. Answer *a* is a one-up response that may be necessary because Mary is refusing to participate in making a decision that must be made at that time. Answer *b* is a one-up response that may be necessary because her immediate safety is at stake. Answer *d* is also a one-up response that may be necessary because Mary is so language delayed and cognitively impaired that she can't yet participate in shared decision making. With regard to *c*, the best staff response might be sharing the dilemma and asking for help. Staff might also use an I-statement such as, "Mary, I'm worried about the house not being clean. If I ignore that, I'm not doing my job. What can we do together to solve this?"

4. Answers *a* through *e* are all different types of one-down stance. Response *f* is a kind of one-up stance.

5. Staff members have raised all of these concerns about working one-down.

Sample Answers to Practice Exercise 5.2: One-down vs. one-up

a. Client is threatening to cut himself.
   One-up: "Don't cut yourself!" "If you cut yourself again, you will be restricted to the program."
   One-down: "I'm curious how you feel when you cut yourself. Does it help in some way? Would you be willing to explore if there is another, safer way to get the same feeling?"

b. Client pushes another person.
   One-up: "You are pushing people again. That's not safe! We are dropping your level because of unsafe behavior."
   One-down: "What happened? Joe says you pushed him? Is that true? This is making me worried. You know what I'm worried about? What happens when you push people? How do they respond to you?"

c. Client refuses to go to work.
   One-up: "You have to go to work. It's in your service plan. If you don't go to work, you will lose your job."
   One-down: "How come you don't want to go to work today? Are you just tired or did something happen at work? If you skip work, what may happen to you? Is that what you want?"

d. Client won't help clean her apartment.
   One-up: "I won't take you out shopping until the apartment is clean."

One-down: "Can I ask you some questions? How do you feel living in an apartment that is so dirty? What makes it hard for you to clean? Can I help you with this? I'm worried that if the apartment gets this bad, you will get mice. You might also get evicted. Do you worry about that?"

e. Client refuses to pay her rent, a requirement for living in the residence.
   One-up: "If you don't pay your rent, you will not be able to stay here."
   One-down: "What will happen if you don't pay your rent? Will you be able to stay here? Is that what you want?"

Bibliography

Anderson, H., & Goolishian, H. (1992). The client is the expert: A not-knowing approach to therapy. In S. McNamee and K. J. Gergen, *Therapy as social construction*. Newbury Park, CA: SAGE.

Berg, I. K. S., & Dolan, Y. (2001). *Tales of solutions*. New York: W.W. Norton & Company, Inc.

Glickman, N. (2009). *Cognitive behavioral therapy for deaf and hearing persons with language and learning challenges*. New York: Routledge.

Greene, R. (1998). *The explosive child*. New York: HarperCollins.

Greene, R. W., & Ablon, J. S. (2006). *Treating explosive kids: The collaborative problem-solving approach*. London: Guilford Press.

Meichenbaum, D., & Biemiller, A. (1998). *Nurturing independent learners: Helping students take charge of their learning*. Newton, MA: Brookline Books.

Meichenbaum, D., & Turk, D. (1987). *Facilitating treatment adherence: A practitioner's guide*. New York: Plenum Press.

Regan, K. (2006). *Opening our arms: Helping troubled kids do well*. Boulder, CO: Bull Publishing Company.

Schein, E. H. (2013). *Humble inquiry: The gentle art of asking instead of telling*. San Francisco, CA: Berrett-Koehler Publishers, Inc.

Questions Are Better than Answers

Introduction

In treatment/recovery settings, it is almost always better to ask good questions than it is to provide good answers. Likewise, it is far more powerful and useful to help people evaluate themselves than it is for you to evaluate them.

This lesson is about what Donald Meichenbaum calls "the art of questioning" (Meichenbaum 1994, 2001). The most effective mental health counseling occurs when counselors ask questions *intentionally designed* to help people come up with their own answers. But, even more than finding answers, asking questions respectfully and skillfully engages people in their own recovery.

This lesson introduces the kind of questions that mental health practitioners can use to better understand—and help those they serve to better understand—why problem behaviors occur and, more importantly, what can be done about them. These questions are different from the skill- and strength-based questions that you learned about in Lesson 3.

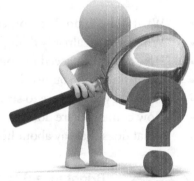

Figure 6.1 Questions
©iStock.com/abluecup

The Role of Questions in CBT

You are engaged in the process of helping people to assess themselves and guiding them to come up with solutions to personal challenges. Asking questions skillfully will prompt this critical self-evaluation and self-exploration. If you can get people to ask themselves these questions, they will be ready for CBT; indeed, they will be doing CBT!

Many of the questions used in CBT focus on identifying the factors (from the environment and from inside the person) that set the stage for a problem behavior or symptom to develop. By asking these practical questions, you are in a position to help the individuals you are working with discover possible solutions to their problem behaviors.

Questions should be presented in a spirit of helpful curiosity. As you learned in Lesson 5, questions flow from a one-down stance. Skilled mental health workers are curious:

- When someone receiving services does something well, skilled mental health workers want to understand *how* they did it, and in particular, what skills the person used.

- When someone exhibits a problem behavior or symptom, skilled mental health workers want to understand *what* triggered and supported it.
- Skilled mental health workers want to understand all of the forces that came together to promote or reinforce those behaviors and symptoms.

This curiosity does not mean mental health providers want to pry into other people's private lives or gain power over them. We are curious because we want to help people find better solutions. In particular, mental health workers are curious about:

- Why does a problem keep happening?
- What can the person do about it?
- What is the person already doing that helps?
- How could the person do even better?
- How can I support the people I'm serving in this effort?

You want to encourage a similar curiosity in the people you serve.

Strength-based Questions

In Lesson 3, you learned about strength-based questions. As you'll recall, strength-based questions help people discover their skills and strengths. They help people discover how and why they are doing so well *in spite of* what has happened to them. This type of question is usually a variation on one of these themes:

- "What did you do that worked?"
- "What are you already doing well?"
- "How did you succeed in doing that?"
- "What skills did you use?"
- "How did you manage to stay in control or handle that situation?"
- "How come you are doing so well in this difficult situation?"
- "What does that say about how you are changing and growing?"

Bright idea 6.1: In mental health work, asking good questions is almost always more helpful than providing good answers.

Bright idea 6.2: The most skillful questions:

- Guide people to identify and reflect on specific positive actions that they took.
- Guide people to think about how well they did in spite of the challenges they are facing.
- Help people to attribute these positive actions or skills to their own decision-making process.
- Guide people to develop a sense of personal agency, a self-story that says, "I can do it!"
- Invite people to consider new behaviors, skills, or ways of thinking that may be helpful.

Practice Exercise 6.1: What is the most skillful response?

Compare three possible interventions to the same situation (see Table 6.1). As you read each response, think about which one you think helped Michael to recognize that he successfully used skills to stay safe in this situation.

TABLE 6.1 Which Intervention Works Best?

Michael lives in a group home. He is feeling very stressed. He doesn't feel well and is worried about money. His housemate Paul has been bothering him. Although Michael has sometimes reacted violently in the past, he is clearly trying to stay safe today.	**Intervention 1**: "I see you are staying safe today. Good job."
	Intervention 2: "I see that you are stressed today. It looks like you don't feel well and Paul seems to be bothering you. But I noticed you are using a lot of skills. You walked away from Paul. You didn't blow up at him. You went to your room and did something to distract you. Now you're expressing your feelings. Lots of good skills. Great!"
Michael walks away when Paul provokes him and goes to his room where he begins to play games on his iPhone.	**Intervention 3**: "I'm seeing you use some skills. Really impressive. Can I ask you a few questions? How are you feeling now? Are you worried about something? Did Paul do something to bother you?"
Later, Michael comes out and asks to talk to a staff member.	*Michael explains.*
The staff member welcomes the opportunity and takes a minute to consider three possible interventions.	"So, you are stressed and a bit angry, but I notice you used several coping skills. Did you notice that? What skills did you use?"
	They discuss the skills Michael used.
Which intervention would you choose?	"What do you think about the fact that you are stressed and you are using skills? This says some good things about you. What does it say?"

Which intervention do you think was most effective? Which would you choose? Actually, all three interventions are strength-based. Each is good in its own way. However, they are *not* equally effective.

Assuming that the goal is to help Michael recognize the skills he used, *Intervention 1* was the least effective. The mental health worker recognizes that Michael had done something well and provided positive feedback. However, simply saying "good job" isn't particularly helpful because it doesn't offer concrete feedback about what, exactly, Michael did well. Intervention 1 gets a C.

Intervention 2 is more effective than Intervention 1 because the mental health worker gave detailed feedback about his observations, the stressors that he witnessed and the skills Michael used. The worker noticed and named specific skills that Michael already has and offered praise. This is a much more helpful response than a vague "good job" for the equally vague accomplishment of "staying safe" that was offered in the first option. This is a competent intervention, but it's not the most effective one. Unfortunately, this is still a one-up response because the mental health worker used his authority to *tell* Michael what was good and bad. While Michael received valuable feedback, the mental health worker failed to guide Michael to figure this out on his own. Intervention 2 gets a B+.

In mental health counseling, the most skillful intervention occurs when you ask questions that help people figure things out on their own. *Intervention 3* gets an A. In this response, the mental health worker uses a one-down style of Socratic questioning to guide Michael to discover his own abilities. It is only after Michael discovers and names his own skills that the counselor offers a reinforcing "Great!"

Using Questions as Part of Behavioral Analysis

A behavioral analysis is a technique designed to help someone understand why they engaged in a particular problem behavior, such as self-harm. It is also called a "behavioral chain analysis" or "functional analysis." A counselor conducts a behavioral analysis by asking a series of questions that leads the person to understand what happened before, during and after a behavior occurs. Behavioral chain analyses are a prominent part of dialectical behavior therapy, or DBT (Linehan 1993). They are also the main way in which cognitive behavioral therapists answer the question, "why did this happen?" In both CBT and DBT, behavioral analyses guide counselors and clients to figure out ways to lessen a problem behavior or symptom.

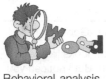

Behavioral analysis

Definition 6.1: Behavioral analysis: A series of questions designed to identify all of the variables that contribute to the occurrence of a problem behavior, as well as interventions that could lessen or prevent the problem behavior.

Example of behavioral analysis: Amanda, a staff member, sits down with Moses, a resident, to figure out why he continues to cut himself. They start with Moses' most recent cutting incident. Amanda asks a series of questions about what led up to it, how he felt and what he thought during the cutting and what happened afterwards.

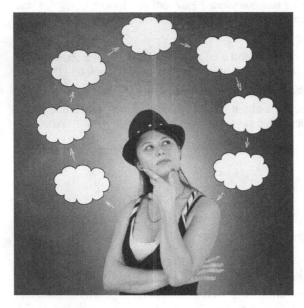

Figure 6.2 Behavior Analysis: What leads up to, supports, and reinforces a problem behavior?

©iStock.com/Mathias Rosenthal

Scenario 6.1

The following scenario presents a situation where behavioral analysis can be used to help identify the underlying issue.

Charlotte lives in a group home with several other residents. Betty, a staff person, has built a strong empathetic relationship with Charlotte. Charlotte didn't sleep well last night and woke up in a bad mood. She drank more coffee than she normally does and had an argument with a roommate. Betty notices Charlotte sitting at the kitchen table with her head in her hands. Shortly after, Charlotte goes out with Betty to do some raking in the yard. She picks up leaves and sticks and puts them in a wheelbarrow. However, the wheelbarrow falls over and everything spills out. Charlotte kicks the wheelbarrow, swears and screams, "This stinks! I can't do anything right!" She marches back into the house and goes straight to the kitchen where she grabs a few cookies. She then goes outside and smokes a cigarette. Finally, she goes up to her room and goes back to bed. Betty continues to do the raking by herself.

Charlotte's reaction to the wheelbarrow tipping over seems extreme. Why do you think Charlotte kicked the wheelbarrow, yelled, and left her chore? A behavioral analysis can be used to uncover several possible reasons and possible solutions.

The questions used in a behavioral analysis are not strength based. The goal isn't to ask why or how a person did something well. Rather, the goal is to learn why or how a person did something badly. These types of question are designed to provide guidance on how the person, and those around the person, could do better.

Tell Me What Happened

A behavior analysis is essentially an attempt to pull from the person a detailed story that describes exactly what happened in a specific situation. It always starts with identifying a specific behavior that will be discussed, followed by asking the person to tell their story.

A behavior analysis is never about something broad like "aggression," but about a specific instance. For example:

"Yesterday, at 2:00, you punched Solomon on the arm."
"This morning, while waiting for staff to arrive, you took 10 extra pills."
"Sunday, after dinner, you went to your room and cut yourself deeply on your thigh."

Problem behaviors that might be analyzed include a specific act of aggression or self-harm or a specific instance where a problem symptom reappeared. If you are having trouble doing a behavior analysis, it may be because you are not starting with a specific behavior at a specific time and place.

Good stories share some common elements. A good story:

- Has a beginning, a middle and end.
- Is linear (proceeds forward in time in an organized way) and includes things like cause and effect. For example: *The wolf chased Red Riding Hood into grandmother's house. (Cause) She felt afraid and hid from him. (Effect)*
- Clearly identifies what happened and who was involved, specifically who did what. For example: *The wolf chased Red Riding Hood, not the other way around.*
- Reveals feelings. In a mental health program, these details can provide excellent clues into the reasons why something happened.
- Includes important details that are essential to the story and omits details or information that isn't essential.

However, what happens to a person's ability to share their story when he or she has experienced extreme language deprivation? How can a person share their story when environmental or neurological factors interfere with their language development? What happens if someone has had poor or minimal schooling, poor language models, or problems learning language? Any of these factors may make it extremely difficult to tell a clear story.

When we can't get the full story, we strive to get as much of the story as the person can tell. We strive to help people tell their story as fully and clearly as they can.

Your job involves helping people tell better stories. The more language deprived a person has been, the more help they will need telling their stories. Regardless of what else is going on, when working with people with language and learning challenges, you are always attempting to help them develop better language and thinking skills. You can do this by helping people tell clearer stories.

A good way to begin is by asking the Deaf-friendly question, *"Will you tell me the story?"* This shows interest and curiosity: *"How did this happen? I really want to understand."* Because we all love stories, the invitation to "tell me the story" is a friendly, probably universal, way to engage people in this process. Hopefully, you recognize that asking this question shows curiosity, one of the hallmarks of working one-down.

Once you have invited the person to share their story, you can assist them by providing "structuring questions," such as:

"When did this happen?"
"Who was there?"
"What was going on?"
"What happened first? Then what? Then what?"
"How were you feeling?"
"What were you thinking?"
"What did the other person [people] say and do?"
"How did it end?"

Language development occurs at the same time as the development of thinking skills. When working with individuals who have language and learning challenges, you must assess, match, and promote language and cognitive development while simultaneously working on emotional and behavioral challenges. The following scenario illustrates how language limitations can lead to challenges in a therapeutic setting. It also shows ways that staff can help the individual develop communication skills as a crucial part of any intervention plan.

Scenario 6.2

Diego is a young Deaf man. He grew up in a third-world country where he had only minimal formal education. When he came to the United States at age 15, Diego had little formal language skills in either spoken or sign language. He was placed in a signing Deaf residential school where he was very far behind his peers in terms of both language development and academic skills. At school, Diego frequently became aggressive with his peers and teachers. He pushed, punched, and kicked people and damaged property. Managing this aggressive behavior was difficult for the school, but the situation became even more challenging when Diego touched a female peer on the breasts and gestured that he wanted oral sex. The girl was frightened and went to authorities. Diego, by now 19 years old, was arrested, brought to a psychiatric emergency room and admitted to a psychiatric hospital. He eventually was transferred to another psychiatric hospital with a Deaf inpatient unit.

While he was in school, Diego had picked up some simple ASL so he could make many of his basic needs known using signs and sign phrases. However, it remained difficult for even very skilled Deaf signers to understand him fully. Diego frequently signed BOTHER-ME, for instance, without saying who, what, when, where, or why he was bothered. He would sign UPSET or MAD but could not elaborate. This left the people working with him to guess what had really happened.

Diego's sign language completely lacked any tense or time markers and offered no context for his statements. If he signed HIT, for instance, it wasn't clear whether he had hit someone, was planning to hit someone, or wanted to hit someone. The sign also could be interpreted that someone had hit him, threatened to hit him, or he had seen one person hit another.

On the Deaf inpatient unit, Diego continued to show physically and sexually aggressive behaviors. One day, Angela, a female peer, came running to the nursing staff, crying and claiming that Diego put his hand on her crotch. Staff offered her an evaluation and support. She was not physically harmed, but she was frightened and confused. Angela had better language skills than Diego. She could give a reasonably clear account of what happened (how Diego came to touch her and how she touched him back but she was less skillful at communicating to others (Diego or the staff) whether or not she was consenting to this sexual activity. She seemed anxious and confused, but more about whether or not she was in trouble than over Diego's (and her) behavior.

When staff asked Angela questions, they learned that part of the problem was that neither Diego nor Angela was communicating well about what they wanted or agreed to. Angela appeared to passively go along without really indicating consent until it went too far and she panicked. Staff assured her she wasn't in trouble, separated her and Diego, and began working with her on assertiveness. Staff saw from Angela's account that while she may have pressured to have sexual contact she didn't want, part of what she needed was stronger abilities to communicate yes or no.

It was much more difficult for staff to get a clear story from Diego. For three hours, staff and Diego gestured, role played, drew and used toy figures in an attempt to elicit a rough approximation of Diego's account of what happened. According to Diego, as best staff could understand, he and Angela had kissed each other and touched each other's genitals. He seemed to believe they both wanted this. He certainly wasn't attending to how she felt and had no real understanding about consent. It might well be that, as people feared, he was a sexual predator; but what staff saw was a person without any of the abilities, including basic language skills, needed to understand what he was feeling and negotiate relationships with another person.

As they were talking with Diego, the Deaf staff did the best they could to model for Diego how to sign what he appeared to be saying. This was challenging because they didn't want to lead Diego to say something he didn't mean. They also made it clear to him, through signing and role playing, that Angela had not agreed to that sexual contact. He had not asked her clearly, and she had not responded clearly. She may have touched him because she was afraid (this wasn't too hard to role play). In any case, they could not behave that way in the hospital. This was a complicating factor. Both Diego and Angela understood rules (no sexual contact in the hospital) better than they understood negotiation and consent. The easier path for staff was to talk to them about rules. The much tougher task was to engage them in learning skills.

Staff role played and signed with both what consent looked like. They also role played that if Diego touched someone's private areas when that person didn't consent, the police might come and Diego could go to jail. They used the sign FORCE, gave examples of FORCE SEX such as FORCE KISS, FORCE TOUCH BREASTS, FORCE INTERCOURSE. With these examples, they also taught him the concept and sign for RAPE.

The staff signed and gestured that they were worried about Diego, and asked him what he thought they should do, as well as what he thought he should do. Diego signed that he would apologize to Angela and stay away from her. Angela, with staff support, was able to meet with Diego and hear his apology and promise. She told him she just wanted to be friends. Staff also increased supervision on both during their hospital stays.

While attempting to find out what had happened, staff members working with Diego and Angela were also asking questions that are part of a behavior analysis. Mostly, they were working on the basic task of getting a clear story. From Angela, they learned that part of the problem was that neither had good communication skills for negotiating something like sexual activity. Angela had enough language to tell the story, but she was unskillful at communicating her feelings and wishes, especially if she felt pressure to consent.

Diego's language skills were more limited, but the process of attempting to get the story from him showed the staff some of what they needed to do. They had to help him develop better language, including important concepts like forced sex and consent, and they also needed to teach him to ask for and obtain clear consent before initiating sexual contact. This wouldn't be easy. Diego's language deprivation meant he was facing adult challenges with the mind of a preschooler.

Fortunately, Diego had been arrested previously and feared going to jail. Staff were able to use the realistic possibility of arrest and jail to motivate him. If the police or courts had just dismissed his behavior and excused him, it would have been far more difficult to engage him. Diego does need to face negative consequences for sexual offending, but the consequences should be imposed by legal, not mental health, authorities.

Bright idea 6.3: When you are counseling someone with language and learning challenges, you are always working on language development. You can't assume that people have the language they need in a situation. You have to help them develop it. Indeed, with persons who have very little language, language development is bound to be a primary therapeutic task, no matter the other mental health or behavioral issues.

Bright idea 6.4: Language development is cognitive development. Someone who has poor language skills may have difficulty with structures like linear time, establishing a topic clearly, moving from topic to topic, conveying cause and effect, and relating behavior to feelings and thoughts. They may have difficulty establishing context: "Yesterday, while it was raining, this is what I did." When you teach language, you are also teaching the thinking structures that make problem solving possible.

As a staff person trying to understand why something happened, your job is to pull out the best, most complete story that you can. Sometimes, the story will be very simple. Sometimes, you will be able to get only part of the story. It is important for you to know what a good behavior analysis looks likes so you can ask as many questions as the person has the ability to understand. While your goal is to do a thorough analysis, you need to take into account the language and conceptual abilities of the person you are serving. The complexity of the behavior analysis must match the complexity of the person's language and storytelling abilities.

Elements of a Behavior Analysis

A good behavioral analysis has six key elements. Let's look at each more closely.

We will use Charlotte's situation (Scenario 6.1) to help explain these elements. As you'll recall, Charlotte was helping staff with outdoor chores when she became frustrated, kicked over the wheelbarrow, and ran into the house. The specific behavior we want to understand is this particular "blow-up," which consisted of kicking, screaming, leaving her job, and storming off. Again, we are not analyzing blow-ups in general, but this *specific instance*.

Take a moment to review Charlotte's story before examining each.

Element 1: Vulnerability

When do you think that Charlotte's blow-up began? It wasn't at the moment when she kicked the wheelbarrow. Remember, Charlotte hadn't slept well and woke in a bad mood, drank more coffee than normal, and argued with a housemate.

These factors indicate that she was "primed" for a problem behavior. She was vulnerable to a relapse of her problem behavior of having tantrums. There may have been other vulnerabilities that we don't know about.

For example, was Charlotte in pain or distress? Was she preoccupied or dwelling on something negative? Was she sick?

It is important and relevant to identify Charlotte's vulnerabilities. How has she been feeling generally and how well is she taking care of herself generally, before this particular problem happened? Problem behaviors are much more likely to show up when a person is stressed, sick, in pain, tired, or in a bad mood. Some skills that can be addressed in CBT are critical self-regulation skills such as: sleeping, eating, exercising, recreating, and managing stress. A person is going to be able to manage any problem behavior better if they take good care of themselves.

This makes sense. Imagine how you would feel if you were up all night drinking alcohol, coffee, and smoking cigarettes. Then, the next morning, a family member left the kitchen a mess. You respond by yelling at him and tossing the dishes into the sink, breaking a glass. What primed you to respond like this? You were physically exhausted. Maybe you were experiencing a hangover. Because you were more vulnerable, something that might normally have led to a calm discussion resulted in a more extreme reaction.

Questions that you can use to better understand if a person was more vulnerable to a recurrence of a problem behavior include:

1. How have you been sleeping?
2. How have you been feeling? What's your mood been like lately?
3. Have you been in any pain or physical distress?
4. How have you been taking care of yourself (e.g., diet, exercise, recreation, etc.)?
5. Have you been struggling with cravings or other reactions to addictive substances?
6. Before this happened, do you think were you feeling at your best?
7. When you are really feeling good, what do you do? Would this have happened if you were really feeling good that day?

Can you see how these kinds of question could be important for a treatment plan?

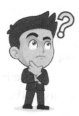

Questions to ponder 6.1: Even without proceeding further with the behavior analysis, can you see how these questions alone might help a person come up with a plan to avoid problem behaviors? Don't we all cope better at some times than others, depending in part on how well we are taking care of our basic needs?

Element 2: Triggers

Charlotte's outburst appears to have been triggered when the wheelbarrow tipped over. But, is it possible that her outburst was triggered by an earlier event or situation, such as too little sleep or the argument with her roommate?

Almost anything can be a trigger and what bothers one person may not bother another person. As you'll recall from Lesson 1, a scene from the movie *Temple Grandin* was used to explain the importance of sensory-based coping skills. In that scene, Temple's overwhelming anxiety is triggered by a combination of things—a piece of paper that has floated to the floor, the rustling of curtains, the sounds of a metal fan turning, the shadow of the fan as it circles the wall. In treatment programs, people's problem behaviors are often triggered by interactions with peers or with staff. Some common triggers are:

- Staff behaving in an overly directive, controlling or one-up manner.
- Staff saying "no" in what the client feels is an arbitrary or disrespectful manner.
- Another person's failure to empathize well.
- An insensitive or invalidating comment.

- Perceived or real criticism
- Stressors associated with being dependent on others.
- Stressors associated with being unable to get what the person wants.
- Having to wait—not getting immediate satisfaction or an immediate response.
- Perceived unfairness—the belief that somebody else seems to be getting something that you are not getting.

The point is that environmental triggers do not *cause* problem behaviors. Someone saying "no" to you does not cause you to hit him. While it may trigger or provoke a feeling and a behavior, it does not cause the behavior. As we will discuss in Lesson 9, what causes the behavior is how you think and how you choose to respond. Of course, people aren't always aware that they are choosing to respond in a negative way. You can help the people you serve notice their choices by discussing times when they responded differently. Take Charlotte's situation, for example:

Charlotte kicked the wheelbarrow today, but yesterday, when the power went off during her favorite television program, she didn't *kick the television. She went to talk to staff and waited patiently for the power to come back on. She experienced two different triggers, but responded differently to each. Staff can ask questions to help her see that triggers and stressors are everywhere, but sometimes she copes with them better than she does at other times.*

You can start a conversation about triggers simply by inquiring, "What happened?" and showing you appreciate that this might be a big deal to them, even if it strikes others as no big deal. In other words, a conversation about triggers will be much more effective when you show *empathy*. For example, the staff member could say something like the following to Charlotte:

"You must have felt so frustrated when the wheelbarrow tipped over again. You seemed to want to do a good job, and then all the sticks fell out, and you had to start over again."

This conversation follows a simple formula. First, you identify the trigger (*"the wheelbarrow tipped over"*). Second, you validate and empathize (*"That must have been hard. I can see why you'd feel frustrated."*). Finally, you separate the trigger from the response to the trigger. (*"You kicked the wheelbarrow and went to your room."*)

When you identify the moment by moment details leading to the problem behavior, it's like you are watching what happened in slow motion. In the process, it's easier to show how the person's behavior was not inevitable. The person could have chosen to behave differently.

Note that the concept of "trigger" may be unfamiliar. You may have to teach what this means. In Lessons 11 and 12, we discuss teaching strategies from Deaf mental health care. One of these strategies is providing lots of examples and stories to illustrate the concept. You may need to teach the concept of "trigger" by providing lots of examples.

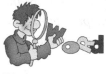

Trigger

Definition 6.2: Trigger: An act or event that serves to start, stimulate or provoke a reaction or series of reactions.

Example of a trigger: Alejandra saw her friend drinking a beer, which triggered her to get herself a beer also.

Element 3: Physical Reactions

Before she went out to rake, Betty, the staff member, noticed Charlotte sitting at the kitchen table with her head in her hands. Could this have been a moment at which Betty could have helped her? People, like other animals, often give away their emotions through:

- Body posturing.
- Movements.

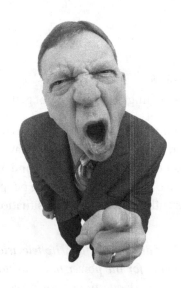

- Facial expression.
- Breathing.

Sometimes it is useful to ask questions including:

1. How were you sitting/standing?
2. What was happening with your hands?
3. Did you notice how you were moving around?
4. Did you notice your breathing?

Breathing, in particular, is worth noticing because emotional arousal is often accompanied by *short, shallow* breathing. *Changing posture* and *facial expression* can be clues to changing emotions and behaviors. As a result, *recognizing these changes* can be helpful.

The following scenarios illustrate how recognizing physical symptoms of stress and using other, most positive physical strategies can help a person manage their response to a trigger.

Figure 6.3 Forgetting to breathe?
©iStock/com/sdominick

Scenario 6.3

Bjorn is a staff person in a day treatment program who is leading a group on coping skills. Today, the group is talking about how to respond to a staff person they don't like. Bjorn uses role-play exercises to help members of the group notice how they walk, talk, move, and breathe, as well as how their faces and bodies look when they are angry. He teaches them to tense and relax different muscles. He asks them to stand in stiff, tense postures followed by standing in loose, relaxed postures. He then asks them to describe how they feel based simply on their posture. They also practice responding to the staff person they don't like just by breathing, standing, and moving differently.

Scenario 6.4

Abby is a deaf patient in a psychiatric hospital who has very poor self-soothing abilities. She becomes agitated and aggressive very easily, based on stressors that most people find insignificant. Susanne, a staff member, is helping Abby prepare for a meeting with her case manager where the case manager will deliver the bad news that Abby can't return to her previous program. Staff members are not optimistic that Abby will be able to cope with this kind of trigger.

Abby has very little ability to do a personal behavior analysis, but she has been able to calm herself down when staff guide her through simple yoga postures, and slow, diaphragmatic breathing. Susanne prepares Abby for the meeting by doing the postures and breathing with her. They also agree that, if needed, Susanne will prompt Abby to stop and breathe by tapping her lightly on the arm to get her attention and then modeling the breathing. Susanne also has alerted the case manager that they might use this strategy in the meeting.

Element 4: Feelings and Coping Skills

A key part of every behavior analysis is gathering information around the question "What were you feeling?" Before she went out to rake the leaves, Charlotte may have been sad or angry. Her comments, "This stinks," and "I can't do anything right," suggest she was likely feeling more upset with herself than the fact that the wheelbarrow has tipped over.

"How do you feel?" is probably the most common question asked in the mental health field. This question has many purposes. One is to help people notice and name internal experiences, an especially important skill for persons with language delays and gaps. In a behavior analysis, you should always ask, "What were you feeling?" *after* a trigger and *before* a problem behavior occurred, as a way of helping the person connect their feelings with their reactions. Sometimes, when a person has very weak analytic abilities, the resulting behavior analysis may have only two or three components.

Using Charlotte as an example, she might answer the question "What were you feeling?" as follows:

The wheelbarrow tipped over. ➡ I felt frustrated and angry. ➡ I kicked the wheelbarrow.

Even this very simple behavior analysis provides vital information. It tells us that Charlotte has trouble coping with feelings like frustration and anger. If she were better able to cope with those feelings, she wouldn't have kicked the wheelbarrow. The goal, then, is to help her learn to cope better.

Questions about feelings can open up questions about coping. For example:

"When you felt frustrated, how well did you cope?"
"Did you use any coping skills?
"Did the coping skills help?
"What coping skills might you have used?"
"If you had used those skills, what would that have looked like?"
"Could we practice that?"
"Do you want to learn any other coping skills?"

Element 5: Thoughts

Charlotte may not be aware of her thoughts, but the interaction offers several clues about what she was thinking. She expressed, "This stinks," and "I can't do anything right." These are thoughts. Usually before people engage in some problematic behavior, they give themselves permission to do it with statements they say to themselves. However, they are usually unaware of how they are doing this. For example, before drinking a can of beer, Julien may think, "I'll just have one," or "I deserve it." Before punching someone, Stephan may think, "That jerk deserves a punch in the face." Neither Julien nor Stephen is aware of how they are giving themselves permission to behave in these ways.

People with language and learning challenges often have a great deal of difficulty noticing their thoughts. You need language to think abstractly—in other words, you need language skills in order to be able to think about thinking. Lessons 8, 9, and 10 contain strategies that you can use to help people with language and learning challenges notice their "self-talk"—what they say to themselves and the impact it has on them. When people can begin to notice what they think, you will have many more tools to help them feel and behave differently.

Element 6: What Happened After?

It is important to understand and take into account what happens *after* a problem behavior occurs, particularly how other people reacted.

After Charlotte left the job, she went into the house, and rewarded herself with some cookies and a cigarette. She then went up and slept, which may have served as an additional reinforcement of her behavior. The staff person, Betty, completed the yardwork herself. Thus, Charlotte was able to avoid doing yardwork at her own house.

Traditional behavior therapy pays close attention to whether behaviors are reinforced or punished. It assumes that people use more behaviors that are reinforced and fewer behaviors that are punished. This is a good principle to remember, even if one isn't doing behavior therapy strictly speaking. You could help Charlotte understand what happened and how others reacted to her outburst by asking questions along these lines:

"After you went inside, what did you do?"
"How did the cookies make you feel?"
"How did the smoking make you feel?"
"How did going back to bed make you feel?"
"Did you notice that Betty finished the work?"
"You were able to avoid doing the raking. How do you feel about that?"

These questions are intended to identify things that reinforce the problem behavior. You might be able to help Charlotte change her behavior by agreeing with her to reinforce her successes. This might include setting up a plan that Charlotte and staff members will do something fun together after Charlotte completes her chores. This type of reinforcement plan must be done with her knowledge, participation, and agreement. Behavior modification without the informed consent and active participation of the person receiving services is a one-up intervention in which staff try to control someone they serve. That approach is *not* part of this pre-therapy program. But using reinforcers with the person's informed agreement, especially if it is decided after a process of discussion and negotiation, may be very helpful.

"Why Did it Happen?"

When you use behavior analysis to understand why a behavior happened, you are really asking *how* it happened. By getting answers to the question "how," you begin to view the behavior in its full context. You need to consider and gather information related to what happened *outside* the person, in the environment:

* What happened before the behavior?
* What happened after the behavior?
* Was the behavior reinforced in any way? If so, how?

You also must be aware of what is happening *inside* the person. To understand this, you must depend on the person's ability to label and identify internal states:

* What were they feeling?
* What were they thinking?
* How did they show their thoughts and feelings in their bodies and behaviors?

You may have to teach people to recognize and label their inner experiences. Sometimes you may have to literally give them the words.

You don't need try to look for causes in things that happened long ago. For example, someone may remind you of your father and your reaction to this person may echo the way you behaved with your father when you were a child. While what happened long ago may be relevant to a full understanding of your reactions, the behavior analysis focuses on what is happening *right now*, and what you are feeling and thinking *right now*. You will find the causes of a behavior by looking at all of the factors that are present immediately before, during and after the behavior. You will be better able to influence and change these factors as opposed to something that happened long ago.

Thus, when trying to answer the question "Why did this happen?" you will likely answer in one of the following ways:

* The person was vulnerable and, therefore, easily triggered. (Example: The person didn't get much sleep or wasn't feeling well.)
* A particular trigger occurred. (Example: A staff person scolded the person or staff behavior triggered a traumatic memory.)

- The person's thinking encouraged the behavior. (Example: The person thought, "Joe is a jerk. I will hit him.")
- The person couldn't cope with a strong emotion or environmental stressor. (Example: Poor ability to manage anger, anxiety, sadness, or cravings.)
- The person was unable to cope with symptoms associated with trauma, mental illness, and/or substance use.
- The person lacked adequate communication, coping, conflict resolution, and other psychosocial skills.
- The behavior was reinforced, even if unintentionally. (Example: Bullying behavior resulted in staff giving the person what he wanted.)

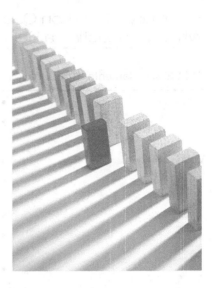

The concept of behavior analysis can be illustrated with a row of dominoes, with each domino representing a moment in the chain of events that surround a person's response in a situation. When working with an individual, keep a set of dominoes on hand to help explain the chain reaction that often accompanies a problem behavior. You can remove dominoes from the chain to illustrate how the result could have been different. For example, you can remove a domino (see Figure 6.4) to represent attending to a particular moment, such as breathing better, and point out how that could stop the chain reaction.

Figure 6.4 Dominoes reflecting a behavior analysis

©iStock.com/hansslegers

Scenario 6.5: The Domino Effect

Before talking with Charlotte, Betty pulled out a box of dominoes. Then, the two sat down to talk about what happened. Betty listened as Charlotte told the story of her tantrum. Each time Charlotte mentioned a different moment in the chain of events. Betty handed Charlotte a domino and asked her to line it up with the others.

The first few dominoes represented her vulnerability: *Charlotte was not sleeping well prior to her argument with Betty and was in a bad mood.*

The next domino represented the trigger: *The wheelbarrow falling over.*

After this came Charlotte's physical reactions: *Her muscle tension, rapid and shallow breathing.*

The next dominoes represented her feelings *and* thoughts: *She felt frustrated with herself and thought: "This stinks," and "I can't do anything right!"*

Then came the domino representing her problem behavior: *She kicked the wheelbarrow, screamed, stopped working on her chore, and stormed off.*

The final dominoes represented how she reinforced *herself with cookies and a cigarette. With all the dominoes lined up, Betty asked Charlotte to knock them over. Betty then explains to Charlotte that all of this chain, from the first domino to last, is called a "relapse." The relapse was not just the tantrum, but everything that led up to, came with, and followed it.*

The use of dominoes also provides a concrete illustration of how a relapse can be stopped. At any point in the chain of events, Charlotte could have prevented the relapse. For example, Charlotte might have been less vulnerable if she had taken care of herself better. She might have used breathing skills to calm herself down. She might have used other coping and social skills, like talking with Betty. She might have rewarded herself for positive behaviors instead of negative ones. If any of these had occurred, one domino would have been pulled out, disrupting the chain. The domino cascade would have been interrupted, just like a relapse would be interrupted.

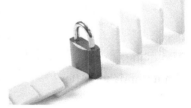

Figure 6.5 An interruption in a relapse as represented by dominoes

©iStock.com/Devonyu

When you are able to ask these kinds of question skillfully, you are well on your way to helping people develop some type of relapse prevention plan. This will be discussed more in Lessons 11 and 12.

TABLE 6.2 Elements of a Behavior Analysis

Story	• Can you tell me the story of what happened?
	• How did it start? What happened next, and next and next?
	• Please tell me the details, like we are watching a movie in slow motion.
Vulnerability	• How have you been sleeping?
	• How have you been feeling? What's your mood been like lately?
	• Have you been in any pain or physical distress?
	• How have you been taking care of yourself (e.g., diet, exercise, recreation, etc.)?
	• Have you been struggling with cravings or other reactions to addictive substances?
	• Before this happened, do you think were you feeling at your best?
	• When you are really feeling good, what do you do? Would this have happened if you were really feeling good that day?
Common Triggers	• Staff behaving in an overly directive, controlling, or in a one-up manner.
	• Staff saying "no" in what the client feels is an arbitrary or disrespectful manner.
	• Another person's failure to empathize well.
	• An insensitive or invalidating comment.
	• Perceived or real criticism
	• Stressors associated with being dependent on others.
	• Stressors associated with being unable to get what the person wants.
	• Having to wait—not getting immediate satisfaction or an immediate response.
	• Perceived unfairness—the belief that somebody else seems to be getting something that you are not getting.
Physical Reactions	• How were you sitting/standing?
	• Was your body tense or relaxed?
	• How were you moving?
	• How were you breathing?
	• What was your facial expression?
Feelings and Coping Skills	• At that moment, what were you feeling?
	• Where did you feel it in your body?
	• How did you cope with that feeling? What did you do?
	• Did you use any coping skills?
	• Did the coping skills help?
	• Could you have done something else that would have helped more?
	• How could you have stayed calm/safe?
	• Do you want to learn any other coping skills?
Thoughts	See Lessons 8–10
What Happened After?	• After you did x, what did you feel?
	• After x happened, what did you do next?
	• How did other people respond to you?
	• Did anything good/bad happen next?
	• Do you want people to respond to you the way they did?
	• How could people have helped you better?

Bright idea 6.5: Instead of asking someone why they did something, help them to tell the story. Use dominoes, blocks, or other physical items to create a visual chain of events to illustrate your behavior analysis. Ask questions that draw out vulnerabilities, physical reactions, feelings, skills that were used or missed, thinking, and what happened after the problem behavior occurred. This will help create a more complete answer to the question: Why did this happen?

Practice Exercise 6.2

1. Read Scenario 6.6.
2. Answer the questions that follow the story.

Scenario 6.6: Isaac's Story

Isaac is a 22-year-old deaf male with Usher Syndrome, a hereditary condition that causes gradual vision loss. He has trouble seeing at night or when lighting is not excellent and he's starting to experience tunnel vision. Isaac's life was stressful enough before he began to experience this vision loss. He's experienced neglect, and physical and sexual abuse at the hands of various caretakers. He also has delayed language development, reads at a first grade level, and has conflictual relationships with most people.

Lately, he seems to be experiencing a crisis nearly every day. He isn't sleeping or eating well. He reports depression and says that demons in the house are trying to kill him. He's fought with his roommates because he believes they are sloppy and leave things for him to trip over. He also says he's furious with anyone who doesn't show support to him as a deaf-blind person.

On Monday morning, Alice, a staff person, arrives wearing a sweater with a complicated design on it. Isaac already wasn't fond of Alice, but when he saw her wearing this sweater, he screamed at her, in voice and sign. He said that she was mean because she wore clothing that made it difficult for him to focus. He signed angrily to Alice that she "didn't care about deaf-blind people." Then, he knocked over a chair, frightening Alice and his roommates. He threatened to file a human rights complaint against Alice and gave her the finger as he went back to his room.

An hour later, after he had calmed down, Alice tried to talk to him. She knew he had used some skills (he didn't hit her or anyone else and he did eventually go to his room) and she was prepared to apologize for wearing clothing that made it difficult for him to focus. She asked him if he was willing to talk to her and he said yes. She then added that there needed to be some ground rules about how they talk to each other. Could he come up with some rules? This seemed to engage him, and they started to talk.

Now answer these questions:

1. Which of Isaac's behaviors do you think should be targeted by the behavior analysis?
2. Did the problem behavior have a clear starting point?
3. Where do you think the analysis should start?
4. Did Isaac have vulnerabilities that primed him for this aggression? If so, what were they?
5. Can you identify clear triggers?
6. What do you think Isaac was feeling?
7. Do you know anything about what he was thinking?
8. What happened after the aggression?
9. What aspects of Alice's approach to Isaac do you think helped engage him?

10. What would a good conversation between Isaac and Alice look like?
11. Do you think that Alice's stance with Isaac is likely to increase or decrease his use of aggression with her? Why?

 Practice Exercise 6.3

In this exercise, you will conduct a behavior analysis of one of your own behaviors that you consider a problem (e.g., overeating, smoking, yelling, fighting, watching too much television, etc.). You will need a set of dominoes to complete this exercise:

1. Choose a specific, recent example when you exhibited the problem behavior. Remember, you are not analyzing a general problem like overeating, but one specific instance of the problem (e.g., yesterday, at 6:00, after getting home from work, I . . .).
2. Tell the story of how you came to show this behavior. Be sure to include any relevant details.
3. Look back to *before* the behavior happened. Ask yourself if you were vulnerable to relapsing. Consider your sleep, diet, health, stress, pain, mood, or anything else that may have "primed" you to relapse.
4. Identify your triggers.
5. Identify how your body responded. How were you breathing? Describe your posture. How did you move? What facial expressions, if any, did you show?
6. What were you feeling? Try to identify specific emotions, then rate the intensity of these emotions using a scale of 0 to 10.
7. What were you thinking? Is there any way in which you gave yourself permission for behaving this way, even though you weren't fully aware that you were doing so?
8. What happened after the behavior? How did other people react to it? How did you feel afterwards?
9. What may have reinforced the behavior?
10. Use dominoes to lay out all of the facts in your story as a series of specific events.
11. Was there anything you or another person could have done, at any step of this process, which would have decreased or prevented the problem behavior?

 Practice Exercise 6.4

In this exercise, you will conduct a behavior analysis on another person. You will need a set of dominoes to complete this exercise as well:

1. Ask a person who is not a client to help you with this exercise.
2. Ask the person to choose a specific, recent example where they exhibited a behavior they consider a problem (e.g., overeating, smoking, yelling, fighting, etc.).
3. Ask the person to tell the story of how he or she came to show that behavior. Be sure they include any relevant details.
4. Ask the person whether they felt they were vulnerable to relapsing. Ask them to look back to before the behavior happened. Be sure they consider their sleep, diet, health, stress, pain, mood, or anything else that may have "primed" them to relapse.
5. Ask them to identify any possible triggers.
6. Ask them to describe how their body responded. How were they breathing? Ask them to describe their posture. How did they move? What facial expressions, if any, did they show?

7. Ask them to try to identify specific emotions, then rate the intensity of those emotions using a scale of 0 to 10.
8. Ask if they think there was any way in which they gave themselves permission for behaving this way, even if they weren't fully aware of doing so.
9. Ask them to describe what happened after the behavior. How did other people react to it? How did they feel afterwards?
10. Ask them to identify forces that may have reinforced their behavior.
11. Use dominoes to lay out all of the facts in their story as a series of specific events.
12. Explain what each domino in the chain represents.
13. Ask the person if there was anything another person could have done at any step of this process that would have *decreased or prevented* the problem behavior.
14. Ask the person what forces he or she thought may have *increased* the likelihood that the behavior would occur.
15. Consider each step in the chain. What do you think the other person might have done to decrease or prevent the problem behavior from happening? What do you think the other person do in the future to decrease or prevent the problem behavior from happening?

Lesson 6 Skill Sheet

- Participants demonstrate skills in asking questions that help people notice what skills they use.

- Participants demonstrates skills in asking questions that are part of a behavior analysis. Specifically, participants ask about vulnerabilities, triggers, bodily reactions, feelings, thoughts, and environmental reinforcers.

- Participants ask questions with a spirit of caring and helpful curiosity. Participants are attuned to and respect people's willingness to respond to questions.

- Questions are used to engage people in a process of identifying the forces that push them to behave as they do and think about ways to promote more skillful behaviors. Participant realizes that the purpose of asking these questions is to look for possible ways to avoid or decrease the problem behavior.

Lesson 6 Quiz

1. Sandra lives in a group home. She is upset with her roommate, Stacey, because she took Sandra's soda from the refrigerator. It appears that Sandra is about to hit Stacey but stops herself and goes to her room. Kenneth, a staff member, observes this and approaches Sandra later. Rank Kenneth's possible responses from least to most effective:

    a. "Seems you just used the red, yellow, green skill we talked about. Good job."

    b. "Good job."

    c. "Sandra, I'm glad you didn't hit Stacey but why didn't you come to staff to talk about it?"

    d. "Sandra, I saw what happened between you and Stacey. You used some awesome skills. Did you notice the skills you used?"

2. Why are good questions generally more effective than providing answers? (Check all that apply.)

    a. Questions help people find answers themselves.

    b. Questions flow from a one-down style of relating to people.

    c. Questions are less likely to trigger angry responses than directives are.

    d. Questions are usually more likely to engage people than directives.

    e. Asking good questions helps people develop problem-solving skills.

3. Which of the following are parts of a behavioral chain analysis? (Check all that apply.)

    a. Understanding vulnerabilities.

    b. Use of a token economy.

    c. Understanding triggers.

    d. Understanding thoughts.

    e. Understanding emotions.

    f. Providing positive feedback.

4. Which of the following are possible triggers to an angry response in a therapeutic setting? (Check all that apply.)

    a. Staff members behave in a bullying manner.

    b. Staff members or peers behave in a way that reminds the person of someone in their family or their past.

    c. The person watches a television program in which an angry person shoots people.

    d.   The person gets staff attention after he person blows up.

    e.   The person notices that something he loves is missing.

5.   Which of the following could make someone vulnerable to a behavior problem? (Check all that apply.)

    a.   Not enough sleep.

    b.   Hunger.

    c.   A sunny day.

    d.   Being in pain or physical distress.

    e.   Feeling sick.

6.   Our approach focuses on developing skills. We don't pay attention to reinforcers (rewards or punishments) of behaviors. True or False?

Lesson 6 Questions for Discussion

1.   Are good questions really better tools for helping people than good answers? What do you think?

2.   How often and how well do you and the people you work with encourage clients to evaluate themselves?

3.   There is an art to questioning, especially using the Socratic method. How skillful are you in asking questions that guide people to find their own answers?

4.   Are there bad or unhelpful kinds of questions? What are some examples?

5.   Can you ask good questions in an unhelpful manner? What would that look like?

6.   Which of the following questions is more helpful? Why?

    a.   Why did this happen?

    b.   How did this happen?

7.   A behavioral chain analysis can range from simple to complex. What would a simple analysis look like? What would a more complex analysis look like? What level of analysis do you think the people you are working with are capable of?

8.   How does a good behavioral analysis lead to ideas about ways to help a person avoid a problem behavior?

9.   Review the list of common questions and considerations for conducting a behavior analysis at the end of this lesson. Which do you think are the easiest parts of a behavior analysis to understand and answer? Which are the hardest? Would even a partial behavior analysis be helpful to you and the person you are serving?

10. Consider the people you are serving. What kinds of question, if any, can they answer without difficulty? Which will be more challenging for them?

11. How do you think a good behavior analysis can guide you in developing a relapse prevention plan?

Lesson 6 Quiz Answers

1.   Starting with the most effective, the answers should be ranked *d*, *a*, *b*, and *c*. Answer *d* is the best response because it used questions to help Sandra discover her own skills. Answer *a* is the next best because it identifies specific skills Sandra used. Answer *b* is the next most effective because it offers positive feedback albeit vague and non-specific. Answer *c* is the least effective. While it involves asking a question, the question focuses on a problem/skill deficit, not an ability.

2. All five answers are good reasons.

3. Answers *a*, *c*, *d*, and *e* are all parts of a behavioral chain analysis. Answer *b*, use of a token economy, has nothing to do with behavior analysis. A token economy, in which a person earns tokens for good behaviors, is part of a traditional behavior modification program, not part of a behavior analysis. Response *f*, providing positive feedback, is also not part of a behavioral analysis. You might want to provide positive feedback, but a behavioral analysis is an assessment procedure, not a reinforcement plan.

4. All of these things could be discovered through a behavioral chain analysis and could be determined to be part of the reasons for a problem behavior. Response *d* would not be considered a trigger because a trigger happens *before* a behavior, not after.

5. Responses *a*, *b*, *d*, and *e* are most likely to create vulnerabilities. It is unlikely that a sunny day would make most people vulnerable to a relapse. However, a sunny day could cause someone with light sensitivity to become stressed, and, as a result, more vulnerable. We'd have to know what a sunny day means for this particular person.

6. The correct answer is False. Even in a skill-based program, we pay attention to reinforcers. When seeking an answer as to why something occurred, you are looking mainly for skills or skill deficits. But, you also are asking whether the environment "pulls" or motivates the person to fall back into problem behaviors. You also engage the person you are serving to help you put in place rewards that make sense. However, this should only be done when the person understands and agrees with the plan.

References

Linehan, M. (1993). *Cognitive behavioral treatment of borderline personality disorder.* New York: Guilford Press.

Meichenbaum, D. (1994). *A clinical handbook/practical therapist manual for assessing and treating adults with post-traumatic stress disorder.* Waterloo, Canada: Institute Press.

Meichenbaum, D. (2001). *Treatment of individuals with anger-control problems and aggressive behaviors: A clinical handbook.* Clearwater, FL: Institute Press.

Promoting Self-Assessment

Introduction

In this lesson, many of the concepts and techniques that you learned earlier will come together in a focus on helping people assess themselves. Lesson 7 teaches how good questions promote self-assessment. You'll also learn how you can help people to feel more comfortable taking a critical look at their own behaviors by asking themselves important questions like "What am I doing right? What am I doing wrong? Is what I'm doing helping me get what I want? What can I do better?" The goal is to help people answer these questions for themselves rather than have you and other authorities answer them.

Some important tools from the CBT world that help with self-assessment are self-monitoring forms on which people record or rate their own behaviors, feelings, thoughts, symptoms, etc. Self-monitoring forms can be adapted fairly easily for people who do not read well. This will also be discussed in this lesson.

The people you serve are ready for CBT when they are open to considering the possibility that they need more help or new skills. Your pre-therapy job is to help them get to this point.

Quick Review

So far, you've learned a lot about the importance of asking good questions. You've learned about:

- Asking questions from a one-down stance.
- How good questions can be used to help engage people in the tough work of personal change.
- How strength-based questions help people notice skills they already have.
- How questions from a behavior analysis help people discover how problem behaviors happened and how they could be avoided.
- How using questions to pull out a story helps people develop language and cognitive abilities.
- How staying grounded in an empathic understanding of the other person is likely to make anything you do more successful.

As you'll recall, some people cope with distress in unhealthy ways, such as abusing alcohol or drugs, smoking, overeating, cutting, or other self-destructive behaviors. People who have experienced abuse and other forms of trauma may have learned to survive in the moment by using coping strategies, such as shutting down emotionally, which may not be healthy for them in the long term. These coping strategies become harmful when people are not able to turn them off. Even positive coping skills, like distraction, can be weak and ineffective tools in some situations. People could do better if they are willing to learn more powerful skills.

Our strength-based orientation is designed to engage people, but we know they need help. They would not be in special schools and treatment programs if the skills they had were sufficient. We want the questions we ask to pull them into a process of exploring, "How can I do better?"

Reality Therapy

Reality therapy is a form of CBT that was developed by William Glasser and refined further by Robert Wubbolding (Wubbolding 2000). It uses a unique style of questioning designed to help people evaluate whether their behaviors are helping them achieve their goals.

Reality therapy can be very helpful in preparing people for learning new skills. People who serve individuals with language and learning difficulties can borrow four helpful questions from reality therapy. You can use these questions to guide the people you serve to evaluate how well they are doing and encourage them to be more willing to consider healthier or more positive alternatives. A reality therapy-style of questioning is particularly useful for engaging "difficult to serve" persons in self-evaluation. In terms of pre-therapy work, this style of questioning is appealing because it focuses on practical problem-solving and decision-making skills, rather than abstract concepts.

Bright idea 7.1: The coping strategies that people use make sense to them even if they are self-destructive like drinking, drug use, and self-harm. It's often helpful to validate how these strategies helped them survive. Follow that, if you can, with questions like, "Do these strategies have a negative side? Do they have a cost? Is the cost so heavy that you are ready to learn something new?"

As you do this, keep in mind that you are working to build some thinking skills. In particular, you are building the ability to consider pros and cons. This is a foundation tool for much problem solving.

The basic format for reality therapy, as described by Wubbolding in his book, *Reality therapy in the 21st century*, takes this form: **W**ant, **D**o, **E**valuate, **P**lan (**WDEP**). The core questions are:

1. What do you want?
2. What are you doing?
3. Is what you are doing helping?
4. Can you make a better plan?

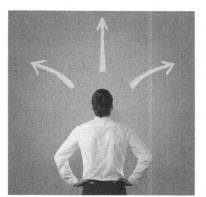

Figure 7.1 What do you want?
©iStock.com/Nastco

You can ask these questions in many ways. Remember, many people who fall into the category of "difficult to serve" resist directives that come from authorities. To overcome this challenge, you can use a one-down approach that puts the person receiving services in the role of problem solver. People who come up with answers themselves are more likely to follow their own advice.

Let's look at each of the WDEP theme questions more closely.

WDEP: What do you *WANT*?

The word "want" refers to the person's stated goals. Some common examples:

"I want to be independent."
"I want to move to my own apartment."

"I want to be discharged."
"I want a girlfriend."

It also may refer to goals a person *doesn't* want. For example:

"I don't want staff to keep watching me."
"I don't want to go to jail or get in trouble."
"I don't want to stay in this stupid program for the rest of my life."

Wubbolding recommends asking each person they are serving about his or her full array of wants, including what the individual wants:

- For him or herself, now and in the future.
- For the people they care about.
- For the world around them.
- For other people they have to deal with.
- In terms of school, work, or meaningful activity.

You also may find that some of the people you serve may have very general goals. These need to be broken down into smaller components. For instance:

- People in residential programs often talk about wanting to be independent without seeing the connection between independence and life skills related to self-care, managing their environment, establishing and following a budget, solving everyday problems and staying safe.
- People who are hospitalized commonly talk about being discharged without appreciating what they need to do certain things in order to show they are safe enough to be discharged.
- People who are supervised closely because of their unsafe behaviors often want the supervision to stop but need help understanding the behaviors they need to show before staff will feel comfortable backing off.
- People may want jobs without appreciating that they have to develop employment skills that are attractive to an employer.

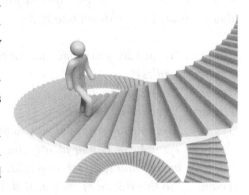

Figure 7.2 Goals and steps
©iStock.com/ayzek

A significant amount of counseling time may be devoted to helping people break goals down into steps that the persons themselves can take. Again, this is often best done through good questions.

Here are a few examples:

"You said you wanted to be independent. What skills do you think you need to be independent? Is learning to budget, shop and cook part of independence? If you are independent, how will you handle this if no staff members are around? Do you want to learn that now?"

"You don't want to have staff with you all the time. Do you remember why staff members are with you? Maybe we could start by letting you be without staff for short periods of time. What would be a first step, a small goal? How could you show that you are safe to try this out? How will we know if you are not ready for this?"

"You really want a job. That seems like a very important goal. I know you want to mow some lawns. How can you get some customers? What do you think the customers will ask you? How will you get more business? How will people decide if you are doing a good job? How will you know if you are doing a good job?"

"People looking for jobs have to sell themselves. How would you sell yourself to an employer? How could you convince people you will do a good job?"

Setting goals and breaking them down into specific steps is a common problem-solving strategy. This can be very difficult for some people. Depending on the person, you may need to devote considerable time to teaching this abstract idea. A good teaching strategy is to offer practical examples. One effective strategy is to repeat the goal and then follow up by asking what steps the person would need to go through in order to achieve their goal. For example: *"You said that your goal is to prepare a meal. What steps are involved?"* If even this is too abstract, or the concept of "steps" is unfamiliar, you could break this down further. *"What would you do first? Then what? Then what?"*

Keep in mind that there is no better way to teach this concept than to use the strength-based approach of pointing out to people how they have already broken down goals into steps. For example, you could point out how they broke down a task like making a meal, cleaning a room, or planning a party into steps; and how this process is just like what they need to do now with some new goal.

Scenario 7.1

Tyson, a staff person working in a group home, is working with Lamar, a resident with mild developmental disabilities, on his goal of becoming independent. Tyson frequently invites Lamar to learn specific skills, like taking a bus or preparing a shopping list, but Lamar usually states he is too tired or "it's boring." However, one day Lamar did make himself a cheeseburger. After he finished eating it, Tyson asked him leading questions to help him appreciate that goals are broken down into steps.

Tyson:	*"Wow. I see you made that cheeseburger yourself."*
Lamar:	*(smiles)*
Tyson:	*"How did you do it?"*
Lamar:	*"I cooked it."*
Tyson:	*"No, I mean, what did you do first, then next, then after that."*
	Tyson helps Lamar identify the concrete steps in making a cheeseburger: planning, shopping, getting the meat, onions, cheese, and rolls, making the meat patties, etc.
Tyson:	*"So this is kind of complicated. How many steps do you think you had to do?"*
Lamar:	*(without counting) "Many! Ten!"*
Tyson:	*"Yeah, at least 10 steps. I wonder if that is how you learn something, one step at a time."*
Lamar:	*"Ok."*
Lamar:	*"So what else did you want to learn? What about taking the bus to your family's house? Does that have steps too?"*

People who have grown up dependent on others often believe that a goal is met when *another person* does something, rather than when *they* do something. For example, if the person wants someone in authority to give them something or allow them to do something, the person may not see the relationship between the desired outcome and their own behaviors. It can be hard to help a person break this thought pattern if:

1. You remain in authority (one-up) roles and they are never brought into the problem- solving or decision-making process.
2. You don't help them connect their goals with their behaviors.

Bright idea 7.2: Don't assume that it is easy to establish goals and break them down into steps. The task may be difficult for several reasons. First, the concept of breaking goals down into steps is abstract and may be hard for the person to understand. Second, it requires the person to understand that you achieve goals through *your own* behavior. Third, some very protective environments don't support clients in learning decision making, even around easy and safe matters.

You may find that you are going to have to devote considerable time to teaching this critical idea.

WDEP: What are you *DOING*?

This question focuses on a person's behaviors, not environmental stressors, and sets the stage for self-evaluation. Reality therapy is about helping people to take responsibility for their choices. This often requires helping the person recognize that they have actually made a choice. Asking "What are you doing?" easily leads into asking the person about skills. For example, "Did you use skills in handling that problem?" By asking variations on this question, you are already helping people move towards self-evaluation.

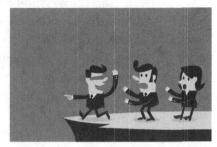

Figure 7.3 What are you doing?
©iStock.com/monkik

This question also challenges a person's passivity, dependence on others, and inability to see themselves as capable of influencing their own future.

Many people served in residential programs believe that going to staff is their only option when they face problems. Sometimes, staff members promote this belief by telling clients to "come to staff" when they have problems. Although it may be necessary at times to use a one-up approach to settle problems, this should be your last recourse, not your first. It's much more skillful to think, "How can I help the people I serve see themselves as capable of solving this problem?" The following scenario illustrates why this approach offers more potential for long-term growth.

Scenario 7.2

Joseph lives in a group home. He has a mild developmental disability and many behavioral challenges. He attends a work program during the day. He argues with peers and staff often. His most frequent complaint is that someone bothered him. Staff members are finding it difficult to remain patient with him because this complaint never seems to go away. A routine has developed in which Joseph complains about someone bothering him and staff responds by telling him to ignore the person. While Joseph has a limited range of skills for solving conflicts, staff appears to have an equally limited range of skills for helping him deal with them. No one is growing—not Joseph and not members of the group home staff.

As difficult as it may be, the only way forward has to be to help Joseph develop new coping skills besides "telling staff." He also needs conflict resolution skills besides "ignoring the person."

Joseph has a broad goal of "independence" and brings it up all the time. He is not good at seeing the relationship between how well he can cope and manage conflicts and how independent he can become. Staff members need to help him see this connection, even if it requires daily review for a long period. This can be accomplished by asking questions in the reality therapy style.

Staff acting from a one-down stance: "Joseph, I'm puzzled. Can you help me?"
Joseph: "What?"
Staff: "I'm puzzled. I'm confused. I don't understand. Can you help me?"
Joseph: "OK."

Staff:	"You tell me every day that you want to be independent, right?"
Joseph:	"I want to be independent."
Staff:	"Well, you want to be independent but every day you come up to me and ask for help. You say that this person or that person is bothering you. You want me to make them stop bothering you. But if every day you ask me to solve your problems for you, how are you becoming independent? I don't understand."
Joseph:	"Sam bothers me all the time."
Staff:	"I understand. Sam bothers you all the time. When Sam bothers you, what do you do?"
Joseph:	"I tell staff. Sam won't stop bothering me."
	(Note: This conversation often continues quite a while.)
Staff:	"Do you think you are doing a good job of solving your conflicts with Sam?"
Joseph:	"I ignore him."
Staff:	"Are you really ignoring him? What did you do when he bothered you just now?"
Joseph:	"I pushed him."
Staff:	"Is pushing him the same as ignoring him?"
Sam:	"It's hard to ignore him."
Staff:	"Yes, it is hard. But, I wonder . . . I'd like to ask you a hard question, okay?"
Joseph:	"What?"
Staff:	"Is your ignoring skill strong enough? Can you do it all the time? Does it work all the time or are you still upset a lot?"
Joseph:	"I'm still mad. Sam bothers me."
Staff:	"Well, I wonder, do you think it would it make sense to learn some new skills besides ignoring? I could show you some new skills and we could practice them together. Then you can tell me if they help or not. What do you think?"
Joseph:	"OK."

This kind of conversation can be much more difficult to pull off when people have limited language and reasoning abilities. The staff person will most likely have to keep in mind a "template" for the way he or she hopes the conversation will go. He or she will probably have to try out numerous versions before Joseph is actually ready to learn something new. It is important to remember that Joseph is a slow learner with well-established patterns of behavior. Otherwise, Joseph probably wouldn't be participating in this program. In other words, staff members should be prepared to repeat this conversation over and over again.

Regardless of Joseph's intelligence, staff members' challenge is to get him to buy in to the process of learning new skills. It would be easier for staff to just tell him that he needs to learn new skills. But, Joseph has a *greater chance of learning and using new skills* if he comes to this conclusion himself.

Socratic questioning will be more helpful than giving a directive like "you need to learn new skills." As you learned in Lesson 5, Socratic questioning is a one-down approach that requires much more confidence and skill from staff. Initially, staff may believe that this style of work makes them look weaker. However, the opposite is true. Staff members who can use Socratic questions to guide people to draw their own helpful conclusions exhibit exceptional teaching and counseling abilities.

WDEP: *EVALUATION*—Is it HELPING?

In Lessons 1 through 3 of this workbook, you learned about noticing and labeling skills that people already have. Once a skill has been noticed and labeled, you can now expand your questions to encourage the person to evaluate the effectiveness of

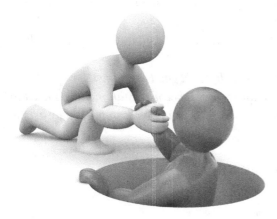

Figure 7.4 Is it helping?
©iStock.com/Palto

these skills. For example, after asking the individual to name the skill he or she used, you can follow up their response with more questions, such as:

"Are you happy with the skills you used?"
"Are your skills strong enough?"
"Do you want to learn more skills?"

Remember, these skills may be very weak and you may have to search hard to find evidence of them. The skill-building process begins with identifying skills for two reasons. First, identifying and naming specific skills gets the person talking about skills. This helps to establish a schema around skill building. Second, naming skills encourages the person to start talking in a positive way about what they already do well. By adding self-evaluation to the discussion, you help the person you're serving move beyond simply noticing existing skills to questioning whether or not their skills are enough and, finally, whether they need to learn other, stronger skills.

Reality therapy questions are designed to help people evaluate their behaviors in relation to their personal goals. If you know a person's specific goal (e.g., becoming independent, leaving the hospital, making a friend, staying safe, feeling happy, etc.), you can ask a variation of the question, "Is it working?" to help them consider whether they have enough skills to achieve this goal. For example: *You say you want to make friends. Does yelling at people help you make friends?* This includes questions like "Is what you are doing now working to get you to this goal?" and "Are the skills you have so far strong enough or would it help you to learn something new?"

People can become defensive when they are asked to correct a problem. But, for most people, the idea of learning a new skill isn't particularly threatening. Asking if they might want to learn new skills, and then offering to show/teach them these new skills, is a gentle way of inviting them to move forward. Couching your question in everyday language, as opposed to clinical language, also helps take away negative emotions associated with what might be perceived as criticism.

Letting the person evaluate his or her own behaviors also can take the sting away. Very often, people know that what they are doing isn't working and will acknowledge this if you give them the chance. Questions that lead to self-evaluation often follow these lines:

"Is this skill enough?"
"Can you do better?"
"Is that working?"
"Do you want to do better?"
"Are you willing to work at doing better?"
"Will you let me help you do better?"
"What would 'doing better' (using more skills) look like? Can we give it a try?"

Scenario 7.3, Part A

Doreen is a young woman with a history of severe sexual abuse. She frequently engages in self-harming behaviors such as cutting herself. While she has learned about coping skills, she tends to focus only on the most concrete coping skills such as distraction skills ("I watch TV. I play a game"). These skills work at times but are not strong or solid enough to really help keep her from harming herself. As a next step, staff would like to help her learn some sensory-based grounding skills such as:

- *Running cold water over your hands.*
- *Stretching and simple yoga poses.*
- *Jumping.*
- *Dancing.*
- *Playing with toys in sand.*

A quick Internet search on "grounding skills" uncovered a long list of sensory grounding skills that staff thought Doreen might find helpful. Staff members also know that it isn't the particular skills themselves (e.g., using sand or clay to ground oneself) that matters, as much as the sense of personal agency (e.g., I can do something to help myself) that exploring skills together promotes. To engage Doreen in the process of exploring skills, staff members have to help her decide if the skills she currently has are sufficient.

Staff: "Doreen, I have a question for you. Is this a good time to ask you?"
Doreen: "What?"
Staff: "It's a hard question."
Doreen: "What?"
Staff: "I notice that you use a lot of distraction skills. You watch TV. You play games. You do puzzles. I'm impressed by your distraction skills."
Doreen: "Thanks."
Staff: "But I also notice that you still cut yourself a lot. Do you notice that too?"
Doreen: "Yeah. Sometimes, I still want to cut myself when I'm watching TV."
(Note: Staff may want to draw out this discussion because it might be an opening for Doreen to volunteer how and why she thinks her skills aren't adequate.)
Staff: "Oh? What do you mean?"
Doreen: "I still need to cut myself. I feel better after I cut myself."
Staff: "The urge is just really strong."
Doreen: "Yeah."
Staff: "Well, there are many, many other kinds of skills you haven't tried yet. I wonder if they would help."
Doreen: "What do you mean?"
Staff: "There are lots and lots of kinds of skills. There are probably hundreds of skills. How many do you use?"
Doreen: "Uh, I don't know."
Staff: "Well, you watch TV, play games, and use puzzles. Anything else?"
Doreen: "I go for a walk."
Staff: "That's right. So, how many skills is that?"
Doreen: "Four."
Staff: "Four. But there are hundreds of others. How could you find out about them? Would you be willing to work with me to learn more and try them out?"
Doreen: "I guess so."
Staff: "Great!"
Doreen: "I don't think they will help."
Staff: "How do you know?"
Doreen: "I just feel it."
Staff: "Could we explore this together and find out?"
Doreen: "Yeah."
Staff: "How would we do that? Do you have any ideas?"

In this scenario, the staff person is trying to involve Doreen in working together to find a process of investigating what works. This is a very common style of work in both reality therapy and CBT. In both therapies, the goal of the questioning is to engage Doreen in the process of:

1. Thinking about her own goals and behaviors.
2. Helping her become an agent in her own recovery.
3. Engaging her in trying out new approaches and evaluating for herself whether they are helpful.

Notice that Doreen expressed a belief that learning new skills will not help. If Doreen has the ability to notice her thinking, we may be able to help see that this belief is tied to symptoms like depression and to self-defeating behaviors. But many people with language and learning challenges have trouble looking at their thoughts. Our next three lessons will address ways to make a person's thinking more visible to them as well as some simple strategies for changing their way of talking to themselves.

WDEP: What Would be a Better *PLAN*?

A better plan is likely going to involve a willingness to use different skills or draw on different social supports. If you have already established a large vocabulary for coping and conflict solving skills, you will be better prepared to suggest new skills. Your knowledge of skills will expand quickly as you study different forms of CBT. In most cases, the best plans will involve:

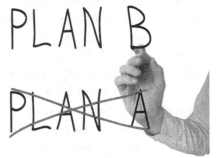

Figure 7.5 Plan B
©iStock.com/matspersson0

1. A willingness to learn newer, more powerful *coping* skills. For example:
   • Using a sensory strategy (e.g., deep breathing, physical activity and exercise, using hot or cold substances, or deep rubbing for grounding).
   • Learning a cognitive strategy, such as self-talk.
   • Using a problem-solving strategy, such as weighing the pros and cons in a situation.
   • Using a mindfulness-based practice such as meditation or yoga or practicing "noticing without judging."
2. A willingness to learn new, more powerful *social* skills. This usually means moving beyond simple "ignoring" or "shield" skills to better, more complicated communication skills, such as:
   • Expressing feelings safely.
   • Listening.
   • Taking turns talking.
   • Understanding how other people feel.
   • Negotiation and compromise
   • Seeking out social support or participating in some social group or event.

A new plan may also be less about skills and more about using resources differently. For instance, the new plan might be to attend an AA meeting, talk to someone, or join a planned recreational activity. Or, it can be about taking better care of one's body and health in order to be less vulnerable to stress. These activities can always be framed as skills (e.g., "go to AA meeting" skills, "seek help" skills, "go to YMCA" skills, etc.). Remember, however, to always adjust the level of the language you are using to reflect the language of the person or people you are working with. Otherwise, you will sound like a parrot.

Some questions that may help encourage people to try something new include:

"Do you want to practice this skill to make it stronger?"
"Do you want to learn some other skills?"
"What else could you do?"
"What does _____ do when he faces this problem?"
"If your friend had this problem, what would you tell her to do?"
"Are you willing to try something new? A little? Some? A lot?"

Scenario 7.3, Part B

Let's see how the dialogue with Doreen might continue with this new information.

Staff:	"Do you think we could we explore this together to find out?"
Doreen:	"Yeah."
Staff:	"How would we do that? Do you have any ideas?"
Doreen:	"I don't know."
Staff:	"Are you willing to do a little work to find out?"
Doreen:	"I don't know. It depends."
Staff:	"It sounds like you are not sure about this plan. Part of you is curious but part of you doesn't want to try something new. Is that right?"
Doreen:	"Yeah, I think so."
Staff:	"Which part of you should I talk to now? Can I talk to the part of you that is curious and might be willing to give it a try?"
Doreen:	"What do you mean?"
Staff:	"It seems like there are two Doreens."
	The staff member takes out a piece of paper and draws two stick figures.
Staff:	"This Doreen says, 'Can't learn anything new. I'm stupid.' This other Doreen says, 'Hmmm. I'm curious. Maybe I can try this out.' Does that make sense?"
Doreen:	"Yeah" (laughs).
Staff:	"So which Doreen should I talk to now?"
Doreen:	"Oh. This one, the one that is curious."
Staff:	"OK. Do you know what grounding means?"
Doreen:	"I'm not sure."
Staff:	"Grounding skills are great if you have anxiety. Grounding skills can help you calm down and feel solid like a tree in the ground. Can we try one now?"
Doreen:	"Sure."
Staff:	"Wow. I really am talking to the curious, willing Doreen. I like that Doreen!"
	Doreen smiles.
Staff:	"OK, great. First, can you tell me how anxious you are on a scale of 0 to 10? I have this scale here."
	The staff member pulls out the diagram shown in Figure 7.6.
Staff:	"Can you use this scale to tell me how anxious are you right now?"
Doreen:	"Hmm. I guess about a 5."
Staff:	"Can you color the thermometer in, up to the five line?"
	Doreen colors in the thermometer.
Staff:	"A five. OK. Now, we want to do something together to see if it makes a difference. Are you willing to do something with me?"

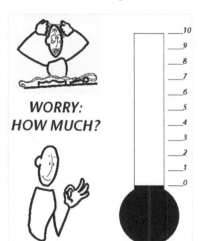

Figure 7.6 Worry thermometer

Doreen:	"It depends."
Staff:	"Oh, I'm confused. I thought I was talking to the curious, willing Doreen."
Doreen:	"That Doreen went away."
	Staff laughs.
Staff:	"Well, I don't know how to talk to the other Doreen. She's very stubborn. She's hard to help."
Doreen:	"What do I have to do?"
Staff:	"Go for a walk with me. It's nice outside. Let's go for a walk in the park."
Doreen:	"Oh, that's okay."
Staff:	"Then when we get back, you can fill in a new thermometer. I'm curious if you will still fill in to the five line or if you will feel different."
Doreen:	"That doesn't sound too hard."
Staff:	"No, and I'd enjoy it too. But the important thing is you are willing to try out new skills. That's the only way we can find out what works."

Practice Exercise 7.1

In this exercise you will use Socratic questions to help the person in each situation begin to evaluate their own behavior:

1. Review each scenario.
2. Identify some questions you might ask the individual to encourage them to evaluate their behavior. Follow the WDEP format.

Scenario 7.4

Jason lives with two roommates. He likes his roommates and wants to be their friend. However, he keeps eating all of the food in the refrigerator.

_____

_____

Scenario 7.5

Joshua and Alice are boyfriend and girlfriend. They talk about getting married. However, they argue every day. Today, they are arguing because Alice wants to go shopping and Joshua wants to stay home. When they argue, they insult each other. Sometimes Alice hits Joshua who then shoves her back.

_____

_____

Scenario 7.6

A staff member accompanies Simon whenever he goes into the community because Simon often approaches young children and touches them. Although he is not trying to harm them, Simon is a large adult and this behavior frightens the children as well as the adults with them. He constantly asks to be "independent" and resents when staff go with him.

_____

_____

 Practice Exercise 7.2

1. Read through each of the following situations.
2. Practice asking questions using the WDEP format.
3. If you find yourself telling people what to do (giving directives), stop and notice. Then try to reframe it as a question.

Scenario 7.7

Stephanie is an inpatient on a psychiatric hospital unit. Every day, she complains about hating being there. She has a clear goal to "get out of this damn place." However, she continues to make suicide attempts. She tried to strangle herself with some sheets. She hid a knife in her mattress (for an unclear purpose). When she got some off-grounds privileges, she went to the pharmacy and purchased a large bottle of aspirin and smuggled it back on to the unit with the apparent intention to use it to overdose. She complains about how unfair and mean staff is to her and that they control and abuse her.

Stephanie has had moments where she has used positive skills. She's had several good conversations with staff and shows some insight at times. She is sometimes very active and engaged in treatment groups. Stephanie also has helped a peer with more physical disabilities to eat and clean herself.

Imagine that you are a mental health worker on the unit. The nurse has asked you to talk to Stephanie to try to engage her in recovery efforts. You start with a one-down stance of confusion and worry (e.g., "I'm confused Stephanie, and I'm a little worried too. I'm hoping you can help me"). You ask permission to talk to her. After she agrees, you explain why you are confused and worried. (e.g., "I'm confused because your behaviors seem to conflict with your goals. Do you see that? What is your goal? What are you doing? I'm worried because I don't know how you will get out of this damn place if you continue these behaviors. I don't know how to solve this without your help").

What questions can you ask that will help Stephanie explore a relationship between her goal of "getting out of this damn place" and what she is actually doing? Write your answers in the space provided.

_____

_____

Scenario 7.8

George acknowledges that he has a drinking problem. He says that he wants to be sober but is drinking again. His previous sobriety plan was "I won't drink." George refuses to go to AA meetings ("I don't want to be with those losers") and won't work on a relapse prevention plan ("I don't want to dwell on the past").

What questions can you ask that will help:

- Remind him of his goal of sobriety.
- Uncover what led to the relapse.
- Ask him if he remembers his previous plan to stay sober.
- Help him evaluate whether this place was strong enough to help him stay sober.

Write your answers in the space provided.

_____

_____

Scenario 7.9

Jacob lives in a group home and wants to be independent. His individual treatment goal focuses on learning budgeting and cooking skills. However, each time staff members approach him to work on these skills, Jacob says he's too tired. Yesterday, when Sarah approached Jacob about it, he yelled at her and told her to "stop bothering" him.

What questions can you ask that may help Jacob question whether his behavior matches his goal? Write your answers in the space provided.

_____

_____

Adapting WDEP

You may be thinking that WDEP works only with people who have good language skills. While it is true that counseling strategies work better when someone has the language and cognitive abilities to fully understand them, sometimes you can select pieces of a strategy that are easier to understand. For example, you may just talk about goals. Or, perhaps you can focus on asking the person "What are you doing?" and "Is that helping you?" It also may be that the person is so unprepared for this kind of self-exploration that all you can do right now is wonder out loud and invite:

"Hmmm. I wonder if you are using the best skills for this."

"I wonder if you are happy with the progress you have made."

"Some people get better when they are willing to try something new. Are you willing to try something new?"

It can also be very helpful to spend a lot of time on the question, "Are you willing?" You might say, *"Are you willing to learn a new skill?"* The person might well say, "no," but the question makes it clear she is making a choice. You could respond, *"Ok. Good saying 'no' while staying safe. I'll ask you again later."*

Remember, skills building is a long-term, developmental process. Sometimes you must work on helping people develop skills in smaller increments, bit by bit. Often you are planting seeds and setting the stage for later work. If you are discouraged, stop and ask yourself, "What part of this can I work on with this person *now*?"

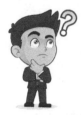

Questions to ponder 7.1: You are learning to ask good questions. You are learning to guide people to draw conclusions by asking questions that lead them through a decision-making process. You are modeling and teaching problem-solving skills. These are difficult counseling skills to acquire.

As you learn this new set of skills, pay attention to your own thoughts about it. Are you thinking, "This is too hard." or "This will never work with my clients." Or, are you thinking, "Well, this may take some time but I'll learn this bit by bit." Hopefully, you're thinking, "Let's see how much of this I can do with this individual."

The way *you* think about this work is going to play a significant role in your effectiveness. Pay attention to your own self-talk!

Self-Monitoring

Self-monitoring is a common CBT technique. For instance, suppose that a person comes in to see a counselor because he wants to stop smoking, change some eating habits, improve his mood, or stop having panic attacks. Counselors with a CBT orientation will often begin by asking clients to simply keep track of their current behaviors, emotions, or symptoms. In other words, the counselor starts by asking the client to "stop and notice" what is going on.

Think back to Doreen's situation. Did you notice that the staff member used a "worry thermometer" to help Doreen measure her level of anxiety? Rating scales like this are superb tools for self-monitoring. They are particularly useful when working with individuals who have language or learning challenges because they are easily adapted to meet the language abilities of people.

The core principle behind using a rating scale is that a person must stop and observe a problem before he or she can change their behavior. In other words, you have to *notice something before you can change it*. For example, you will not be able to quit or cut back on smoking if you don't recognize your smoking habits. You

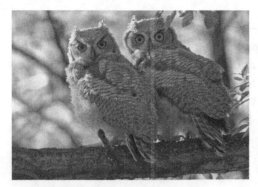

Figure 7.7 Stop and notice

©iStock.com/Frank Leung

have to begin to notice when, where and why you smoke, as well as what comes before, during, and after you smoke. Indeed, one of the best ways to devise strategies to stop smoking is to begin with a behavior analysis. You ask yourself, what are all the forces that promoted your smoking yesterday at a particular time?

Practice Exercise 7.3

We use self-monitoring in CBT and we also use it in pre-therapy. Indeed, the less prepared someone is to work actively on some skill-building, change strategy, the more inclined we are to *not* ask them to change, but instead to just ask them to notice.

1. Stop reading.
2. Think about how much energy you feel right now. Rate your energy using the scale in Table 7.1.

TABLE 7.1 An Energy Rating Scale

0	No energy; very tired
1–3	Low energy
4–6	Just right amount of energy (5 means, "I am alert and able to focus fully on what I am doing")
7–10	Too much energy (10 means "I have so much energy that I can't focus on this. I have to go out and do something active right now")

3. Select your rating. Write it in the space provided: _____
4. Do some type of physical exercise (e.g., stretching, jumping, sit-ups, walking in place, etc.) for one or two minutes.
5. Re-rate your energy level. Write it in the space provided: _____
6. Did the number change?

Realistically, you probably didn't do the activity. Right? So, what was the point of "wasting" time doing the activity? There is a deeper, more important point to this exercise. If the connection between activity and increased energy seems obvious to you, that's probably because you take it for granted that you have the power to *do something* to change how you feel. In other words, you have a strong sense of personal agency.

But, many of the people you work may not have a sense of personal agency. You may need to help them discover that what they do impacts what they feel. This is an essential part of engaging the person in the work of *getting better*. Asking them to use a rating scale before and after an activity is a clear, concrete way to help the person make these connections.

Scenario 7.10

Diane Trikakis was a long-term occupational therapist on the Westborough State Hospital Deaf Unit who was largely responsible for bringing sensory movement strategies to the program. She was also an expert at using self-monitoring to help people in the unit discover their own abilities. One day, she was trying to persuade Clare, a very depressed young woman, to engage in an art activity with her. Clare declined and expressed the usual negative self-talk associated with depression and helplessness: "I can't do it." "I'm not good at art." "I stink at this." "I don't feel like it." "I'm too tired . . ."

Using the one-down stance of curiosity, Diane said to Clare, "I'm wondering if you'd be willing to rate your self-esteem right now, on a scale of 0 to 10, with 10 being excellent self-esteem." Clare gave herself a rating of "1." Diane then asked Clare if she would participate in the art project for Diane's sake, because she would be helping Diane. Clare was willing to participate as long as doing so meant she was helping someone else.

Within a very short time, Clare became engaged in the project and actually produced something she seemed proud of. She showed it to several other people and received a lot of praise. Seeing Clare beaming, Diane asked her what her self-esteem rating was now. Clare said "8" without hesitation.

Diane, in a beautiful, one-down style that would have made Columbo proud, commented: "Hmm. You were able to get your self-esteem rating from 1 to 8 in just one hour using one activity. What do you think about that?"

Clare: "I guess I should do more art."

Diane: "Well, it does make me wonder if doing more art would make a difference? How would we find out?"

Clare: "Try it, I guess."

Diane: "But how would we measure it?"

Claire: "I guess we could do the same thing, 0 to 10."

Diane: "Hmmm. What a great idea. I have one other question for you. Are you ready?"
(Notice this variation on the "ask permission skill.")

Clare: "What?"

Diane: "You've been very depressed, but in just one hour you were able to do something to change your self-esteem and, I think, change your mood, right? What does this suggest about your ability to do something that changes how you feel?"

Clare: "Maybe doing art or other stuff will help me feel better."
(Note: While Clare was able to answer this without difficulty, other people might not be able to and would need even more concrete guidance to come to this more abstract conclusion.)

Diane: "How would we find out whether doing more art or other stuff would help you with your mood?"

Clare: "I don't know."

Diane: "I don't know either. Could we explore it?"

Clare: "Sure."

Diane: "How would we do that?"

Clare: "I don't know."

Diane: "How did you find out that doing this art work helped you?"

Clare: "Oh. I could try different things."

Diane: "You could try different things, like what?"

Clare: "I don't know."

Diane: "Well, what's on the activity schedule for today?"
They look at the activity schedule together and consider what Clare could join.

Diane: "And what about all these skills we keep talking about? I wonder if you would want to consider practicing any of them."

Clare: "They are stupid. I can't do them."

Diane: "Really? Like art is stupid? Not worth your time?"
Clare smiles.

Diane: "How could you find out if a skill is stupid or worth your time?"

Clare: "I don't know."

Diane: "Really? I seem to recall you doing something to measure your self-esteem."

Clare: "Oh, I could do that 0 to 10 thing."

Diane: "Yes, you could do that 0 to 10 thing. Wow! Now you're thinking like a pro."

Rating Scales

Rating scales range from simple to complex. They can be used to monitor one thing or multiple things. You can use a formal scale created by someone else or create your own. The goal is to find or create a scale that the person you are working with can understand. Possible options include:

Yes or No.

A scale from 0 to 10.

Thumbs up, thumbs middle, thumbs down.

Pictures of faces. (This rating scale uses picture or pictographs of various emotions to help an individual identify the emotion he or she is feeling. These are similar to the "emojis" that many people incorporate into text messages.)

Fill in the blank. (The person writes or draws their description of how they feel.)

Do something creative! There are lots of different ways to create a rating scale. The important thing is to find or create one that works for the individual you are serving. For example, in Lesson 10, you will learn about creating pictures of monsters that represent negative emotions and symptoms. If you are trying to help someone who struggles with anger, you could ask the person to draw a picture of an anger monster, or other representation of the anger, and then draw a picture of themselves (this strategy will be explored more in Lesson 10). You could also use clip art that they find on the Internet. Ask the person to show, right now, how large the anger monster is, and how large the person is. The relative size of each shows how strong each feeling is.

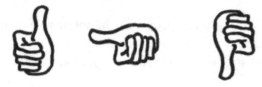

Figure 7.8 Thumb rating scale

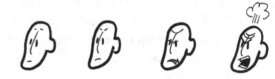

Figure 7.9 Faces rating scale

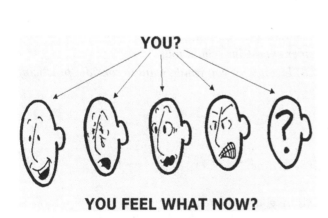

Figure 7.10 "Draw your emotion" scale

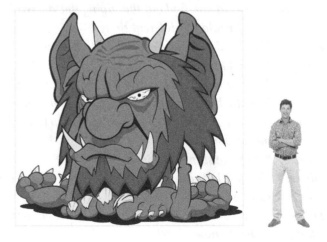

Figure 7.11 The anger monster vs. you

©iStock.com/artychoke98;
©iStock.com/Troels Graugaard

The kind of rating scale you use doesn't really matter as long as the person doing the rating accepts it as valid. You can devise a rating scale by asking questions like:

"How do we know how big x is?"
"How do we know how well you are doing in fighting x?"
"How can we tell if this works? How can we measure it?"
"Here are some examples of how people measure this. Which do you like?"

What Should You Monitor?

You can monitor anything that might provide useful information. Mental health workers often monitor the following:

- Behaviors, feelings.
- Thoughts.
- Attitudes.
- Symptoms.
- Skills.

Note that if you have the technology, biofeedback can also be incorporated helpfully into self-monitoring. For instance, Biodots or similar technology that change color reflecting stress levels are a concrete and appealing way for people to stop and notice their own reactions. Biofeedback has obvious appeal as an approach to help persons with language and learning challenges notice and attend to their "inner world."

Behaviors are easiest to monitor because they are external actions and, therefore, more easily observed. Monitoring feelings and thoughts are more advanced skills that require the person to be able to recognize and label them. In many cases, monitoring symptoms can be extremely challenging because it requires the person to be able to not only understand what a symptom is but also be able to recognize the symptom when it occurs.

Figure 7.12 is a picture of hallucinations that could be used with a client who cannot read beyond simple words. The picture is used to illustrate the concept of hallucinations and help the person rate the symptom. As you learned earlier, rating scales can be adjusted to reflect the individual's abilities. For example, a rating scale of "None? A little? A lot?" can be understood and used by many people with language or learning challenges.

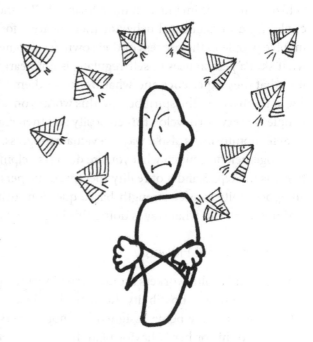

Figure 7.12 Hallucination? None? A little? A lot?

Developing a Self-Monitoring Form

Once a person has been introduced to the idea of self-monitoring, many individuals enjoy creating their own self-monitoring forms by drawing or searching for relevant pictures. This is a great activity to do with the individuals you serve.

Follow these steps to help someone to design a self-monitoring form:

- *Step One: Decide what to monitor.* Choose from the list above or add something else that interests to you.
- *Step Two: Create or choose a rating scale.* If possible, discuss different rating formats with the person to find an option that appeals to the individual. Be sure to consider how complex to make the rating.
- *Step Three: Decide how the self-monitoring tool will be used.* Common purposes include:
  a. Getting baseline measures before doing something to compare what is being measured against measurements taken some time later (e.g., rate your mood before starting your therapy or skill building program).
  b. Gathering information to find out if something you are doing is having an impact (e.g., rate your anxiety level before and after doing breathing exercises).
  c. Tuning in to aspects of a person's experience—or your own experience—that aren't obvious, like attitudes, beliefs, or thoughts.
  d. Evaluating your skill level and whether or not you are improving.
- *Step Four: Decide when the self-monitoring will be done.* Some possibilities include:
  1. At a particular time of day.
  2. After a particular behavior is done or skill is practiced.
  3. When certain meetings occur (for instance, before and/or after meetings with counselors).
  4. After particular events (e.g., after being with family, taking medicine, or joining particular activities).
- *Step Five: Talk about the results.* Self-monitoring is a tool. There is little point in doing it if you don't talk about what you've learned.

Self-monitoring is included in most forms of CBT though it often goes by other names. For instance, the "diary cards" used in dialectical behavior therapy are a form of self-monitoring. The intention of this process is to involve people in the process of their own development. Exactly what a person chooses to monitor, like exactly what skill a person uses to self-regulate, is not nearly as important as the fact that they are actively investigating what they experience and what works for them. We are using this procedure to help people discover things about themselves. The spirit behind this work is one of curiosity. What's going on? What will help? We want the people we serve to develop this curiosity and then realize there are some tools that will help them find answers.

Self-monitoring is also a way to evaluate progress. You ask a person to measure, using the tool you have created together, how much what you are doing is helping. If the person says, "it isn't helping," you explore alternatives, as in Steps 3 and 4 of reality therapy. If the person's evaluation shows that "it helps a little," then you have an opportunity to ask a strength-based question such as, "You rated this as helping 3 on a 5 point scale. Why 3 and not 2 or 1? In what way is doing this helping a little?"

Concerns about Honesty

Some mental health workers are concerned that the persons they serve will not be honest in their self-ratings.

Lying is always a possibility. Realistically, what would the person gain from lying? After all, these are *self-ratings*, not a rating being assigned by another person. A person would have reason to lie if the self-ratings were part of his or her behavior plan, however, *we are not using self-monitoring in that way.* The goal of self-monitoring here is to promote self-assessment. There are no "right" or "wrong" answers.

Perhaps they rate themselves too high because they think this is what you expect or want. Most likely there is a thought behind that like, "I need to give a high rating or my counselor will be upset with me." If you can, explore their expectations and clarify that you are looking for an honest response. You can say, "There is no right or wrong answer. We are just trying to learn what helps. If this doesn't help, we want to know that."

A more common problem is that people don't really know how to rate themselves. As a result, they rate themselves too high or too low because they are not used to thinking in terms of degrees. If that is the case, a simple "yes" or "no" or "thumbs up, thumbs down" scale can be used. Even better, teach the person to think about gradation. For some people, learning to evaluate themselves as mid-range on a scale (4 to 7 on a 10-point scale) can show an advance in their thinking skills.

As people become more comfortable with self-monitoring, many are able to move from a very simple two-point "yes" or "no" scale to a 10- or even 100-point rating scale. If the goal is to engage the person in more complex cognitive therapy at some point, he or she will need to be able to think in terms of degree, not all or nothing. This skill will be vital to evaluating progress towards goals.

Scenario 7.11

Bill, a staff person, asks George to complete a pictorial rating scale every day. George is a client with language and learning challenges who also has a history of aggressive behavior. Staff are working with him on simple skills like "cooperate" and "expressing feelings safely." With George's help, staff developed a rating scale (Figure 7.13) that included:

1. *The four principal emotions (happy, sad, angry, nervous).*
2. *Pictures of aggressive behaviors (throwing things, slamming doors, hitting, biting).*
3. *Pictures of some skills he was working on.*
4. *Which therapy groups he joined.*
5. *What skills he used.*

The plan also called for George and Bill to sit down at the end of each day to complete the form together. This created a structure for a daily check-in that both Bill and George found helpful, especially when Bill used this time to connect with George emotionally and not just complete a task because he was told to do so.

George began by always giving positive answers. He denied any aggressive behaviors, said he was happy, and checked off all the skills. Bill knew this was often not true. Sometimes Bill observed George acting aggressively, only to have George deny it when he completed the evaluation form. George always checked "Happy." Bill wondered whether George thought this was the "right answer." Bill also considered the possibility that George wasn't yet able to identify and rate emotions.

Bill understood that there were two goals. One goal was to engage George in more honest self-evaluation; the second goal was to teach him how to do it. Bill would gently try to challenge George's obviously incorrect assessments, always using a one-down stance of curiosity. Bill would also use the "ask permission" skill to decrease the chance that any confrontation could lead to violence.

One afternoon, George gave his usual "all is good" rating even though he had slammed the door and threatened a staff person just an hour previously. Bill used the afternoon check-in to teach George about honesty.

Bill:	*"Can I ask you a question?"*
George:	*"What?"*
Bill:	*"I want to ask you a question. First, right now, are you safe? Are you going to hit me or can we have safe talk?"*
George:	*"Safe talk."*
Bill:	*"OK. Great. Here is my question. Are you ready?"*
George:	*"Yes."*
Bill:	*"You checked off 'Happy 10, Mad 0'. But, what did you do an hour ago?"*
George:	*"Nothing."*
Bill:	*"Nothing? I was here, remember? Did you slam the door?"*
	George looks down and nods "yes" weakly.
Bill:	*"You are being honest now. Great. Good 'being honest' skills. What else happened?"*
George:	*"I was mad."*
Bill:	*"Yes, you were mad. You slammed the door? Did you do anything else?"*
	George looks tense and appears to be becoming angry. Bill is starting to feel anxious.
George:	*"I don't want to talk."*

Bill: *"You don't want to talk. That's 'clear communication' skill. Also 'expressing yourself safely' skill. Terrific. I think you are also being more honest now, right?"*
George relaxes a bit.
George: *"Yes."*
Bill: *"So let's stop now. Good job being honest. Good job expressing yourself safely. I will ask you again later or tomorrow, okay?"*
George: *"Yes."*
George walks away.

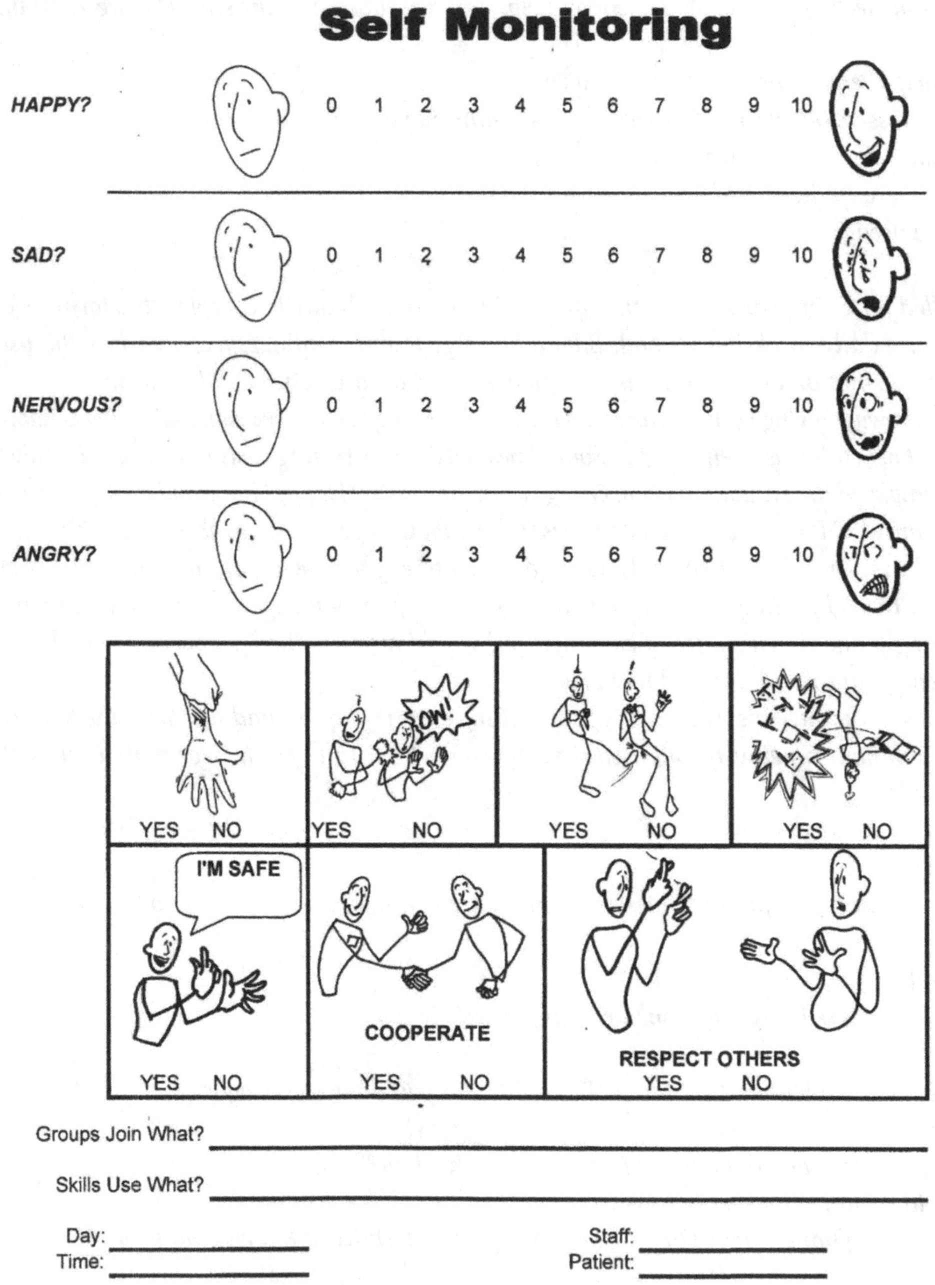

Figure 7.13 George's self-monitoring form

Certainly one wishes George could have gone further. Bill wants and needs to address his threatening behaviors. If Bill were using a traditional behavior plan, George would have not met criteria for reinforcers and Bill would have had to confront him directly about his threatening behaviors and say something like, "You didn't earn your points." Not only would that discussion likely push George away but it also could trigger additional aggression. Instead, Bill is working skillfully to engage George. It's slow and difficult, but no real progress will happen until George is ready to work with Bill.

Since the arrival of smartphone technology, there are many apps for self-monitoring and more appear every week. It is now very easy to find ready-made electronic self-monitoring forms for just about anything. Simply search "self-monitoring" and see what you can find!

Bright idea 7.3: Use self-monitoring forms and questions as part of a one-down stance with clients. Remember, your immediate goal is not client honesty. Rather, it's a higher level of client engagement. After that, you are using this to teach people to evaluate themselves.

Bright idea 7.4: You've now learned three kinds of questions: Strength-based questions, behavior analysis questions, and reality therapy questions. There are many other kinds of helpful questions. The kind of questioning strategy that you choose isn't as important as the ultimate goal: engaging people. Asking good questions is more effective at engaging people than telling them what to do. And, it is far more useful to help people evaluate themselves than for you to evaluate them.

Practice Exercise 7.4

In this exercise, you will develop a self-monitoring form for your own use. Even if you can download one or obtain a relevant app, it is important to do the work of creating a form yourself:

1. Decide what you want to monitor.
2. Choose or create a rating scale.
3. Decide how the scale will be used.
4. Decide when you will use the scale.
5. Talk with someone else about what you learn.
6. Repeat the process with someone else, preferably a person you are serving in your program. Be sure to involve the person in every step of the process.

Lesson 7 Skill Sheet

- Participants understand the value of helping the people they serve to evaluate themselves.
- Participants ask about goals and break down goals into steps.
- Participants ask people what they are doing and whether their behavior supports their goals.
- Participants ask people whether the skills they have now are strong enough to meet their goals.
- Participants help people develop new plans.
- Participants design a self-monitoring form for their own use.
- Participants assist another person to develop a self-monitoring form.

Lesson 7 Quiz

1. Which of the following is not a question that is routinely used in reality therapy?

    a. What do you want?

    b. Why did you do that?

    c. What did you do?

    d. What is your plan?

2. How can reality therapy questions fit into a CBT model? (Check all that apply.)

    a. Reality therapy questions engage people in skill development.

    b. Reality therapy questions promote staff–client collaboration and problem solving.

    c. Reality therapy questions are primarily attuned towards helping people cope better with their environments, rather than changing the environments.

    d. Reality therapy questions can set the stage for skill-building activities.

    e. Reality therapy questions probe for deeper unconscious meanings in client behaviors.

3. Simon has said many times that he wants to be independent. However, he lacks many of the key skills he needs for independence, such as managing a budget, shopping, menu planning, cooking, cleaning, using public transportation, and medication management. Even more worrisome, he has poor judgment about other people. For instance, he will do whatever anyone asks of him. He has fallen for multiple Internet scams where he has sent away his money.

    Which of the following questions reflect a reality therapy framework that might help Simon? (Check all that apply.)

    a. What does independence look like?

    b. What skills do you need to become independent?

    c. How well are you learning independent living skills, like following a budget?

    d. How good a job are you doing at making sure you have enough money?

    e. How could we help you become more independent?

    f. Are you willing to make a new plan?

4. A self-monitoring form is a tool that can help someone notice which of the following: (Check all that apply.)

    a. What they are doing.

    b. How they are feeling.

c. What they are thinking.

   d. Their symptoms.

   e. Skills they are using.

   f. Their attitude.

   g. How they view the helpfulness of other people.

5. There are many different self-monitoring tools available online. True or False?

6. Which of the following are good reasons to use self-monitoring forms? (Check all that apply.)

   a. It can help engage someone in the process of self-evaluation.

   b. It is a way of evaluating whether or not something you do is helping.

   c. It is a way of evaluating how serious a symptom or behavior is.

   d. It can be a great way for staff to check in with people they serve.

   e. Self-monitoring can help people discover their strengths and weaknesses.

Lesson 7 Questions for Discussion

1. Patrick is a 30-year-old male with a history of depression, self-harm (head banging, scratching, and cutting himself), and perceptions that other people are trying to harm him. He doesn't want to hurt himself but sometimes feels compelled to do so. Staff wonders out loud to him what else might be going on at times he hurts himself. They ask him if he would be willing to complete a log each day of his moods and when he hurts himself. He asks them to clarify what that means. What might a self-monitoring form for Patrick look like? What do you think Patrick would be willing to monitor?

2. What are some ways you might you use this form to help Patrick?

3. In Lessons 3, 6, and 7, you learned about three kinds of questions: strength-based questions, behavioral analysis questions and reality therapy questions. Which of these kinds of question do you think are most useful?

4. Are there other kinds of questions that are also useful?

5. What would be an *unskillful* way to ask these questions?

6. Have you used self-monitoring in your own life? Has it been helpful?

7. What do you think of the WDEP model of questioning used in reality therapy? Who do you think would respond well to these kinds of question? Who might have difficulty with these questions?

8. Notice that in all of this work, the focus is on helping people develop a sense of personal agency so that they can make a difference in their own lives. When people are triggered or stressed, for instance, you are trying to help them respond more skillfully. We are not trying to create stress-free environments for people but rather to help them respond more skillfully to stressors that they face in their current environment.

   In this way of thinking, mental health programs differ from vacations. Vacations are designed to provide a break from stress while mental health programs are designed to build up people's abilities to manage their own lives competently:

   • Do you agree with this perspective?

   • How much should mental health programs focus on shaping environments? That is, how much should mental health programs try to shape a person's environment so that it is stress free?

   • How much should they focus on helping people respond to their environments more skillfully?

   • If you are designing a mental health program, you must think about this issue. How much of your focus is on shaping the environment, and how much is on building a person's ability to cope with the environment? Where is the emphasis in your program? Are there some persons for whom the focus really needs to be mostly on shaping the environment to minimize stress, as opposed to teaching skills?

9. What have been some of the most helpful questions that people have asked you in your life?

10. What if someone has a goal that you don't support? For example, suppose Solomon's goal is to become the most successful drug dealer in his city and he wants help becoming more skillful at negotiating drug deals. How should mental health providers respond if they don't agree with the goals of the person they serve?

Lesson 7 Quiz Answers

1. All of the questions *except b* could be asked as part of reality therapy. Reality therapy does *not* ask, "Why did you do that" questions. The focus of reality therapy is on helping people evaluate whether their own behaviors are helping them move closer to their goals.

2. Reality therapy fits within a larger CBT framework in all of the ways cited *except e*. Neither CBT nor reality therapy is directly concerned with the idea of unconscious thinking. CBT pays a lot of attention to helping people understand their underlying beliefs and thinking patterns. However, the idea of "unconscious thinking" fits better with psychodynamic therapies.

3. These are all good reality therapy questions.

4. A self-monitoring form could focus on any of these things. The list also could include a rating of how the person views the helpfulness of other people. Strictly speaking, ratings of other people aren't truly self-monitoring. However, these ratings may provide helpful information and decrease a person's defensiveness or reluctance to self-rating.

5. True. What doesn't have an app these days? If you have a smartphone, search "self-monitoring" and see what you find.

6. These are all good reasons to use self-monitoring.

References

Self-monitoring is such a widely used CBT practice that it is difficult to find a CBT book that does *not* include it. You will probably find the most creative uses of self-monitoring in works focused on using CBT with children. The use, for instance, of colorful thermometers to measure moods is found in practically every such book and, again, is all over the Internet.

Wubbolding, R. (2000). *Reality therapy for the 21st century*. Bridgeport, NJ: Brunner-Routledge.

Thoughts and Self-Talk

Introduction

Lessons 8, 9, and 10 address the cognitive or thinking part of cognitive behavioral therapy. These lessons focus on teaching people with language and learning challenges to pay attention to their "self-talk." In other words, they are designed to help people *stop* and *notice*, and eventually *change*, how they think and talk to themselves. Lesson 8 is just about noticing thinking. Lesson 9 is about helping you see the connections between thoughts, emotions, and behaviors so you can help the people you serve see these connections, as far as they are able. Lesson 10 presents some simple strategies for helping people change how they talk to themselves. As pre-therapy, these lessons are designed to help you help people who don't easily recognize thoughts become more aware of them and start to practice talking to themselves differently and intentionally.

The Connection between Thinking and Feeling

The way a person thinks affects them in many ways. Thinking shapes how you feel. Some people go so far as to say that your thinking *causes* your feelings. Similarly, the way a person thinks contributes to, and sometimes causes, their behavior. The ability to recognize and solve problems is closely connected to how flexibly and creatively a person thinks. When someone repeats the same behaviors over and over, it is often because they are stuck thinking the same thoughts over and over. This is why noticing and understanding a person's "self-talk" is so critical.

Up to this point, this workbook has emphasized skill building—the "B," or behavioral, part of CBT. Now, we are beginning to explore the "C," or cognitive part, of CBT.

Cognitive skill building is a critical part of successful CBT. The most basic cognitive skill is *noticing*:

First, noticing *that* you think.
Second, noticing *what* you think.
Third, and far more advanced, noticing *how what you think, feel,* and *do* are related.

Noticing thoughts is difficult for many people. It is especially difficult for people with language, learning, and other cognitive challenges. Like the coping and conflict resolution skills discussed in earlier lessons, the cognitive skill of noticing thoughts *develops*. When people are able to notice their thinking and can intentionally practice thinking differently, they have access to a wealth of new tools that can help them achieve the kind of life they want.

Thinking about thoughts is a very abstract process. Take a moment to consider this. You don't need language to think about things you can directly see. For instance, you don't need language to visualize birds sitting in a tree. However, you do need language to ponder meaning. To consider questions such as, "What is a bird?" and "Why can birds fly but humans can't?" you need language. When we think about thinking, we are taking a step back from our thoughts to consider what they mean. How would this be possible without well-developed language abilities?

CBT works most readily with people who can think abstractly, rationally, and analytically without much difficulty. CBT therapists will explain the CBT model of how thoughts, feelings, and behaviors are related, something we will cover in the next lesson. The idea may be new for people, but the expectation is that, once explained, people will readily grasp and use it. A cognitive behavioral therapist working with clients who can't identify thoughts, much less analyze them, can be like someone trying to steer a boat without a rudder or paddles. The process can just come to a halt. Rather than freeze, we anticipate this problem. We don't assume that people can identify thoughts. We test it out. When people can't, perhaps because their language and thinking skills are not well developed, we realize our task must be to promote this foundation. We'll do this with a few strategies.

First, we're spend more time just noticing thoughts and feelings, labeling them, and saying them back to people. We'll point out to people *that* they are thinking and *what* they are thinking. We will give it a name, *self-talk*. We focus on *noticing*, not *changing*.

Second, we help people see their thoughts better by writing, or drawing them in thought bubbles. We also use a process called externalizing, explained in Lesson 10, whereby we put these thoughts into the minds of creatures who talk to us.

Third, we don't concern ourselves with higher level processes of analyzing thinking patterns but rather we focus on the simpler skill of talking to yourself differently.

Fourth, in addition to using visual aids, we will do a lot of role playing.

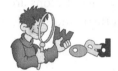

Definition 8.1: Self-talk: The act or practice of talking to oneself, either out loud or silently.

Example of self-talk: Betsy was feeling very depressed and thought to herself, "I really am a total loser!" She doesn't realize how that this self-talk just made her feel even worse.

Bright idea 8.1: Before you can change the way you think, you have to *notice* how you think. This comes so easily for many people that they may assume everyone can do this just as easily. In fact, for many people, this skill is very elusive.

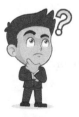

Questions to ponder 8.1: Are the people you serve prepared to think about thinking? Can they identify a thought or belief? Can you? How skilled are you at identifying your thoughts and distinguishing them from your feelings?

Thoughts vs. Feelings

What is the difference between a thought and an emotion? It's worth spending some time learning to distinguish between them.

We commonly say that thoughts occur in the brain while feelings occur in the heart but actually both thoughts and feelings occur in the brain. We have feelings that are emotions, such as the primary emotions of happiness, sadness, anger, fear, surprise, and disgust. We also have physical feelings such as being tired, energetic, nauseous, in pain, or sexually aroused. While our brain interprets these feelings, we experience them as in our bodies.

We experience our thoughts, when we attend to them, as in our head. Usually, we experience thoughts as an inner voice, as if we are talking silently to ourselves. We can also think in pictures. People vary in how much of their thoughts are language based and how much are picture based. We may presume that people with poorer language skills think more in pictures, but it is likely this varies from individual to individual.

My experience has been that people who have poor language skills have difficulty putting thoughts into words, saying, "This is what I think. This is what I believe." That would seem to make them poor candidates for cognitive therapy, which focuses on helping people think differently. Actually, it means we have to select simpler cognitive therapy strategies and do more of the foundational work of noticing and labeling thoughts.

Practice Exercise 8.1

1. Read each of the following words and statements.
2. Decide if it is a thought or a feeling.
3. Write your answers in the spaces provided.

You will find the answers at the end of the lesson.

- Sad. _____
- Embarrassed. _____
- Nobody loves me. _____
- Joe is ignoring me because he thinks he is better than me. _____
- Men can't be trusted. _____
- Nervous. _____
- Hate. _____
- Everyone drinks on New Year's Eve so I can too. _____
- Just one drink won't cause any problems. _____
- Sexual lust. _____
- My life is a complete mess. _____
- I am a failure. _____
- I feel that you are not listening. _____
- I feel like you hate me. _____

Tips and Techniques

Here are a couple of easy tips that you can use to determine if the person is describing their thoughts or their feelings:

Tip 1: Don't assume that a person is expressing a feeling just because they use the phrase "I feel . . ." as in the last two statements in our list. These are both actually thoughts. In modern American English, it is common to make statements that begin with "I feel that . . ." and then are followed by a thought. For instance, the statement "I feel that people are against me" reflects a thought, not a feeling. However, there is a feeling behind the thought, and it is probably fear or anxiety. Remember, if the word "that" follows the word "feel" ("I feel that . . .") you are about to hear a thought, not a feeling.

Tip 2: Feelings are almost always identified by just one or two words such as you would find on a feelings chart. There are many examples of feeling charts available on the Internet. People with learning and language challenges often find it easier to understand emotions through pictures of people expressing different emotions. Feeling charts are excellent tools (see Figure 8.1).

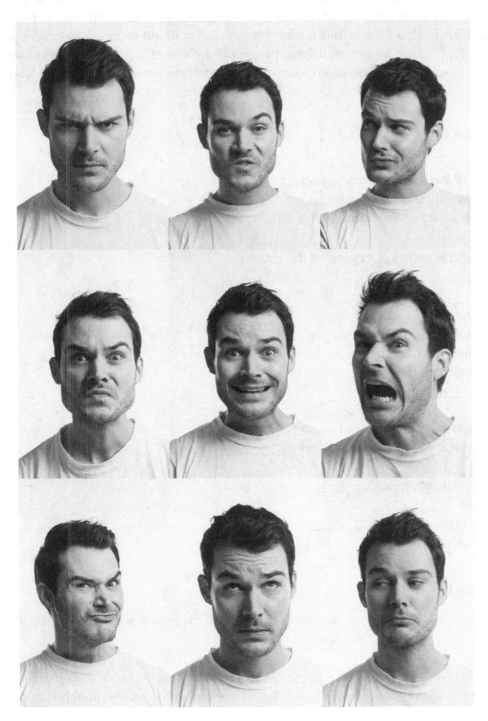

Figure 8.1 A feelings chart

©iStock.com/theo_stock

Tip 3: People show their feelings on the faces. Research by Paul Ekman found that human beings express primary emotions in the same way regardless of culture. In fact, with study and practice, people can become very expert in interpreting even subtle emotions accurately (Ekman 2007). If you look at Figure 8.1, you can probably guess the emotions pretty accurately. The ability to read accurately the emotional expressions and body language of other people is a crucial skill for mental health counselors. It is also a skill we want to help the people we serve develop.

Tip 4: One way to help someone develop the skill of separating thoughts from feelings is to have them look at pictures of human beings expressing emotion and then ask them to guess the emotion. You can also help the individual try to make up thoughts that might fit the feeling and the picture. For example, look at Figure 8.2. Based on the picture, what do you think the person is feeling and thinking?

Possible feelings: Impatient, irritable, angry, hostile.

Possible thought: "I won't put up with this nonsense from you one more minute! Do you understand me?"

Tip 5: You can use thought bubbles to help people pay attention to their thoughts. Whenever possible, help a person you are working with draw a thought bubble and put what they are thinking inside of it. Of course, be sure to adjust this technique to reflect the person's reading ability by selecting words or phrases he is likely to use and know. You may also have to draw the thought bubble yourself and do the writing. Once you have finished, ask the person, "Is this what you think?" This is a good way to validate that you have guessed correctly and also draw the person's attention to their thoughts. In situations where the person has very limited reading skills, you may need to draw pictures rather than use words.

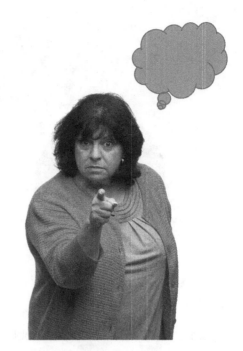

Figure 8.2 Woman with thought bubble

©iStock.com/DRB Images, LLC

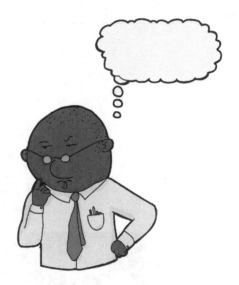

Figure 8.3 Man with thought bubble

©iStock.com/ericb007

Practice Exercise 8.2

1. Examine the pictures in Figure 8.4, 8.5, 8.6, 8.7, and 8.8.
2. What do you think the person in each picture is feeling?
3. Make up a thought that you think goes with the feeling.
4. Write your answers in the spaces provided.

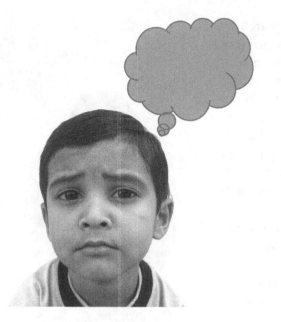

Figure 8.4 Boy with thought bubble

©iStock.com/Aman Kahn

Feeling: _____

Thought: _____

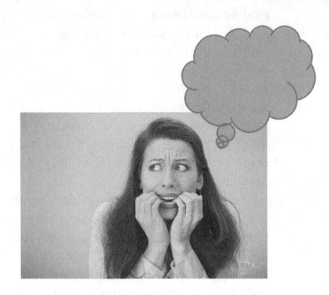

Figure 8.5 Woman with thought bubble

©iStock.com/ATIC12

Feeling: _____

Thought: _____

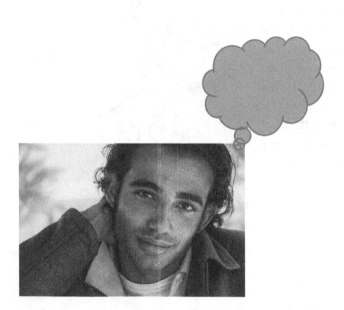

Figure 8.6 Young man with thought bubble

©iStock.com/Kemter

Feeling: _____

Thought: _____

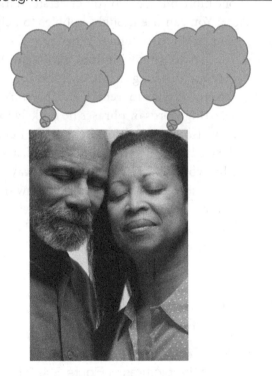

Figure 8.7 Couple with thought bubble

©iStock.com/FangXiaNuo

Man's feeling: _____

Man's thought: _____

Woman's feeling: _____

Woman's thought: _____

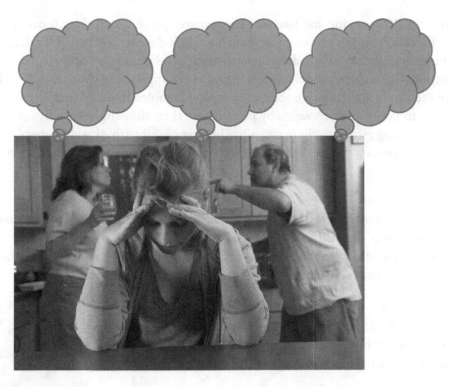

Figure 8.8 Fighting couple and teenage daughter with thought bubbles
©iStock.com/ejwhite

Man's feeling: _____

Man's thought: _____

Woman's feeling; _____

Woman's thought: _____

Girl's feeling: _____

Girl's thought: _____

Connecting Thoughts with Specific Emotional States

Of course, you can't read other people's minds, but you can make some educated guesses about their thinking based on what they say or how they act.

Some thoughts tend to correspond with specific emotional states. Learning these connections will help you to guess what a person is thinking or feeling more accurately. (You will learn about these connections in Lesson 9.)

Four Strategies for Identifying Thoughts and Feelings

As you'll recall, you learned four strategies for finding and naming skills in Lessons 1, 2, and 3. These four strategies can be adapted and used to identify and name thoughts. Let's review these strategies and see how they apply to thoughts and feelings.

TABLE 8.1 Skills and Thinking Strategy 1

Skills strategy 1: Help the person notice and label *skills* they already use, no matter how simple. Label positive behaviors as skills.	**Thinking strategy 1:** Help the person notice and label their *thoughts* they are expressing, even if they don't realize these are thoughts.

As you learned earlier, noticing and labeling skills requires you to have a very broad understanding of what skills look like. This also requires you to understand how skills develop and recognize that adults with language and learning challenges may not have had the opportunity to develop complex skills. In a similar way, the thoughts of a person with language and learning challenges may be very simple, like a child's thoughts. This may be because they don't have the words and language abilities to explain complex thoughts and feelings. You can help them develop the ability to notice their thoughts by pointing out their thinking skills when you find some evidence that the person is thinking productively. In fact, since helping people to think well is one of our prime therapeutic objectives, it is very important that we help people to notice any evidence that they are doing just that.

Scenario 8.1

Jonathan is staying in his room and not coming out to talk with anyone. Solomon, a staff member, goes to talk to him. Jonathan says quietly, "They all hate me. Stupid jerks!"
Solomon draws a thought bubble, writes Jonathan's words in it, and then repeats it back to Jonathan.
Solomon asks, "Is this what you are thinking? Is this what you are telling yourself?"

In this example, Solomon uses the simplest words possible in keeping with Jonathan's reading skills. If Jonathan were not able to read at all, Solomon could still use the thought bubble to emphasize thinking. However, instead of writing words inside the bubble, Solomon could act out Jonathan's thoughts in a role play.

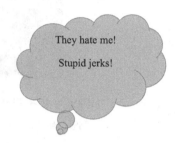
Figure 8.9 Jonathan's thoughts

At this point, Solomon has several options. He can point out that Jonathan is using the skill of "expressing self safely," or "noticing how you think." Example: "*You are expressing yourself. You are telling me how you feel. You are also telling me how you think. And you are doing it safely. Great communication skills.*"

He could also simply empathize with Jonathan's feelings. Example: "*It sounds like you feel angry . . . and maybe sad too?*" Solomon might use empathy to help Jonathan notice his feelings and his thoughts and, hopefully, connect them. For instance, Solomon can point out that Jonathan is using his "express self safely" skills, as well as other skills like "express feeling skills" and "notice thinking skills."

If possible, Solomon could reflect on both the feeling *and* the thought. Example: "*So you feel angry and sad, and you think, 'They hate me! Stupid jerks!' You think this and you feel that. Is that right?*"

For pre-therapy purposes, you're *most interested in helping people notice that they have feelings and thoughts.* You could also call this the "noticing feelings and thoughts skill". When Jonathan can master this, you are ready to start asking some of the harder questions that are part of traditional CBT. For instance, in CBT you would typically follow up by asking questions designed to help people evaluate and change their thoughts. For instance, you might ask:

"How do you know they all hate you?"
"What's the evidence for that belief?"

You would also point out "data" that seem to contradict Jonathan's belief. Example: "*Remember yesterday how Jimmy was playing Uno with you? If he hates you, why did he play Uno with you? Does Jimmy play games with people he hates?*"

TABLE 8.2 Skills and Thinking Strategy 2

Skills strategy 2: Explore the reasons why a problem behavior is absent to find the skill the person is using.	**Thinking strategy 2:** Explore the reasons why a problem behavior is absent looking for the self-talk the person is using.

Asking a person why a problem behavior did *not* occur will often reveal some productive self-talk. Remember, "self-talk" is another term for the way the person thinks.

Scenario 8.2

Sue has a history of hitting other people and biting herself when she is frustrated. When she asks Julia, a staff member, to go to McDonald's, Julia asks her to wait a few hours until a second staff person arrives. Frustration over having to wait sometimes triggers Sue's aggressive and self-harming behaviors. But, today, she goes and sits in front of the television. Julia is impressed and goes over to her.

Julia: "Sue, I'm really impressed with you. Sometimes you get frustrated and then you hit people or hurt yourself. You just asked me to go to McDonald's. I had to ask you to wait until Tim arrives. You didn't blow up. You didn't hurt me. You didn't bite yourself. Wow. How did you do it?"
Sue thinks for a moment.

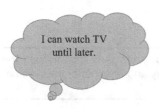

Figure 8.10 Sue's thoughts

Sue: "I can watch TV until later."
Julia takes out a piece of paper, draws a thought bubble, and writes down what Sue said.
Julia: "Is this what you said to yourself?"
Sue nods: "Yes."
Julia smiles in return.
Julia: "Wow. Look how you are talking to yourself. You are telling yourself you can wait. You are telling yourself you can watch TV. The way you talk to yourself is called your self-talk. I wonder. Does talking to yourself this way help you stay calm?"

People will often tell you what they think without having the self-awareness that they are describing thoughts and beliefs. You job is to help them develop this self-awareness *that* they are thinking and *what* they are thinking. When you observe that a person is thinking in a helpful way, point it out to make sure that they are aware of it. You can also find examples of this if you probe with a person for why problem behavior is *less bad* than previously.

TABLE 8.3 Skills and Thinking Strategy 3

Skills strategy 3: Notice when problems or behaviors are not as bad as before and ask why, looking for the skills the person is using.	**Thinking strategy 3:** Notice when problems or behaviors are not as bad as before and ask why, looking for the self-talk the person is using.

Scenario 8.3, Part A

Joyce is a 21-year-old who often cuts herself. She has a very severe history of being abused and says she cuts herself to feel better, not to kill herself. She is unhappy with the scars that are all over her body. Sometimes she cuts herself very deeply, requiring a hospital visit and suturing. One day, she showed Diego, a staff member, some superficial cuts on her upper arm. Diego responded matter-of-factly, as he had been trained. He helped her clean the area and apply ointment, then commented:

Diego: "I notice you didn't cut so deeply this time. Do you see that as improvement?"
Joyce: "Yes, I feel better after I cut myself, but the scars are embarrassing."
Diego: "So how did you keep yourself from cutting more deeply?"
Joyce: "Well, I told myself that just a little cutting was enough."
Diego: "You told yourself that just a little cutting was enough?"
Diego draws the thought bubble (see Figure 8.11).

Diego: "You were thinking this."
Joyce: "Yeah, I guess so."
Diego: "And it helps when you think that?"
Joyce: "Yeah, I guess so."

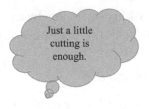

Figure 8.11 Joyce's thoughts

Because Joyce seems to understand the concept of thinking, Diego uses a one-down stance and wonders out loud.

Diego: "I wonder what else you could think that would help."

Hopefully, Diego's question will lead to more conversations about Joyce's self-talk. While Joyce may or may not be ready for this, it is worth trying. You'll explore this kind of conversation in more depth in Lesson 10.

Sometimes you can't find skills in a person's problem behavior, but you can find them later, in the recovery.

TABLE 8.4 Skills and Thinking Strategy 4

Skills strategy 4: Find, point out and discuss the *skills* used in the recovery and repair after the problem event.	**Thinking strategy 4:** Find, point out, and discuss the *self-talk* used in the recovery and repair after the problem event.

Scenario 8.3, Part B

The next day, Joyce cuts herself again. This time, the cut is very deep and requires medical attention. She is brought to the hospital where a physician treats the wound and discharges her. Later, Diego notices that Joyce seems depressed and approaches her.

Diego: "How are you doing Joyce?"
Joyce: "Well, I cut myself again."
Diego: "I know. What happened?"
Joyce: "I just felt that I had to do it."
Diego: "You felt you just had to. I wonder, how do you feel about it now, looking back?"
Joyce: "I'm going to have another scar."
Diego: "Yes, you probably will. Could you have avoided that?
Joyce: "I wish I had remembered that I hate the scars."
Diego: "How could you have reminded yourself?
Joyce: "I could have just looked in the mirror. I could have looked at my arms and legs."
   Diego asks her to draw a thought bubble and write in it what she just said.
   Joyce writes what can be seen in Figure 8.12.
Diego: "You could have told yourself that?"
Joyce: "Yeah."

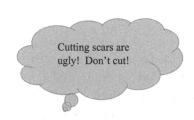

Figure 8.12 Joyce's recovery self-talk

Notice Diego's skillful use of Socratic questioning. He guided Joyce to figure out what she could say to herself that would be more helpful. He didn't give her the answer; he let Joyce come to her own conclusions. Later, he could give her credit for her skillful ability to talk to herself in this more helpful way.

In Lesson 10, you will learn how to turn self-talk into a script. For example, in this situation, Diego could have said, *"What else could you have told yourself? Could we write it down? After we write it down, would you want to post it somewhere in your house where you would see it all the time?"*

Bright idea 8.2: You can often uncover a person's thinking by asking them why a problem behavior did *not* happen or was less severe. You can also uncover their thinking by asking how they were able to behave differently this time.

Practice Exercise 8.3: In this exercise, you will practice noticing thoughts:

1. Ask one or two people to participate in a role play. Person 1 is the staff person and Person 2 is a client. Optional: Person 3, a supervisor.
2. Read through each of the situations.
3. Person 1 (staff person) should help Person 2 (client) explain his or her thinking and write it in a thought bubble.
4. If a third person, the supervisor, is involved, he or she should offer constructive feedback.
5. Write the person's thoughts in the space provided.

Scenario 8.4

Abel lives in a group home and is looking forward to a visit with his family. He expects staff to drive him to his parents' house at 3:00. However, a second shift person called in sick so Abel will have to wait a few hours until a replacement can be found to drive him home. He complains and pouts before sitting down to watch TV until a staff person can take him.

(Person 1 is staff. Person 2 is Abel. Person 3 may be a supervisor.)

_____

_____

_____

Scenario 8.5

Hugo is a young man who lives with his father and receives support services through an outreach worker. Hugo has a fascination with guns. In the past, he has obtained a BB gun and used it to shoot squirrels. His father was furious with him and forbade him to have any sort of gun in their house. Hugo was once arrested for stealing a BB gun from a store, although the only consequence was a stern warning from a police officer about the dangers of guns.

A friend invites Hugo to his home where there is a large back yard. The friend also likes to play with guns for target practice. He offers Hugo the chance to practice shooting his BB gun at the targets in is backyard. Hugo thinks about it. He recalls what his father had told him and remembers the police officer yelling at him. He then goes ahead and shoots at the targets. He tells you about it later.

(Person 1 is staff. Person 2 is Hugo. Person 3 may be a supervisor.)

_____

_____

_____

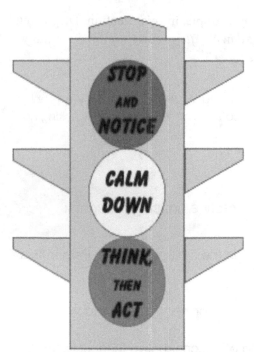

Figure 8.13 The red, yellow, green light coping skill

Scenario 8.6

Shelly is a 50-year-old Deaf woman in a psychiatric pro-gram. She communicates in simple ASL. Shelly becomes confused easily. When she's confused, Shelly sometimes responds by yelling at people and pushing them. Staff have been trying to help her use the RED, YELLOW, GREEN LIGHT (see Figure 8.13) skill to "stop and notice" when she is upset (the red light), sit in her rock-ing chair with pillows and breathe slowly (the yellow light) and tell herself to calm down (the green light). They are working on helping her develop a self-calming script of sentences she can say to herself to help herself calm down.

Shelly is signing to a hearing staff person who doesn't know sign language. The hearing staff person is talking to her but Shelly doesn't understand. Another staff person who does sign notices that Shelly is becoming upset and goes over to talk to her. The staff person reflects that Shelly seems angry. Shelly signs "yes." The staff asks if she is angry because the first staff doesn't sign. Shelly responds in a confused way that doesn't make much sense. The staff person guides her to her favorite chair and models the slow, deep breathing they have practiced. After Shelly settles down, the staff person helps her come up with a few simple phrases that she can say to herself to stay calm.

(Person 1 is the staff person. Person 2 is Shelly. Person 3 may be a supervisor.)

_____

_____

_____

Notice Your Own Thoughts

Just like in the people you serve, your own thinking affects your emotions and behaviors. If you are like most mental health workers, you think about the people you serve and develop theories about why they behave as they do. Your theories influ-ence what you feel, how you react, and even how long you can continue doing this difficult work.

Paying attention to your personal thoughts and beliefs is very difficult; it's a skill you must practice intentionally. You can cultivate more positive ways of thinking in order to foster better stress management and coping. The more you master this skill, the more able you will be to help others learn it also.

Consider the following thoughts that most staff people have at some point in their careers. Do any of these thoughts seem familiar?

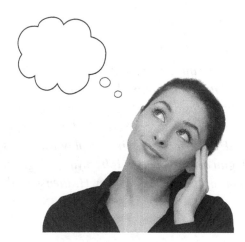

Figure 8.14 Woman with thought bubble
©iStock.com/Nastia11

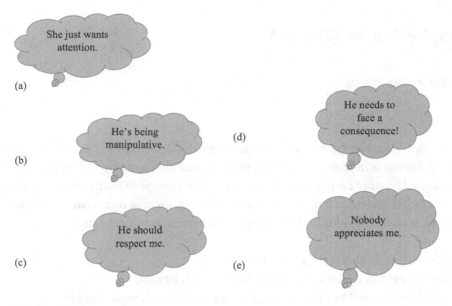

Figure 8.15

Practice Exercise 8.4

1. Read each thought bubble.
2. What emotion do you think goes along with it?
3. Write your answer in the space provided.

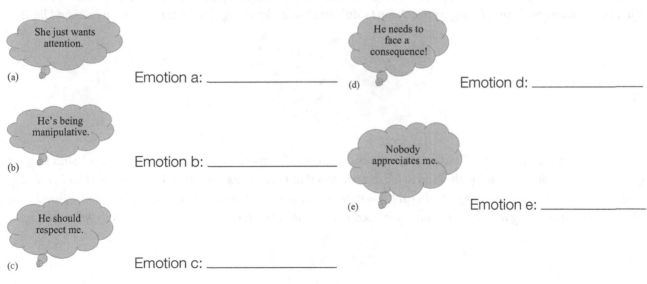

Figure 8.16

Do you see how these thoughts pull for specific emotions? If you have these thoughts a lot, how might they impact your coping and your feelings about your work?

You'll learn more about the connections between thoughts and feelings in the next lesson.

Practice Exercise 8.5, Part A

Read the following introduction.

Scenario 8.7

Treatment staff members on a psychiatric unit have gathered to discuss how to respond to Lauren, a patient who keeps hurting herself. Lauren is hoping to be allowed to go out into the community. However, members of the treatment team are frustrated because Lauren doesn't seem to be safe enough to justify being unsupervised in the community. Each person on the team has a different idea about what is wrong and what should be done. Each person is thinking differently, and the thoughts and beliefs of each person affects their emotions and response to Lauren:

1. Read what each person on this team says about Lauren.
2. Consider how each person explains the difficulty Lauren is having.
3. Put the person's thoughts and key beliefs about Lauren into the thought bubble.

Melissa is the team psychiatrist: "Lauren has been refusing to take her medications for several days. She's actually going through medication withdrawal right now. We need to help her accept that she has to take her medications."

Stephen is the staff nurse: "Lauren is just trying to manipulate us into giving her what she wants. She knows exactly what she is doing. She's just playing games. I don't think we should play along. We have to set more rules and limits."

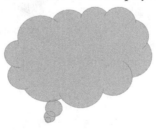

Alicia, team social worker: "That's a really insensitive way of approaching this work. I don't think she's playing games. You are not appreciating the kind of life experiences that Lauren has had and why it is so hard for her to stay safe. You also aren't appreciating how her self-harming behaviors help her cope in the moment. She's suffered a lot of abuse and has a long history of trauma. We need to understand better how her cutting actually helps her cope."

George, team psychologist who is responsible for risk management: "What's causing the behavior doesn't affect whether or not she can have a pass into the community tomorrow. The fact is that she's cutting herself more and more seriously every day, no matter what we do. I'm really afraid of letting her off the unit right now. I think she

will just cut herself even more seriously, maybe even kill herself. We need to keep her on 1:1 supervision. It's just too risky to give her a pass into the community right now."

Colby is a nurse's aide who often speaks up for Lauren: "None of you are giving her a chance. I know her better than you do. She cuts herself because she is mad at us. Maybe we are the problem."

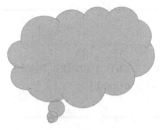

 Practice Exercise 5, Part B

1. Read Lauren's perspective.
2. Write down what you think she's thinking in the final bubble.

Scenario

The team then invites Lauren to join the meeting. The team expresses their concerns about discharging her while she is still harming herself. Lauren replies that she always cuts herself and that it is no big deal. She doesn't want to die, but she does want to get out of this damn hospital. She says that the hospital is making her worse.

 Practice Exercise 5, Part C

Answer the following questions based on the information presented in each of the different viewpoints. Write your answers in the spaces provided.

a. Which member of the team is angriest with Lauren? What makes you think so?

_____

_____

b. Which member of the team is most likely to "burn out" or lose interest in their job first? What makes you think so?

_____

_____

_____

c. Which members of the team are most likely to have the best relationship with Lauren? What makes you think so?

_____

_____

_____

d. Is there a connection between how a team member thinks and his or her ability to form a relationship with Lauren? What do you think it might be?

_____

_____

_____

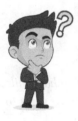 **Questions to ponder 8.2:** Have you ever worked on a mental health treatment team where members had very different ideas about what was going on with a person you serve? Do you remember what your own ideas were about the person?

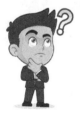 **Questions to ponder 8.3:** What would your own thoughts have been with regard to Lauren? How would you thoughts have affected your feelings about working with her?

In this lesson, we introduced the importance of stopping and noticing *that* you think, *what* you think, and the *impact* of what you think on your emotions and behaviors. If we can help the people we serve notice their own thinking and beliefs, then the C part of CBT will be available to them; and we will have many more tools to use with them. Of course, staff who work with people must have strong abilities to notice and evaluate their own thoughts and beliefs if they are to have any ability to help others with this often challenging skill. In the next lesson, we will draw out some connections between thoughts, emotions, and behaviors. We will see that emotions and moods are reliably connected to certain kinds of thought and belief. We will also see that before you behave in a particular way; for instance, before you hurt someone or pick up an alcoholic drink, you must give yourself permission to do so. Thus how you think paves the way for how you behave.

- Participants are able to distinguish thoughts from feelings.

- Participants can identify their own feelings and thoughts.

- Participants can help the people they serve identify how they are thinking by putting their thoughts into a thought bubble and asking the person to verify that it is what they think.

Lesson 8 Quiz

1. What kind of self-talk is the person in this picture most likely to be using?

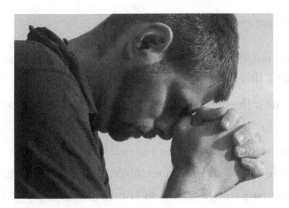

Figure 8.17
©iStock.com/SDannaS

   a. "You bum! I'm sick and tired of all the crap you throw at me!" "

   b. "I wonder why no one likes me."

   c. "What if I lose my job?"

   d. "I can handle this. No problem."

2. What kind of self-talk is the person in this picture most likely using?

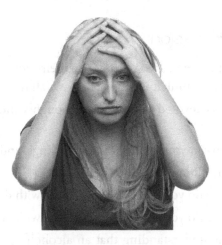

Figure 8.18
©iStock.com/DRBimages.LLC

a. "You bum! I'm sick and tired of all the crap you throw at me!"

b. "What is wrong with me? I keep screwing up!"

c. "I really love you."

d. "I can handle this. No problem."

3. Which of the following are emotions? (Check all that apply.)

a. You bum!

b. I feel like you aren't listening.

c. Curious.

d. Annoyed.

e. Today is the best day I have ever had!

4. Some people who have poor language skills are not yet able to recognize their thoughts. How can staff help the people they serve develop this skill? (Check all that apply.)

a. Reflect back what they hear the person thinking and ask the person to validate that it is accurate.

b. Write the person's thoughts in a thought bubble.

c. Role play and think out loud what the person appears to be thinking.

d. Show people pictures and ask them what they think the people are thinking and feeling.

e. Talk about themselves, saying things like, "Sometimes I think this ___ and then I feel this . . ."

5. Why should staff pay attention to their own self-talk? (Check all that apply.)

a. In order to teach a skill, you must have the skill yourself.

b. Staff will cope with work stressors better if they learn to recognize how their own thoughts and beliefs affect their mood and behavior.

c. Staff may be able to model more effective self-talk through role playing and thinking out loud calming thoughts.

d. Staff members often struggle with many of the same problems as the people they serve so staff also need self-care and coping skills, including positive self-talk.

e. Learning to notice one's thinking is the first step in being able to change one's thinking.

Lesson 8 Questions for Discussion

1. Do you think that teaching the people you serve to notice their thoughts is an important part of preparing them to participate in CBT? Do you think it is important for staff to be able to notice their own thoughts?

2. In CBT, a great deal of attention is devoted to examining thoughts and beliefs. Do you think this is worthwhile? Why or why not?

3. Do you see any connections between your own thinking, feelings, and behaviors?

4. How easy is it for you to appreciate how someone else thinks?

5. What kind of thoughts and beliefs do you think are connected with depression?

6. What kind of thoughts and beliefs do you think are connected with anger?

7. One CBT model is based on the understanding that an alcoholic will give him or herself permission to drink alcohol before actually taking a drink. What kind of "self-talk" do you think alcoholics commonly use to give themselves permission to drink?

8. Have you ever disagreed with a colleague or supervisor about why a person you serve behaves as he or she does? What was your point of view and what was the point of view of the person you disagreed with? Why do you think you both had such different perspectives?

9. How easy is it for the people you serve to notice and identify their self-talk?

10. Can you think of other ways to teach someone with language and learning difficulties the difference between thinking and feeling?

Lesson 8 Quiz Answers

1. The person in the picture looks either depressed or worried. He is most likely to be thinking either *b* ("I wonder why no one likes me.") or *c* ("What if I lose my job?") Answer *a* is more likely connected with anger. Answer *d* is more likely to be associated with successful coping.

2. The person in the picture looks stressed. Her facial expression seems somewhere between depressed and anxious. Response *a* is associated with anger. Response *c* would be associated with love. Response *d* would be associated with confidence and pride. Response *b* is most likely to go along with depression/anxiety.

3. Answer *a* ("You bum!") is a thought that is most likely associated with anger. Answer *b* ("I feel like you aren't listening") is a thought, even though the word "feel" is used. This thought is most likely associated with the emotions of impatience, annoyance or frustration. Answers *c* (Curious) and *d* (Annoyed) are emotions. "Today is the best day I have ever had!" (*e*) is a thought, usually related to the emotion of happiness or exhilaration.

4. All of these are good methods for teaching people to recognize thoughts.

5. All of these are good reasons for learning to recognize your own self-talk.

Answers to Practice Exercise 8.1

- Sad. __Feeling__
- Embarrassed. __Feeling__
- Nobody loves me. __Thought__
- Irritable. __Feeling__
- Joe is ignoring me because he thinks he is better than me. __Thought__
- Men can't be trusted. __Thought__
- Nervous. __Feeling__
- Hate. __Feeling__
- Everyone drinks on New Year's Eve so I can too. __Thought__
- Just one drink won't cause any problems. __Thought__
- Sexual lust. __Feeling__
- My life is a complete mess. __Thought__
- I am a failure. __Thought__
- I feel that you are not listening. __Thought__
- I feel like you hate me. __Thought__

References

The material in this chapter is very basic and isn't associated with any specific CBT author. In his earlier work, Donald Meichenbaum directed the CBT world to focus on self-talk, or what he called "self-instructional training." He developed the focus within CBT to help people coach themselves through stressors. You can find his early discussions of this in the reference below.

Many CBT therapists use thought bubbles as tools. It's so commonly done, in fact, that no one person can claim to have invented this idea. However, the attention we are giving to *noticing* thoughts as a key element of preparing people for CBT is, to the best of my knowledge, unique to this program. More commonly, CBT theoriests assume people can readily do this and place their emphases upon helping people change how they think.

Ekman, P. (2007). *Emotions revealed: Recognizing faces and feelings to improve communication and emotional life.* New York: Holt, Henry & Company, Inc.

Meichenbaum, D. (1977). *Cognitive-behavioral modification: An integrative approach.* New York: Plenum Press.

The Connection between Thoughts, Feelings, and Behaviors

Introduction

In this lesson, you will continue to explore the connection between thoughts (self-talk), feelings (emotions), and behavior.

In Lesson 8, you learned the technique of using thought bubbles to help a person recognize *that* they were thinking and then *what* they were thinking. You will continue to use this tool in Lesson 9. However, now you will ask the person to go a step further—to connect their thoughts with their emotions and behaviors. Some of the people you serve will be able to make these connections easily but others will not. However, mental health workers need to understand and see these connections when the people they serve are showing them even if the persons themselves can't yet see the connections. If you can see how the people you serve are talking themselves into problem mood states and behaviors, you will understand them better, be better able to empathize, and have more tools for helping them.

The Challenge of CBT

This appreciation of the connections between thoughts, feelings, and behaviors is a foundation principle of CBT. A great deal of CBT research is devoted to understanding what these connections look like. Most of the work of CBT is devoted to helping people change how they feel by either changing how they think or changing how they behave.

Aaron Beck, one of the originators of CBT, first identified a relationship between thinking and depression (Beck, Rush, Shaw, & Emery 1979). Beck, his daughter, Judith, and their collaborators went on to show how extreme mood states are related to extreme thinking states. They also identified the relationship between thoughts, beliefs, and most emotions and emotional problems (Beck 1976, 1995). Through their research, they discovered that *people think in predictable ways* when they are depressed, anxious, angry, or abuse substances. People with personality problems also think in predictable ways based on how their personalities are organized. (Beck, Wright, Newman, & Liese 1993; Beck & Freeman 1990). The Becks and their colleagues then developed a number of strategies to help people feel better (or have fewer psychological symptoms) by thinking or behaving differently.

When doing CBT work, you want to:

- Help people understand how their thinking contributes to their problems.
- Help people think in ways that are more constructive.
- Teach thinking skills related to problem solving, coping, and dealing with other people.
- Teach people to use self-talk that promotes recovery from trauma, addiction, mental illness, and other life stressors.

The following scenario shows how focusing on an individual's thoughts can lead to insights into their emotions and behavior:

Scenario 9.1

Latricia is a 35-year-old hearing woman with bipolar disorder and posttraumatic stress disorder. She lives with her two cats in an apartment and receives services from Beth, an outreach worker employed by a social service agency. Latricia has a reputation for being difficult to work with. Before Beth began working with her, Latricia had fired and filed complaints against a string of outreach workers.

Beth made an appointment with Latricia to bring her to the Social Security office at 9:00 a.m. Beth knew about Latricia's history of firing previous workers and left her home early to be sure she would arrive at Latricia's apartment on time. However, on the way to Latricia's apartment, Beth encountered a car accident that brought traffic to a standstill. As a result, she arrived a half hour late.

Before Beth could apologize for being late, Latricia launched into an angry tirade.

Latricia: "I can't believe you're a half hour late! You know this appointment is important to me. Obviously, you don't care about me. You have no respect for me. You want Social Security to cut my benefits! You're just like all the others from that agency. None of you care about the people you work with. You're just in it for the money!"

Beth took a deep breath before responding. Then, she took out a piece of paper, sat down at a table, and started to draw (see Figure 9.1).

Beth:	"I'm guessing that you're angry at me."
Latricia (sarcastically):	"Wow, you're a genius."
Beth:	"Actually, I think I know why you are angry."
	She shows Latricia the thought bubble.
Beth:	"Is this what you're thinking?"
Latricia:	"I just said that."
Beth:	"I know. This seems to be what you're thinking. I arrived a half hour late, and before I could explain what happened, you were already thinking all this about me. Am I right?"
Latricia:	"Yeah, so what?"
Beth:	"Well, it makes perfect sense. If I thought all that, I'd be angry too. This is what you think is going on. You think I don't care about you, don't respect you, just work for the money, and want your benefits to be cut. Of course, you're angry. If this is what you say to yourself about me, I'm surprised you talk to me at all."

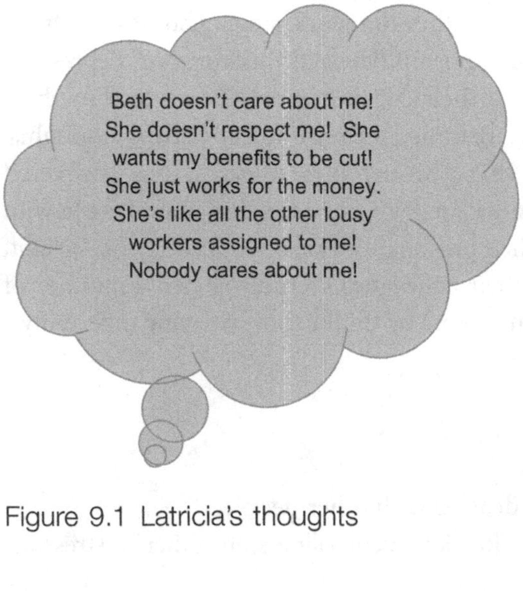

Beth understood that Latricia's anger at her, while unpleasant for Beth, made perfect sense based on how Latricia thought about the reasons Beth was late. Beth was actually able to provide some validation to Latricia (i.e., her feelings makes perfect sense given those thoughts), while still raising the fact that the way she thinks is contributing to her problems. Beth is trying to engage Latricia in the task of attending more closely to her thoughts and then considering how they are affecting her mood and behavior. If she gets this far, she'll next invite Latricia to consider how her interpretation of why she was late is way off-base. She'll try to help Latricia appreciate how she talked herself into a rage because she made assumptions about her that were incorrect.

Understanding the connection between thoughts, feelings, and behaviors allows you to respond better to an individual

Figure 9.1 Latricia's thoughts

whose emotions and behaviors are causing problems. For example, you will be able to notice how a depressed person is thinking and behaving in ways that promote depression. Even more importantly, you will be able to notice when clients think and behave in ways that *promote* recovery and healthy living.

 Bright idea 9.1: There is a saying in the therapy world that "you can only take your clients on a journey as far as you yourself have traveled." If you learn to see these thought-emotion-behavior connections in yourself, you will be prepared to help the people you serve to see them when the opportunities arise.

However, for many people, especially those with language and learning challenges, this is easier said than done. We want to help people understand these connections, but we find that many of the people we work with do not readily notice their thoughts, much less see these kinds of patterns. Much as we want to, we can't jump into the world of CBT. We have to stay longer in the world of cognitive behavioral pre-therapy, teaching such basic ideas as what a thought is and how thoughts and emotions are different. Thought bubbles are one tool to make thinking more concrete and visible, and we will soon learn additional tools.

This lesson is devoted to helping you see these patterns more clearly. Ultimately, we want to be able to ask the people we serve questions like these:

1. When you think that, what do you feel?
2. When you think that, what do you do?
3. When you do that, what do you feel?
4. When you do that, what do you think?
5. Which way of thinking helps you feel better?
6. What do you do that helps you feel better?

These are all abstract questions because they search for patterns. How do we get from this abstract world of CBT into the more concrete world of our clients? One way we do this is by always working with examples. We use examples of particular thoughts, feelings, and behaviors that people are showing. For instance, Beth began her conversation with Latricia by drawing a thought bubble and writing in the specific thoughts that she guessed Latricia had experienced that morning in response to Beth's being late. She didn't say, "You tend to think this way." Rather, she said, "Right now you seem to be thinking this . . . and feeling this . . . Is that right?"

If Latricia knew that, in fact, Beth cared so much about being on time that she had actually left early, would Latricia's emotions change? Would she feel less angry? Would it be helpful to Latricia to understand how drawing the wrong conclusion lead to an unnecessary angry outburst that could damage her relationship with yet another person trying to support her? Would Latricia feel and do better if she learned to notice and question her assumptions rather than jumping to conclusions?

Two Kinds of Story

All the people you serve have at least two kinds of stories (Meichenbaum, 1994, 2001, 2012), meaning they also have at least two kinds of self-talk.

First, they have "problem talk"—the story of their problems and challenges, how hard life is, and how they suffer. Sometimes, the first story takes over and they can only see how bad life is. They forget anything positive, including their struggle for a better life, their own abilities, and the abilities of others to help them. You want to help people notice their problem talk and put it outside themselves in a bubble, so they can begin to question it.

Second, they will also have "recovery talk," which reflects their efforts to fight for a better life. For example, the recovery talk of a person with depression may include things that indicate that the person, the world, or the future has positive qualities. Just as important, the person says things that show they believe they are capable of having an effect on the world. For example:

"I cooked a great meal yesterday. Everyone enjoyed it."
"I'm good with animals. I feel very close to my cat."
"I know my daughter loves me."
"Yesterday wasn't so bad. I had some fun at the movies."
"Yeah. I know how to do that."
"My teacher said I did a good job. I got a B+."

You can put these and similar positive thoughts into thought bubbles and give them a name like "Recovery talk."

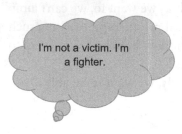

As a staff person, your job is to listen empathetically to the first story ("problem talk") and communicate back to the people you serve that you understand it. You show empathy by demonstrating that you understand how difficult life is for them. At the same time, you listen carefully for the second story ("recovery talk"). When you hear a person make comments that seem to reflect skills and strengths, the ability to respond well to life challenges, you should develop an intense curiosity about these. You will want to say something like, *"Oh, even though you felt so hurt and angry, you were able to stay calm and walk away. That's awesome. How exactly did you do that? Please tell me more."*

Figure 9.2 Recovery talk

For counselors, this means becoming truly expert listeners. We hear a person's pain but we also hear their recovery. The second story reflecting their abilities is almost always there, but it may take an expert listener to hear it.

The Links between Thoughts, Mood, and Behavior

It is important for mental health workers to have a basic understanding of the thoughts related to three main negative mood states:

1. Depression.
2. Anger.
3. Anxiety.

It is also important to recognize the behaviors that commonly accompany these moods. Something happens in a person's mind that *primes* him or her to feel and behave in specific ways. People are usually unaware that they give themselves permission to act in a certain way. An alcoholic, for instance, thinks something like, "I'll just have one," or an angry person thinks, "That creep deserves a punch in the face!" Once someone learns to tune into their thoughts, they can discover and develop a new set of tools for managing their responses to difficult situations.

Bright idea 9.2: Before behaving in a particular way, such as harming themselves or someone else, or engaging in substance abuse, people give themselves permission to behave in that way. The person will have a thought that provides this permission. Helping the people you serve to notice this thought can be very powerful.

We aren't just interested in recognizing self-talk that promotes problem emotions and behaviors. We are even more interested in identifying self-talk that promotes coping, healthy living, and recovery. In strength-based work, you want to be sure to *stop and notice, to catch and label, healthy self-talk* that people engage in. When you see it, ask:

"Is this what you are thinking?"
"When you think that, how do you feel?"
"What else can you think that will be helpful to you?"

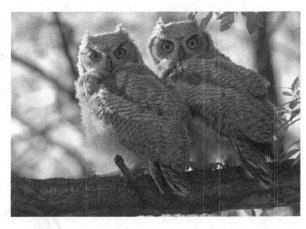

Figure 9.3 So much of our work is just to stop and notice

©iStock.com/Frank Leung

In other words, you must notice the thought-emotion-behavior connection if you are going to be able to help others notice it. The skill, again, is "stopping and noticing."

Moods and Common Thoughts

Predictable ways of thinking accompany every mood or emotion. There's great power in seeing this connection. Here's a personal story that illustrates the thought-emotion-behavior connection.

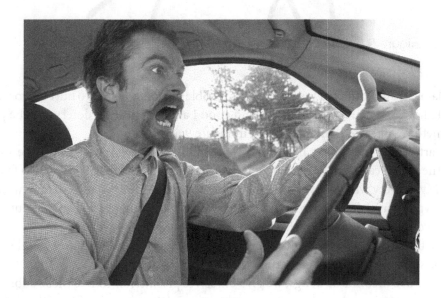

Figure 9.4 An angry driver

©iStock.com/Vladimir Mucibabic

Scenario 9.2

I was in my car at a stoplight, waiting for the light to change when the man in the car behind me began to honk furiously at me. He gave me the finger and made other threatening gestures. I had no idea why he was behaving that way. I considered how to react. I knew that how I would feel would depend on how I interpreted his behavior meant. For example:

    a.   I could blame myself. I could think something like the character in Figure 9.5.
           These kinds of thought will feed depression.

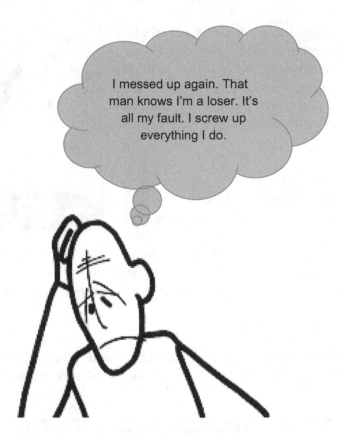

Figure 9.5 Depressed thinking

b. I could blame him. I could tell myself that this terrible person is trying to hurt me for no reason. I could exaggerate how bad he is, how innocent and good I am, and how he deserves to be punished. I could think something like the character shown in Figure 9.6.

c. I could start imagining all the bad things that could happen. I could live in the world of "what if," imaging the worse catastrophes. If I do a lot of this kind of thinking, I'm likely to feel more and more anxious. My anxiety will get even worse if I also breathe in a short and shallow way, and not receive enough oxygen. Indeed, between thinking this way and breathing badly, I could put myself into a state of panic. I could think something like the character shown in Figure 9.7.

d. I could use this man's behavior as justification for drinking or using drugs. I could tell myself that this situation is so stressful, I deserve a drink. (See the character in Figure 9.8.)

Before we use alcohol or drugs, we *give ourselves permission* to use these substances. We think, in some way, that *we should* use these substances. We say something like, "This is so hard. I deserve a drink." We might also say, "This was so easy, I should celebrate with a drink." Whatever we think, we end up giving ourselves permission to drink or engage in whatever addictive behavior we use.

e. Recovery also comes with a predictable way of thinking. When people are in recovery, they are talking to themselves, coaching themselves into more healthy behaviors. With regard to the man in the car behind me, I could think in ways that help me cope and manage this stress. I could think something like the character in Figure 9.9.

Can we help people make these connections? Can we help them learn to talk to themselves in a way that promotes recovery? The first step is that we have to recognize the connections between moods, thoughts, and behaviors ourselves. We also have to notice what kind of thinking appears to help.

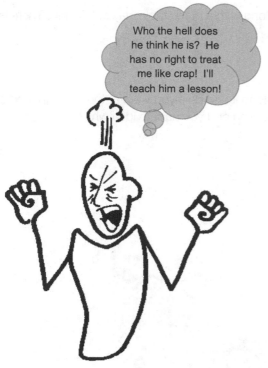

Figure 9.6 Angry thinking

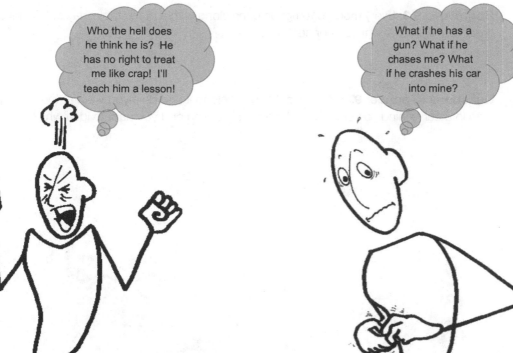

Figure 9.7 Anxious thinking

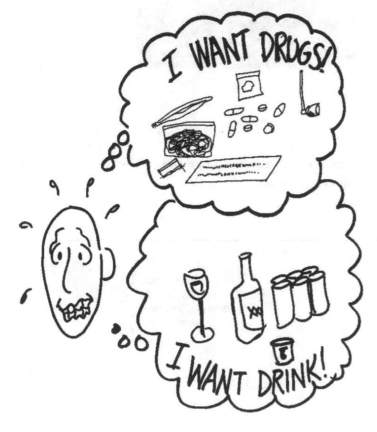

Figure 9.8 Alcohol and drug thinking

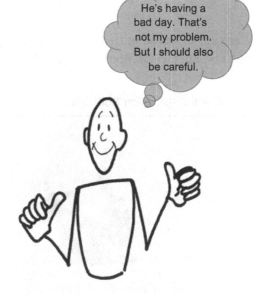

Figure 9.9 Recovery thinking

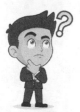

Bright idea 9.3: Every mood or emotion goes along with a predictable way of thinking. There is great power in seeing these connections.

Questions to ponder 9.1: What would you think, feel and do if you were at the stoplight and a man in a car behind you started honking angrily at you and you had no idea why?

Depression

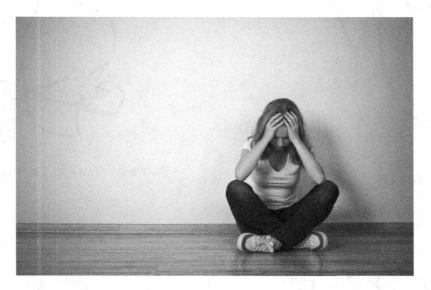

Figure 9.10 Depression
©iStock.com/evgenyatamanenko

The kind of thinking that accompanies depression often reflects a lack of hope and can be warning signs of possible suicide. Common thoughts that feed depression can be seen in Table 9.1.

TABLE 9.1 Depression Self-Talk

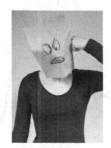

Figure 9.11 Bad self
©iStock.com/Nelosa

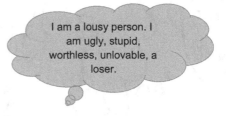

I am a lousy person. I am ugly, stupid, worthless, unlovable, a loser.

Figure 9.12

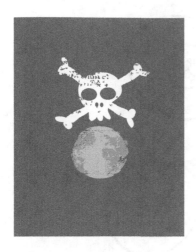

Figure 9.13 Bad world

©iStock.com/Jayesh

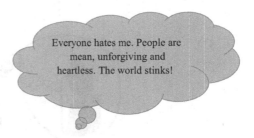

Everyone hates me. People are mean, unforgiving and heartless. The world stinks!

Figure 9.14

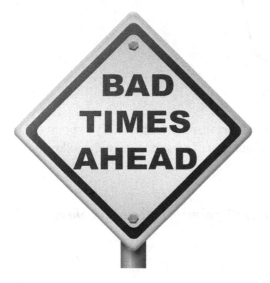

BAD TIMES AHEAD

Figure 9.15 Bad future

©iStock.com/kikkerdirk

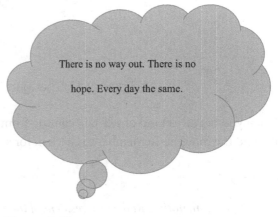

There is no way out. There is no hope. Every day the same.

Figure 9.16

Here are other examples of self-talk that you may encounter in people with depression:

"My life is pointless."
"Nothing matters. No one cares. I don't care."
"Nothing works or feels right."
"Everyone hates me."
"I keep thinking over and over about the bad things that have happened to me."
"My life is just one big ball of misery."

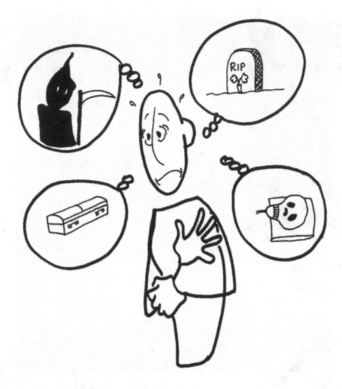

Figure 9.17 Thoughts of death

When you hear this kind of self-talk coming from someone you serve, reflect it back. Try to point out both the feeling and the thought. Remember to check in for accuracy as Julia, a staff person, does in the following scenario.

Scenario 9.3

Julia, a staff person, notices Rodrigo, a resident of the group home, sitting alone in the basement. She approaches him.

Julia: *"You seem sad. What's going on?"*
              Rodrigo shrugs.
Julia: *"Are you sad?"*
Rodrigo: *"Alison broke up with me."*
Julia: *"Oh. Alison broke up with you. I'm sorry to hear that. And you feel really sad?"*
              Rodrigo nods.
Alison: *"Do you want to talk about it?"*
              Rodrigo pauses for a while.
Rodrigo: *"I'll never get another girlfriend."*
Alison: *"You are thinking you will never get another girlfriend?"*
              Rodrigo nods.
Rodrigo: *"Yeah. I will be alone."*
Alison: *"You are thinking you will never get another girlfriend and you will be alone. And when you think that, you feel very sad."*
              Rodrigo nods and starts to cry.

Julia is helping Rodrigo notice his thoughts while empathizing with him. A bit later, she may write Rodrigo's thoughts in a bubble so he can see what he is telling himself. Right now, however, reflective listening (saying back what she heard) is the right response.[1]

In the next scenario, staff person Charlene takes noticing thoughts a step further.

Scenario 9.4

Charlene, a staff person, is working with Jennifer who struggles with depression. Jennifer makes lots of negative comments about herself like, "I'm ugly," and "Nobody likes me." However, throughout the day, she will also make a few comments that suggest she has some pride in herself. For example, when she knit a small hat for her niece and showed it to Charlene, she said, "I think my niece will like this."

Charlene: "Wow. When did you learn to knit so well? I've always wanted to learn to knit but it seems really tough to me."

Jennifer: "It's not so hard."

Later, Jennifer was making a salad and offered some to her housemate, Paul.

Charlene: "Nice salad. It was nice of you to offer some to Paul."

Jennifer: "No big deal."

Charlene: "You can think that, but lots of people around here don't do any cooking for themselves and they certainly don't offer food they made to other people."

She drew two thought bubbles for Jennifer and wrote something different in each one. Jennifer is able to read them. (See Figure 9.18.)

Charlene: "Which of these two thoughts is truer?"

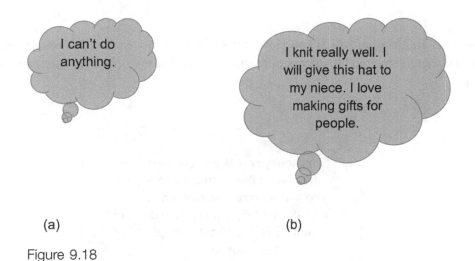

(a)   (b)

Figure 9.18

Notice that in this situation Charlene actually did more than just help Jennifer to notice her thoughts. By asking a good question, Charlene also helped Jennifer evaluate her thoughts. By helping Jennifer to notice and change her thinking, even a little, Jennifer felt better. If Charlene can help Jennifer to connect how changing her thinking changed her mood, she may "hook" Jennifer into doing more of this work, thereby beginning CBT. Right now, she just wants Jennifer to notice the kinds of thing she says to herself. Charlene might also want to ask, and wonder out loud, about how she feels and what she does when she thinks in this more affirming way.

Bright idea 9.4: People always have at least two stories. One is the story of their suffering; the other is the story of fighting back. Often the story of suffering will be dominant. But, if you listen carefully, you will hear the other story also. Skilled counselors learn how to notice and "pull out" the story about recovery.

Anger

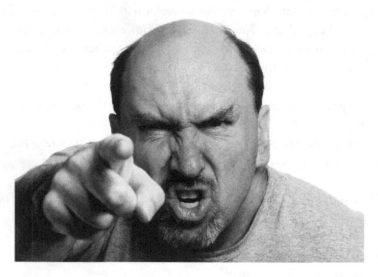

Figure 9.19

©iStock.com/perkmeup

Angry thoughts are those in which you view yourself as an innocent victim. You see yourself as a good person who has been mistreated by other people who are bad. Swear words often intensify this emotion. (See Figure 9.20.)

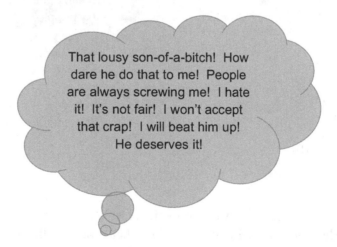

That lousy son-of-a-bitch! How dare he do that to me! People are always screwing me! I hate it! It's not fair! I won't accept that crap! I will beat him up! He deserves it!

Figure 9.20

Here are other examples of thoughts that promote anger:

1. Thoughts that blame another person.
2. Thoughts that magnify how bad you think another person is.
3. Thoughts that convince you that a person is deliberately trying to harm you.
4. Thoughts that convince you that your own honor, integrity, or pride is at stake.
5. Thoughts that a person is not behaving as you think they should, that they are doing something to intentionally cause pain for you or someone you care about.

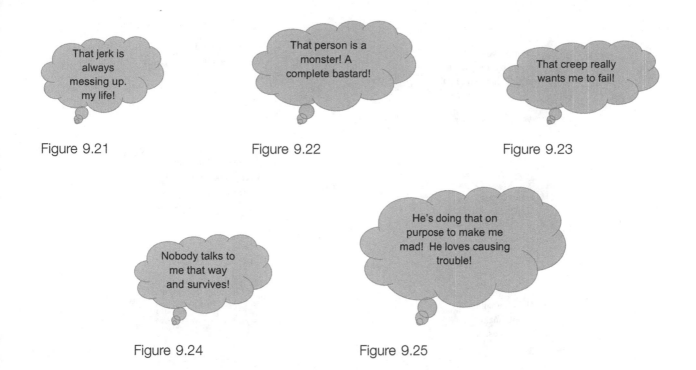

Figure 9.21   Figure 9.22   Figure 9.23

Figure 9.24   Figure 9.25

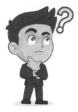

Questions to ponder 9.2: Consider the most recent time you were angry. Can you recall what you were thinking? Were you thinking any of the kinds of anger-generating thoughts just described? Now, consider a time when someone has been angry with you. Could they have been thinking any of these thoughts?

Anger Recovery Thinking

Anger is fueled by the perception that bad people are trying to hurt you *on purpose*, and that, therefore, *they deserve* to be harmed themselves. Thoughts that lessen anger are those that:

- Help someone feel compassion for other people (e.g., "He's only human," or "He's doing his best").
- Challenge the belief about people intending to cause harm (e.g., "It was an accident," or "He didn't realize what he was doing").
- Offer alternative, more understanding explanations (e.g., "Maybe it was all a communication breakdown").

It is not unusual to observe the people you serve become angry and aggressive. It's also not unusual to see them step away from anger. When people who are prone to aggression *don't act aggressively*, or act *less aggressively* then they typically would, some thinking process guided them. Your job is to help people discover the thought patterns that helped them to feel less angry and, therefore, behave less aggressively.

Example anger recovery thoughts can be seen in Figure 9.26.

Whenever a person who commonly behaves aggressively doesn't, or behaves less aggressively, or recovers quickly and strives to repair damage, you should search for the kinds of skill used. Very often there is a thinking skill being used that the person is not aware of. Sometimes you can get clues to the recovery self-talk just by showing curiosity, one-down, and asking: *"You didn't hit me! Thank you. I really appreciate it. I'm wondering how you stopped yourself. I'm wondering how you remembered to stay safe. How did you succeed in staying safe?"*

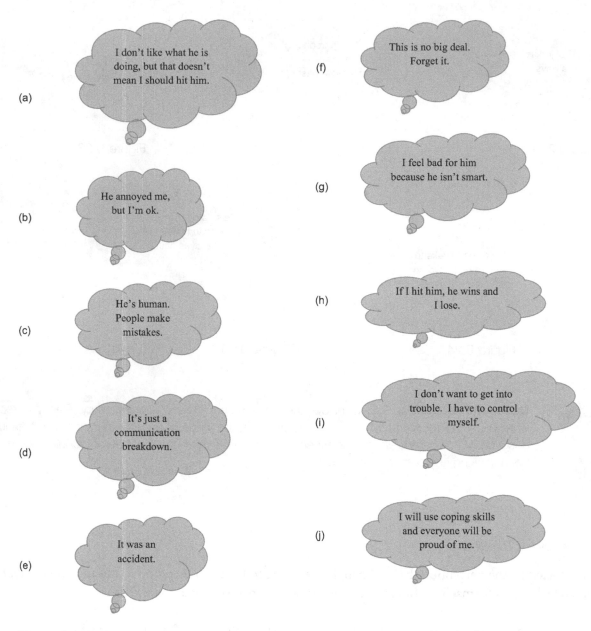

Figure 9.26

Often people with language and learning challenges have difficulty answering abstract "how" and "why" questions. Sometimes we ask these questions not because we expect an insightful answer but because we want to guide people to discover something. We hope to show them how their own thinking affects them for better or worse. We ask the question, "How did you do it?" and then we show them that they succeeded because they used this kind of self-talk.

Scenario 9.5

Simon is a nursing assistant on an inpatient psychiatric unit. As part of his unit checks, he goes from room to room making sure everyone is safe. When Simon goes into the bathroom, he finds Sebastian smoking a cigarette. Sebastian knows this is forbidden on the unit. Simon asks him to put out the cigarette. For a few moments, it looks like Sebastian is going to hit Simon, but Sebastian finally puts the cigarette out and makes a face that shows great annoyance. He angrily walks past Simon and goes to his room.

Later, Simon asks Sebastian if he can talk to him. Sebastian is expecting a lecture on how he broke the rules, but Simon surprises him by offering him thanks.

Simon:	*"Well, I just want to say 'thank you' to you."*
Sebastian:	*"What?"*
Simon:	*"I want to say thank you. I appreciate how you responded to me when I asked you to put out the cigarette."*
	Sebastian doesn't recognize the compliment and, instead, hears some criticism.
Sebastian:	*"What am I supposed to do? I needed a smoke!"*
Simon:	*"I know that. It's really hard to need a smoke and not be able to go out that moment. Can I ask you a question?"*
Sebastian:	*"What?"*
Simon:	*"For a moment, when we were in the bathroom, I thought you were going to hit me, but you didn't. You just put out the cigarette and went out. Thank you for not hitting me. My question is how did you stay in such good control?"*
Sebastian:	*"If I hit you, I'd just get in more trouble. What's the point?"*
Simon:	*"So you talked to yourself. You thought about the consequences and you said to yourself something like, 'What's the point?'"*
Sebastian:	*"Yeah, I guess.*
	Sebastian thinks for a bit.
Sebastian:	*"To tell you the truth, I know you were just doing your job."*
Simon:	*"Wow. Do you see what you are saying? Do you see the skills you are using?"*
Sebastian:	*"What?"*
Simon:	*"You were pissed off, right? Yet you can still talk to yourself, tell yourself it's not worth getting in more trouble. And even more impressive, at that moment, when you were mad at me, you still had some empathy for me. You realized I was just doing my job. I was not trying to give you a hard time."*
Sebastian:	*"Yeah, I guess."*
Simon:	*"It's impressive to me that you have those kinds of skill in you."*

Sebastian appears to have a number of skills, including "perspective taking." His intact language skills also make this work much easier. In this case, Sebastian actually showed how he was thinking; he just didn't identify it as "thinking" until Simon helped him to recognize it.

Of course, it wouldn't be a skill if the person responds with something like, "I will hit you next time." If this happens, staff could respond with empathy (e.g., "Looks like you are still angry.") and ask permission to keep talking (e.g., "Can we talk about it some more? If we talk about it now, can you stay safe?"). With permission, you should return to the strength (e.g., "But you didn't hit me. Again, thank you. I appreciate it. You did something good, something right. You must have used a skill. I'm just trying to help you see it when you do something skillful.").

Practice Exercise 9.1

1. Read each of the following anger-generating thoughts.
2. Think of a believable thought that will help the person calm down.
3. Write your answer in the space provided.

1. "That jerk is always messing up my life."

_____

2. "That person is a total bastard!"

_____

3. "That creep really wants to screw me."

_____

4. "I won't let him walk all over me."

_____

5. "I won't accept that kind of disrespect."

_____

6. "Nobody gets away with treating me like that. I'll show him."

_____

7. "He shouldn't act that way. He's a lousy bastard. He loves causing trouble."

_____

Anxiety

Anxiety is connected to thoughts about the terrible things that might happen and how a person feels unable to control them. Anxiety is also connected to misunderstanding what is happening in your body, believing incorrectly that something is physically wrong.

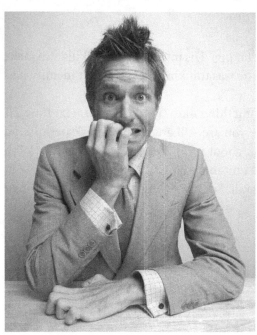

Figure 9.27

©iStock.com/PeskyMonkey

Anxiety is more difficult to notice than depression or anger. It's also easily confused with fear. Fear is a normal human response when faced with real danger. If you are being chased by a lion, you will feel fear. If someone aims a gun at your head, you will feel fear.

Unlike fear, anxiety occurs when there is no real and present danger, only an imagined danger. When you are afraid, you know exactly what you fear. However, when you are anxious, you may have only a vague idea of what is making you feel that way. Thoughts like "I'm going crazy" or "I'm dying" are common. Anxiety is connected to the belief that "I can't cope." The greater the perceived threat, and the less you think you can cope, the greater your anxiety.

You can help the people you serve to recognize the signs and symptoms of anxiety. Many of these symptoms can be easily illustrated with pictures, which can also be incorporated into self-monitoring forms. (See Table 9.2.)

Anxious thoughts take the form of "what if?" People with anxieties live in the world of imagining the worst possible outcome. Albert Ellis, one of the founders of CBT, called this "catastrophizing."

TABLE 9.2 Physical Symptoms of Anxiety

Increased heart rate

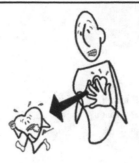

Breathing rapidly (hyperventilation)

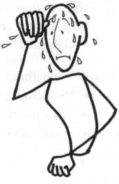

Sweating

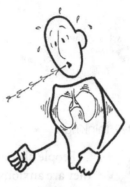

Trembling

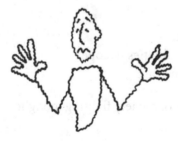

Trouble concentrating or thinking about anything other than the present worry

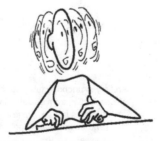

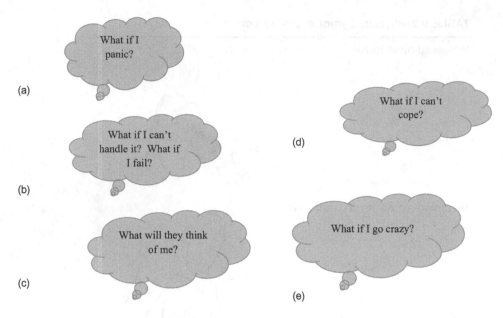

Figure 9.33 "What if?" thinking

People also misinterpret what is happening in their own bodies when they are anxious. They believe they are sick, dying, or going crazy. People with anxiety and panic reactions often end up in emergency rooms because they are convinced their body or minds are failing *right now*.

Basically, they are thinking:

- Something bad is going to happen.
- Something is terribly wrong with me.
- This will be terrible.
- I can't cope.

Figure 9.34

Anxiety Recovery Thinking

Anti-anxiety thoughts:

1. Minimize the threat.
2. Highlight one's own abilities to cope.
3. Are more realistic and fair.

Here are some examples of anxiety fighting thoughts:

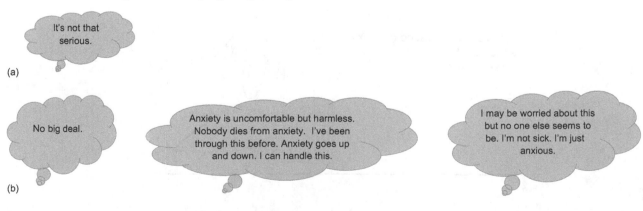

Figure 9.35   Figure 9.36   Figure 9.37

Scenario 9.6

Jorge is a young man living in his own apartment. He calls Susan, a staff outreach worker, when he needs help. However, Susan isn't always available immediately and Jorge gets very anxious when he can't reach her. He starts calling over and over, sometimes calling dozens of times within an hour.

One day, when Jorge couldn't reach Susan, he left five messages instead of his usual 20. When Susan called him back, she noted the progress:

Susan: *"Did you notice how many times you called me?"*

Jorge: *"I know I'm only supposed to call you one time."*

Susan: *"Yes, and it seems you made some progress! How many times did you call yesterday?"*

Jorge: *"I don't know. A lot."*

Susan: *"A real lot. Today, it was much less, just five. You're improving. How did you do it?"*

Jorge: *"I know you don't want me to bother you."*

Susan: *"Thank you for being considerate of my feelings. I want to talk to you but I can't always call back right away. But let me ask you again. How did you cope? You only called me five times. I wonder, did you say something to yourself like, 'Susan doesn't want me to bother her.'"*

Jorge: *"Yeah."*

Susan: *"Did you tell yourself, like we practiced, that this wasn't an emergency. You weren't dying. You were anxious, but you weren't dying."*

Jorge: *"I forgot that."*

Susan: *"Hmmm. You must have said something to yourself to calm down. I wonder what it was. Maybe we can find out and practice that now."*

Susan is working with Jorge to develop a self-talk script that can help him cope with his anxiety. You'll learn more about developing coping scripts in the next lesson.

There are proven coping skills that help people deal with anxiety, such as learning to breathe deeply and slowly, as well as sensory-based grounding skills (e.g., jumping, rubbing, stretching, pushing, pulling, holding or feeling ice, etc.). Remember the story from Lesson 1 of the five coping skills I used to cope with my fears when zip lining. In CBT, we engage people in the process of learning these skills and evaluating their impact.

In this lesson, our focus has been on noticing the thoughts that reliably accompany problem mood states like depression, anger, and anxiety as well as some thoughts that support coping and recovery. Staff who work in mental health programs need to understand these connections so they can help the people they serve notice how their own thinking is effecting their moods, behavior and recovery.

In Lesson 10, we'll discuss some simple ways to make a person's thinking more clear, concrete, and visible to them, and how to begin the CBT work of developing more helpful self-talk.

   Practice Exercise 9.2, Part A

1. Read through each scenario.
2. Identify the likely emotion.
3. Identify possible thoughts connected with it.
4. Identify the skills or strengths the individual used.
5. Ask yourself, what could the person say to herself that would help her cope in this situation?
6. Write your answers in the spaces provided.

Scenario 9.7

Julia is a 19-year-old female living in a group home. She is completing high school. The school district has arranged cab transportation to take her to school in the morning and return to the group home in the afternoon. She likes to sleep late, which means she expects program staff to drive her 45 minutes to her school if she isn't ready when the cab arrives. She also likes to make after-school plans, expecting staff to pick her up wherever she is, regardless of the time or distance from the program. Staff resources are very limited. Program staff have explained this to her and told her that if she misses her ride in the morning, she will miss school. If she misses her ride back, she will have to use her own money to take the train back. Julia doesn't want to hear this.

This morning, Julia overslept again, even though staff tried to wake her. She then came out expecting staff to take her to school. Staff apologized but said they were not able to do that. She could take the train in or miss school that day.

Julia starts screaming at staff, blaming them for not waking her up, saying if she fails school it will be their fault and complaining about the lousy staff that don't "care about me at all." Although she has been assaultive in the past, she manages to go to her room and calm down. Two hours later, she comes out crying, saying that she is failing school and nobody cares.

Likely emotions that Julia is experiencing:

_____

_____

Likely thoughts related to the emotions:

_____

_____

Any skills or strengths you can point to:

_____

_____

Coping thoughts that would help Julia:

_____

_____

Scenario 9.8

Staff and residents of a group home are having a community meeting. Two housemates are angry with Jocelyn, a third housemate. They say Jocelyn never helps out with any chores. She leaves her dishes in the sink, expecting others to clean up after her. She takes a very long time in the bathroom and uses all the hot water. She also takes food out of the refrigerator that belongs to other people and is clearly labeled.

The two housemates bring up these concerns with Jocelyn and staff asks Jocelyn to listen to what they are saying. Jocelyn becomes upset, says that staff and roommates are "ganging up on her," that "it isn't fair," and that she "hates this place." Then she storms out of the meeting.

Two hours later, Jocelyn approaches Mary, a staff person she likes, and starts to cry. She says she feels that everyone at the group home hates her and people have treated her badly all her life. She is upset with staff for "supporting" her roommates against her.

Likely emotions that Jocelyn is experiencing:

_____

_____

Likely thoughts related to these emotions:

_____

_____

Any skills or strengths you can point to:

_____

_____

Coping thoughts that would help Jocelyn:

_____

_____

Scenario 9.9

Chuck is an 18-year-old deaf male who is a patient on a psychiatric inpatient unit for deaf persons. He was hospitalized after numerous incidents of oppositional and aggressive behavior that eventually became more than the staff could handle. On the inpatient unit, Chuck was initially very pleasant and cooperative but, after a few days, he began to complain about the rules and expectations for him.

One night, the unit had a fire drill. During fire drills, all patients are required to get up and go with staff to one of the exits on the unit. Staff tried to wake Chuck up but he refused to get up. Because participation in the fire drill was required, two male staff picked Chuck up out of bed and carried him down the hall to the exit, kicking and screaming as they went.

The next day, the program director asked to meet with Chuck to discuss what had happened the night before. Chuck refused to meet with the program director, called him insulting names, and screamed in sign language that staff members were abusing him.

Likely emotions that Chuck is experiencing:

_____

_____

Likely thoughts related to these emotions:

_____

_____

If Chuck isn't using skills at this moment, where might you find the skills later on?

_____

_____

Coping thoughts that would have helped Chuck:

_____

_____

Practice Exercise 9.2, Part B

1. Think about a time when you *didn't* show a behavior that you normally consider a problem (e.g., You didn't argue with someone; you stopped yourself from drinking alcohol or taking that extra cookie; you forced yourself to act politely with someone you don't like, etc.).
2. Ask yourself what you told yourself in order to get yourself to behave in this new way.
3. Write your self-talk in the space below:

_____

_____

Practice Exercise 9.2, Part C

1. Look for an example of when a client who is often aggressive was either not aggressive or less aggressive.
2. Engage the person in a strength-based conversation about it. Start by asking permission to talk about something positive you noticed.
3. After you get permission, then point out that they *didn't* show the aggressive behavior, or showed less of it.
4. Ask them how they were able to improve so much.
5. While they are talking with you, try to identify the self-talk they might have used.
6. Write your observations below.

_____

_____

Lesson 9 Skill Sheet

- Participant can recognize when he or she feels angry, anxious, or depressed.

- Participant can recognize some of the thinking that occurs when he or she feels angry, anxious, or depressed.

- Participant can notice and identify when another person appears to be feeling angry, anxious, or depressed.

- Participant listens for and helps identify possible thoughts that appear to accompany these mood states.

- Participant can recognize thoughts that appear to help themselves cope better.

- Participants can help another person recognize thoughts that appear to be helpful for coping.

Lesson 9 Quiz

1. Which of the following thoughts are likely to promote *depression*? (Check all that apply.)

   a. "I just can't do anything right."

   b. "I'm ugly. Nobody would ever want to be in a relationship with me."

   c. "My boss keeps giving me a hard time."

   d. "It's not so bad."

   e. "All I see are problems. I can't go on with this lousy life."

2. Which of the following thoughts are likely to promote *anger*? (Check all that apply.)

   a. "He cheated me again!"

   b. "What a bum!"

   c. "I just stink at this job."

   d. "Get the _____ out of my way, you jerk!"

   e. "What if I lose again?"

3. Which of the following thoughts are likely to promote *anxiety*? (Check all that apply.)

   a. "I can't cope."

   b. "I know something bad is going to happen."

   c. "It's all my fault."

   d. "It's all your fault."

   e. "What if I'm having a heart attack?"

4. Which of the following thoughts are likely to promote *coping* and *feeling better*? (Check all that apply.)

   a. "No problem. No big deal."

   b. "Tomorrow is another day."

   c. "All I can do is my best."

   d. "Nobody's perfect."

   e. "If I don't get this done perfectly, I'll lose my job for sure."

5. Why is it helpful to be able to notice your own thinking? (Check all that apply.)

   a. You might be better able to see how you are talking yourself into a bad mood.

   b. You might recognize more helpful ways to think about things.

   c. Your thinking is strongly connected to your ability to solve problems.

   d. Many life problems can be solved or managed by learning to think differently.

   e. If you can notice your own thinking, you can benefit from learning an array of CBT techniques to help you think in more helpful ways.

Lesson 9 Questions for Discussion

1. How hard is it for you to step back and notice your thinking when you are very emotional?

2. Do you have particular slogans or sayings that you use to help you cope?

3. Consider the people you serve in your job. How hard is it for them to connect their thoughts with their emotions? How can you help them make these connections?

4. What are some ways that people give themselves permission to act aggressively towards others?

5. What are some ways that people give themselves permission to harm themselves?

6. What are some ways that people give themselves permission to use alcohol and drugs?

7. Have you ever been able to talk yourself out of a bad mood? How did you do it? What did you say to yourself?

8. Have you ever seen people stuck in a really self-defeating way of thinking and behaving? What are some examples?

9. Use the Internet to find lists of coping statements for particular problems or emotions. What do you find? Are any of these statements helpful to you?

10. Next time you are really upset about something, try to stop and notice what you are thinking. Try to write down your thoughts. Do you see any of the themes for depression, anger and anxiety that were discussed in this module? How easy is it for you to notice your thoughts at these times?

11. Are there any religious or spiritual beliefs that you find helpful in your personal life? What are some of the beliefs that you return to because they help you feel stronger and happier?

Lesson 9 Quiz Answers

1. Answers a, b, and e are thoughts that promote depression. Answers a and b relate to the "bad self" theme; answer e relates to the "bad world" theme. Answer c is more likely to be an anger-producing thought while d is a thought that promotes coping.

2. Answers a, b, and d are likely to elicit anger. Answer c is more likely to elicit depression while e is more likely to elicit anxiety.

3. Answer e is a classic "what if" thought related to anxiety and a possible misreading of bodily cues. Answer a also is likely to be anxiety-provoking. The thought that "I can't cope" often underlies the "what if." Answer b is also likely to foster anxiety. Answer c is more likely to promote depression and answer d is more likely to promote anger.

4. Answers a through d are all thoughts that support coping. Answer e is likely to promote anxiety.

5. All of these are reasons why it is helpful to notice your own thinking.

Note

1. This is not a lesson on assessment or treatment of suicidality, but when someone seems depressed, and especially when they express themes that reflect hopelessness, we ask if they have thoughts or plans to harm themselves. If you are not familiar with procedures for responding to people who appear suicidal, seek consultation immediately (Bongar et al. 1998).

Bibliography

Aaron Beck and his associates have been responsible for much of the research into the connections between thoughts, emotions, and behaviors. Donald Meichenbaum often talks about pulling out "the rest of the story," meaning looking past problem talk to how the person coped with stress or adversity and are moved towards health and recovery. The discussion about people having at least two stories and the need to listen well and help the person amplify the recovery story is based on his work. You will also find that strategy in the narrative therapy of Michael White.

Beck, A. (1976). *Cognitive therapy and emotional disorders*. New York: International Universities Press.

Beck, A. T., & Freeman, A. (1990). *Cognitive therapy of personality disorders*. New York: Guilford Press.

Beck, A., Rush, A., Shaw, B., & Emery, G. (1979). *Cognitive therapy of depression*. New York: Guilford Press.

Beck, A., Wright, F., Newman, C., & Liese, B. (1993). *Cognitive theapy of substance abuse*. New York: Guilford Press.

Beck, J. (1995). *Cognitive-therapy: Basics and beyond*. New York: Guilford Press.

Bongar, B., Berman, A. L., Maris, R. W., Silverman, M. M., Harris, E. A., & Packman, W. L. (Eds.). (1998). *Risk management with suicidal patients*. London: Guilford Press.

Meichenbaum, D. (1994). *A clinical handbook/practical therapist manual for assessing and treating adults with post-traumatic stress disorder*. Waterloo, Canada: Institute Press.

Meichenbaum, D. (2001). *Treatment of individuals with anger-control problems and aggressive behaviors: a clinical handbook*. Clearwater, FL: Institute Press.

Meichenbaum, D. (2012). *Roadmap to resilience: A guide for military, trauma victims and their families*. Clearwater, FL: Institute Press.

White, M. (1995). *Reauthoring lives: Interviews and essays*. Adelaide, South Australia: Dulwich Centre Publications.

White, M. (2007). *Maps of narrative practice*. New York: W. W. Norton & Company, Inc.

Changing Self-Talk

Introduction

As you've learned, it can be difficult for many people with language and learning challenges to notice and change how they think because this skill is abstract and complex. However, being able to notice and change thought patterns is at the heart of even the simplest forms of CBT, and it is a skill we want very much to help people develop.

Lesson 10 introduces some simple strategies to help the people you serve to recognize and change how they think. These techniques are concrete and do not require analytical skills. They focus primarily on the skill of self-talk, not the more advanced skill of analyzing and categorizing thoughts, or searching for evidence of whether or not thoughts are true, that one often does in CBT. We're going to continue to help people take their thoughts out of their heads and visualize them and then practice talking to themselves differently. While the ability to read and write certainly helps, we can do this with simple words, pictures and role playing.

In this lesson, you will:

- Learn how to help the person create monsters or creatures that express the thoughts related to specific moods, such as depression, anger, and anxiety.
- Learn how to help them create recovery creatures that express more helpful thoughts.
- Learn how to create scripts that go along with mood states and recovery.
- Help people practice these scripts in role-playing exercises.
- Continue to practice asking good questions that promote healthier thinking.

As with all clinical work, you can only help other people learn skills that you have mastered personally. Therefore, you own skill development in these areas is an important part of becoming an effective helper for other people.

Externalizing Problems

In Lesson 8, you learned to use thought bubbles to help people with language and learning challenges to notice *that* they are thinking and *what* they are thinking. Putting thoughts into a bubble is an example of *externalizing*.[1]

Externalizing means taking an experience that is inside one's body (internal), such as a thought or feeling or symptom, and putting it outside one's body (external) so that it can be studied more easily.

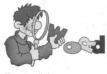

Externalizing

Definition 10.1: Externalizing: Taking an internal experience, one that is *inside* one's body (e.g., a thought, feeling or symptom) and talking about it as if it is *outside* one's body, as if it had an independent life of its own. This allows the person to learn ways to manage the experience more easily.

Example of externalizing: Joseph is a 10-year-old boy with obsessive compulsive disorder (OCD). He repeats certain words to himself over and over and washes his hands for an hour at a time. His counselor helped him to draw an OCD monster. They talked about how the OCD monster was trying to control him by making him think and do things repeatedly. They also discussed how he could fight back against the OCD monster (March & Mulle 1998).

Creating Mood Monsters

If depression, anger and anxiety were monsters, what would they look like? What would they say?

In Lesson 9, you learned some common ways of thinking that are associated with depression. Sometimes it is easier for people to recognize these negative thoughts if they are put into the head of a monster or creature that they have designed. There are many ways to create this "mood monster." The process is very simple.

TABLE 10.1 Creating a Mood Monster

Step 1: Ask the person to describe what they think their mood looks like.	Sample questions to ask: • "What does your depression look like?" • "Could you create a depression monster?" • "What would a depression monster look like to you?"
Step 2: Ask the person what this monster says.	Sample questions to ask: • "What do you think the depression monster says to you when it talks to you?" • "What do you think a depression monster would say?"
Step 3: Ask the person to create a picture of the monster. This can be as detailed or complex as the person wants it to be and is capable of accomplishing.	Options: • Create a simple drawing. • Create a detailed drawing (especially if the person finds art therapeutic). • Find pictures in magazines or other sources. • Download an image of a "mood monster" from the Internet.

There's an example in Figure 10.1.

Note that when the monster is "talking," the bubble looks different from the one used for "thinking." Simply changing the shape makes it easier for the people you serve to tell the difference. For example, compare the thought bubble with the talking bubble in Figure 10.2.

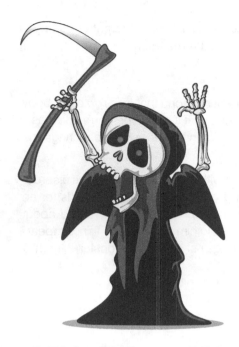

Figure 10.1 Depression monster

©iStock.com/Lee Daniels

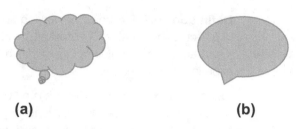

(a)   **(b)**

Figure 10.2 Thought bubble and talk bubble

This procedure can be used to create a monster for any mood state, symptom or problem. Examples of anger and anxiety monsters can be found in Figures 10.3 and 10.4.

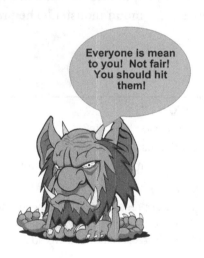

Figure 10.3 Anger monster

©iStock.com/artychoke98

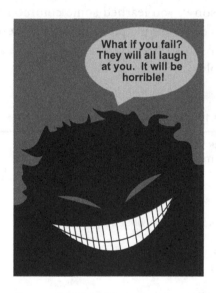

Figure 10.4 Anxiety monster

©iStock.com/sumografika

The following scenario shows how a mental health worker introduced the idea of creating a "mood monster" to a person she is working with on a psychiatric inpatient unit.

Scenario 10.1

Susan, a staff person, is listening as Jeff, a patient, talks about how stupid he is. She knows Jeff struggles with depression. She also knows that depression is associated with that kind of self-talk. Taking a one-down stance, she tries to help Jeff notice this self-talk:

Jeff: *"I'm just so stupid. I get everything wrong."*
Susan: *"I have a hard question for you. Can I ask you?"*

Jeff:	*"What?"*
Susan:	*"It may seem like a strange question."*
Jeff:	*"What?"*
Susan:	*"I'm wondering who is talking, you or your depression monster?"*
Jeff:	*"What do you mean?"*
Susan:	*"Have you ever heard of a depression monster?"*
Jeff:	*"No."*
Susan:	*"Well, could we make one up?"*
Jeff:	*"I don't know."*
Susan:	*"I wonder, could you draw a depression monster? Or, could you find a picture of one? Here's an example. Do you think this looks like a depression monster?"*
	Susan shows him the picture that can be found in Figure 10.5.
	Jeff chuckles.
Jeff:	*"I guess so."*
Susan:	*"Can we use him or would you like to draw your own?"*
Jeff:	*"No, I think he's scary enough."*
Susan:	*"Ok, so here's another hard question. Are you ready?"*
Jeff:	*"Yeah."*
Susan:	*"When you say you are stupid and get everything wrong, who is talking? Are you talking or is the depression monster talking?"*
Jeff:	*"Oh . . ."*
	Jeff thinks for a moment.
Jeff:	*"Maybe both of us."*
Susan:	*"You mean you believe him?"*
	Jeff thinks for a moment.
Jeff:	*"I don't know."*
Susan:	*"I wonder what else he says to you. I wonder what other ideas he's put into your brain."*

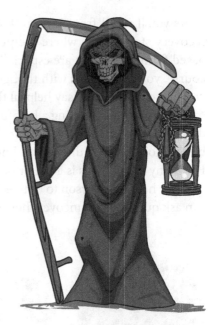

Figure 10.5

©iStock.com/Joe Peragino

Bright idea 10.1: Many difficult emotions or symptoms can be made more manageable by *externalizing* them; that is, putting them outside one's head and having an imaginary creature express those thoughts. This enables you to say, "This is depression talking, not you." It also enables you to help the person come up with strategies to fight the "depression monster" or other mood monster. It can also enable you to recognize and understand the self-talk that goes along with that emotion or symptom.

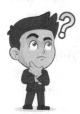

Questions to ponder 10.1: Have you ever invented a monster to represent a feeling, symptom or problem that you have? Have you seen another person do this? Even without creating a monster, have you ever thought of a problem you have as outside of yourself? For instance, have you ever thought, "That's my anxiety talking"?

Recovery Creatures

A person who is trained to recognize the connection between thinking, mood, and behaviors also needs skills to notice when people think in ways that promote better moods and functioning. In other words, they must be able to recognize a person's "recovery talk."

As you'll recall from Lesson 9, everyone has at least two stories: problem stories and recovery stories. A recovery story is one where the person tells about their strength, resiliency, and recovery. Using a strength-based framework, you are especially interested in helping people notice thinking patterns that help them. Of course, you can do this with thought bubbles. But, you can also help someone *externalize* helpful thoughts by creating creatures that say helpful things.

The process for creating a helpful creature is similar to the one used to create a mood monster. The primary differences are that the creature feels kind and supportive, rather than scary. With good questioning, you may be able to learn that the person knows someone or something that they believe would speak kindly to them. For many people, this is a pet or other animal. This is a good place to start.

After helping a person to notice their negative thinking and creating a mood monster that talks to them, you can ask questions to uncover their internal recovery script. For example:

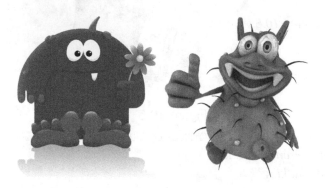

Figure 10.6 Comfort creatures

©iStock.com/Laura Maples;
©IStock.com/julien Tromeur

"If that's your depression monster, what would help you talk back to it? Who could help you talk back to it? Would you want to create a 'recovery creature' or do you already have one? Here are a few pictures other people have used (Figure 10.6).

"Some people don't think of a creature. They think of a person who always tells them something helpful. Some people think of Jesus or God. Some people use a pet or favorite animal."

"What would your recovery creature look like?"

This is a great conversation to have with people you serve. Try to help them:

• Visualize what the comforting voice or presence looks like.
• Ask them to create an image of it. Ask the person to draw a picture, find a photo, if they have identified a pet or a real person, find an image or statue if they use a religious figure like Jesus, the Buddha, etc.
• Find sample images online.

Most people are familiar with the pictures of an angel and devil talking into a person's ear (or signing to them). Usually, the devil is urging the person to do something they shouldn't, while the angel is urging the person to do the right thing. The use of mood monsters and recovery creatures is similar. However, you are not trying to represent good and evil. Rather, the goal is to create images that represent the symptoms, problems, and thoughts associated with problem mood states (the monster) and coping, recovery, and health (the recovery creature). The familiar "angel/devil" picture can help to start this conversation.

The following scenario shows how you might use this familiar image.

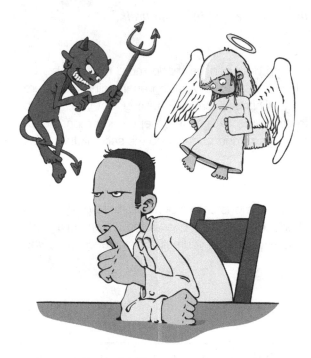

Figure 10.7 Devil talk vs. angel talk

©iStock.com/FP_draw

Scenario 10.2

Alice, a staff person in a group home, is working with a resident named Ahmed. She shows the angel/devil picture to Ahmed.

Alice:	"Have you ever seen this?"
	Ahmed laughs.
Ahmed:	"Yeah."
Alice:	"What do you think the devil is saying to him?"
Ahmed:	"I don't know. Maybe go steal something."
Alice:	"Maybe. What do you think the angel is saying to him?"
Ahmed:	"Oh, the angel says he should be good."
Alice:	"I think you are right. Remember when we talked about the anger monster?"
Ahmed:	"Yeah. I drew the picture."
Alice:	"Well, suppose the devil is really an anger monster. The devil is saying things to the man to get him angry. What would the devil tell him?"
Ahmed:	"I don't know . . . maybe that he should hit someone."
Alice:	"Yeah . . . what else?"
	Alice asks questions to help Ahmed think about this "devil thinking" and compares it to the monster that talks Ahmed into feeling angry. Later, she switches the conversation to focus on what the angel might be saying.
Alice:	"So, what do you think the angel is saying?"
Ahmed:	"Be good."
Alice:	"The angel is trying to help him calm down, not blow up. What would the angel say?"
Ahmed:	"Calm down."
Alice:	"Yeah. How could the angel convince him to calm down? Maybe he's angry and really wants to hit someone."
Ahmed:	"Well, he could say, 'Don't blow up. You'll get in trouble.'"
Alice:	"What else could the angel say?"
	This conversation is the beginning of the process, not the end. By first thinking of words that might come from the angel, Ahmed is starting to learn how to use a script to stay calm. Later Alice helps Ahmed practice using this script to calm himself.

The angel/devil metaphor is widely used so it may be easier for people to understand than putting words into the mouths of imaginary creatures. But some people may not find it hard to imagine what their favorite animal or other comforting creature would say to them. In fact, when people pray and hear the voice of their God or religious figures, they are, psychologically speaking, using a form of externalization. The following scenario illustrates this.

Scenario 10.3

Matthew is a young man with a mild developmental disability and an explosive temper. Matthew also has a strong belief in God and prays each day. His counselor, Richard, understands that these prayers have helped Matthew control his behavior. When Richard asked Matthew what God says to him, Matthew replied that God said, "Control yourself. Be nice to people. Don't hit people."

Richard worked with Matthew to draw this message out even further. Together, they created a script that Matthew could read to himself each day as part of his prayer. This calming script became an important coping skill for Matthew.

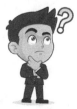

Questions to ponder 10.2: Have you ever created or used a comfort or recovery creature of some kind? Do you have an inner voice that says kind and helpful things to you? Does your religious or spiritual tradition give you such a calming inner voice? Do you imagine the voice of some person who loved you or an animal even? Whoever—or whatever—gave you that inner, calming voice gave you a powerful and wonderful gift.

Practice Exercise 10.1

1. Identify a mood or symptom that is sometimes a problem for you (e.g., depression, anxiety, anger, embarrassment, shame, substance use, aggression, self-harm, etc.).
2. Externalize this problem by finding the image of a monster that represents it.
3. Identify some of the thoughts that this monster might say to you.
4. Write your thoughts in the space provided.

_____

_____

_____

5. Create a recovery script that you could use when faced with the problem you have identified. Tip: An Internet search on "coping thoughts" may provide some ideas. These can be a good starting point but be sure to use your own words.
6. Ask yourself: Would you consider keeping this script in a place where you can access it easily, such as a wallet card? Do you think you will use it when needed? If you are reluctant to use it, why?

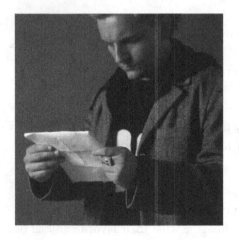

Figure 10.8

©iStock.com/Rasmus Rasmussen

Creating Recovery Scripts

Once you have helped a person to externalize, by creating monsters/ creatures, the thoughts that accompany problem emotions and behaviors as well as recovery, the next step is to help the person elaborate the thoughts that support recovery. Creating a written script of the recovery thoughts is one way to do this. These scripts can be written down or memorized. They also can be very short: A few meaningful phrases are adequate to start.

Some simple recovery scripts can be found in Figure 10.9.

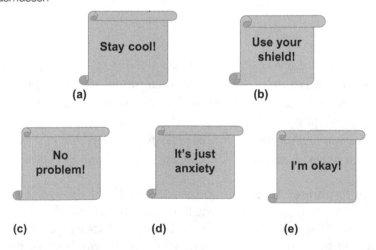

Figure 10.9 Simple recovery scripts

The following scenarios show how this process works.

Scenario 10.4

Joe often becomes aggressive and pushes and hits people. When questioned about his reasons for becoming aggressive, he says other people make him mad. Today, Joe got mad at Emanuel, a staff person. This time, however, Joe just walked away. Later, Emanuel asked Joe's permission to talk and comment on what he noticed. They talked about how Joe felt angry and thought Emanuel was a jerk. Emanuel also helped Joe notice that he told himself to walk away so he wouldn't get in more trouble.

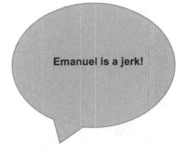

Figure 10.10

Emanuel: "So, let me see if I got this straight. The anger monster we talked about said something like this to you. (He draws and writes the speech bubble. See Figure 10.10.)

Emanuel: "But then Boots, your support dog, also talked to you. And Boots said something like this" (see Figure 10.11).

Emanuel: "Is that right? I wonder if Boots said anything more than that?"

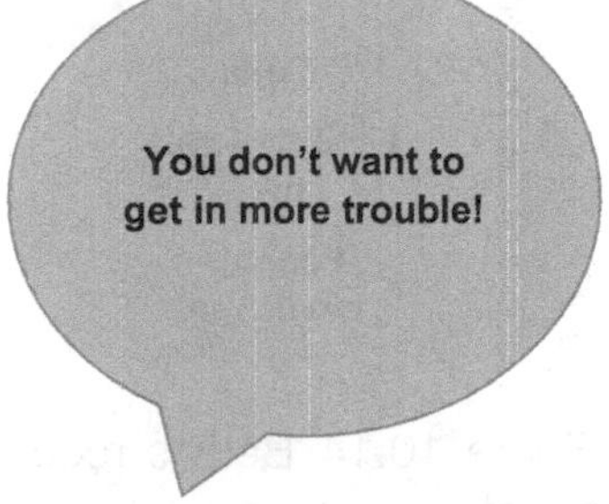

Notice that instead of asking Joe to describe more of the anger monster thoughts, Emanuel asks Joe to focus on the recovery thoughts. Emmanuel is using this approach because his goal is to help Joe create a script of self-talk that Joe can use to help him calm down. Eventually, Emmanual helps Joe write down the script and practice it in a role play. He also tries to expand the script by adding other related thoughts. Eventually, Joe writes down this script (Figure 10.12).

In the following scenario, staff person Martha helps client Betty develop a recovery script for anxiety.

Figure 10.11

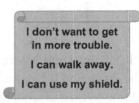

Figure 10.12 Joe's recovery script

Scenario 10.5

Betty is prone to anxiety attacks. Martha, a staff person, has already taught Betty how to notice when she is hyperventilating and to respond by practicing abdominal breathing. Martha is walking with Betty in a mall when she notices that Betty's face has become white. Betty stops and starts to take slow deep breaths. Martha also signs BREATHE very slowly. The signing (or speaking) of the word "breathe" is the beginning of the self-talk.

Martha: "Nice work. You're breathing slowly. Let's do it together."
They breathe together for a few minutes. Then Martha begins to model recovery self-talk. She starts signing to herself, in a way that makes it obvious that she is talking to herself.

Martha: "OK. Breathe slow. I am OK. I just feel anxious. Anxiety goes up and down. It always goes down. Anxiety can't harm me. Breathe, 1-2-3, 1-2-3, 1-2-3."
Martha looks to see if Betty is doing this along with her. However, Betty is just watching, not signing it herself. Martha gently asks Betty to copy her and sign together while they continue to breathe slowly.

Betty signs: "I am OK, I am OK."
Later, when the anxiety attack is over, Betty and Martha discuss what happened.

Martha: "I noticed you were using a few coping skills today. Did you notice them?"
Betty: "Breathing."
Martha: "Yes, you did a nice job of using slow breathing. But not just that."
Betty: "What?"

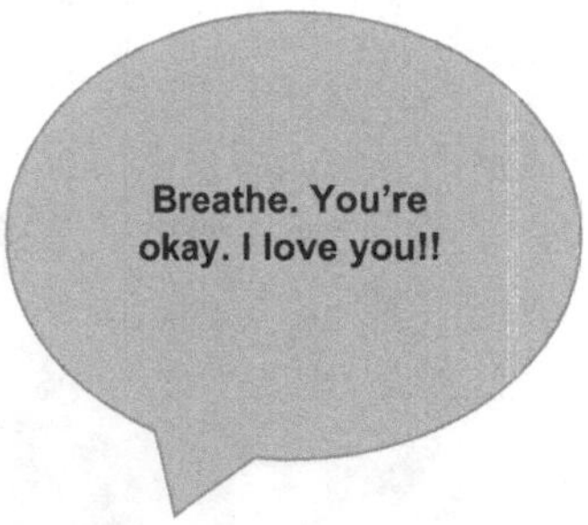

Figure 10.13 Peanuts' coaching of Betty

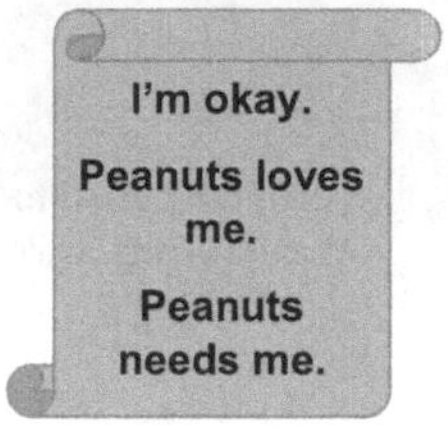

Figure 10.14 Betty's recovery script

Martha: *"Well, first you stopped and noticed your anxiety. Remember, that's the red light skill of stop and notice. Then you decided to do something to help yourself. I wonder if you said to yourself something like, 'I know what to do.'"*

Betty: *"I don't know. Breathe."*

Martha: *"Well, you breathed. Maybe you thought something like, 'I can breathe now.' Then we breathed together. Then you said, 'I'm OK. I'm OK.'"*

Betty: *"Yeah."*

Martha: *"Remember we talked about your anxiety monster and your comfort voice. You said your comfort voice comes from your cat, Peanuts. Maybe Peanuts was helping you talk to yourself by saying, 'I'm OK. I'm OK.' I wonder, could we figure out what else Peanuts might say to you to help you calm down? What does Peanuts say to you?"*

Betty: *"He says, 'I love you.'"*

Martha: *"So Peanuts says, 'Breathe. You're OK. I love you.' Let's write it down (See Figure 10.13)."*

Martha: *"What else would Peanuts say? I wonder if we could make a script together of everything he would say. Can we try?"*

Eventually, they create a script that Betty uses to talk to herself and remind herself of Peanuts' love (See Figure 10.14).

Both Emanuel and Martha are trying to help the people they work with to flesh out a recovery script. Some individuals find it helpful to learn a script that they can repeat when they are in distress. This can be a useful addition to their arsenal of coping skills. Self-talk also balances well with sensory-based grounding skills, such as physical exercise, applying pressure, or rubbing something. There is no question that being able to read and write helps but it isn't essential. What's most important is that the person is learning to talk to him or herself in order to achieve a desired response.

Scenario 10.6

Brian is a young deaf man who can read and write simple words and phrases. An outreach worker, George, works with Brian in his own apartment. Brian tends to become very anxious whenever he has to wait for what he wants or needs. Staff have observed that he handles his anxiety by becoming demanding, then threatening and insulting. Over time, staff drew out a behavioral analysis with him have helped him see this pattern:

Want something now ➡ *Nervous* ➡ *Must wait* ➡ *Angry* ➡ *Threaten and insult staff*

They've also discussed how staff react, and how he then reacts to them.

Staff afraid ➡ *Staff don't want to see Brian* ➡ *Brian more alone and unhappy*

George has helped Brian see this pattern, even though it took months of hard work. George also shared the dilemma that staff members have when working with Brian—staff want to help Brian, but they aren't always available the minute he needs them. In addition, when staff feel afraid, they don't want to see him, and they may be less friendly. Because Brian wants and needs staff to work with him, he agreed to work on various coping skills. He also *agreed to work on a simple script that he could write down and put on his refrigerator to read when he feels nervous. Brian and George developed this script together (Figure 10.15).*

A script can be as simple or complex as the person using it needs it to be. There are lots of good sources for coping statements. A quick Internet search on "coping statements for . . ." will generate many examples. In addition, most books on anger or anxiety management, for example, routinely include helpful self-talk. However, the complex English that some of them use may be difficult for people with language or learning challenges. Often, simple scripts with just a few words or phrases work best. For example:

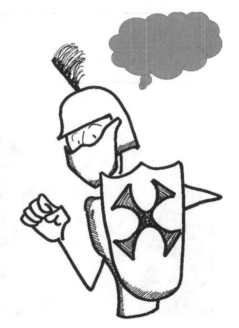

I nervous. I want staff attention. Staff busy now.

I can wait. Nervous is OK. I not die.

I breathe slow. I watch TV. I go out walk.

Later talk to staff. No yell. No threat.

Figure 10.15 Brian's recovery script

- Calm down. No hurt people.
- I can wait.
- I am okay.
- No one hurt me.
- I stay safe. Staff (or important person) proud.

This can also be done using pictures alone, although this is more difficult. In this case, additional role playing will be needed to help the person remember the script. For instance, the following picture can be used to help a person remember to use self-talk associated with the "shield" skill, as shown in Figure 10.16.

Again, because this is pre-therapy work, you are primarily trying to do two things:

Figure 10.16 Shield self-talk

1. Establish the concept of helpful-self talk.
2. Engage the person in developing a recovery script that they use.

If the person is seeing a therapist, hopefully the therapist also will help the individual build on this skill. Once the concepts are established, anyone working with the individual can help the person to elaborate on their coping, recovery thoughts. Once the person learns to examine their thoughts, they may be ready to benefit from more advanced cognitive therapy techniques.

Bright idea 10.2: Sometimes it helps to develop a formal script of words, phrases or sentences that you find helpful for coping with particular problems. Many people use slogans like "this too shall pass" or "no big deal." Alcoholics Anonymous is famous for its use of recovery-oriented slogans like "one day at a time" to combat the "stinkin' thinkin'" that leads to drinking problems.

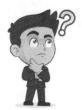

Questions to ponder 10.3: Do you have favorite phrases that you say to yourself to help you cope? Does the person you are working with already have such phrases? If so, use them to form the beginning of a recovery script. What else could be part of your own recovery script? Can you help the person you are working with find more helpful phrases?

1. Identify a comforting person, creature or presence that represents a healthy response to the problem you identified in the first exercise 1.
2. Create or find a picture that represents this creature.
3. Identify some of the thoughts that this creature might say to you.
4. Develop a coping and recovery-oriented script that would be associated with this creature.
5. Read it to oneself. Say or sign it "out loud."
6. How do you feel when you do this?

_____

_____

_____

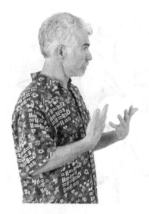
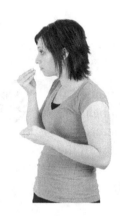

Figure 10.17 Role playing

©iStock.com/Lokibaho

Modeling and Role Playing

Some people who don't read or write well may have trouble understanding and using thought bubbles and scripts. Although it is more difficult, this work can be accomplished without writing anything down by clearly modeling the self-talk. Sometimes, you may need to explicitly ask the individual to "repeat after me." If the person can't write a script down and read it, you will likely need to rehearse it with them more often in order to help them remember it. Active role play practice is essential in almost all circumstances, whether or not the person is able to read.

Scenario 10.7

Sherry is another staff person who works in outreach with Brian, the young man you met in Scenario 10.6. Sherry is role playing with him on how to talk to himself. Unfortunately, Brian doesn't seem to remember what he learned in his previous work with George.

Sherry: "George told me about the anger coping script you are working on. Sounds awesome to me. Can we practice it together?"
Brian: "I don't know. I forgot it."
Sherry: "Oh. Did you write it down? George told me you put in on your refrigerator."
Brian: "I lost it."
Sherry: "Oh well. Can we try to make a new one? I thought it was a brilliant idea. Was that your idea?"
Brian: "Uh, I don't know."
Sherry: "It starts when you want staff but staff are busy, right?"
Brian: "Yeah."
Sherry: "You want staff, but they are busy. How do you feel?"
Brian: "Mad!"

Sherry:	*"Yeah, mad. But I think something else comes before mad. Do you get nervous first, then mad?"*
Brian:	*"Yeah."*
Sherry:	*"So you notice you are nervous, then you are mad. Then you talk to yourself to calm down. What do you say to yourself?"*
Brian:	*"I don't know. This is boring."*

At this point, Sherry realizes she has to re-engage Brian in this work. She does this by expressing:

- *Confusion. (e.g., "Oh, I thought you and George had already done this.")*
- *Then worry. (e.g., "I'm worried about you blowing up again at us and losing your team. I want to help you, but I need to feel safe too.").*
- *Then asking for help. (e.g., "Can you help me so that I can feel safe and then I can come and be here with you?")*

Despite her efforts, Brian is not interested today. Sherry tries again the next day. Eventually, Brian agrees to work on a script and then finds the paper that he and George had worked on.

Brian:	*"Here is the paper."*
Sherry:	*"Great! So can we role play this? How about if you be George, and I'll be you. Okay? Can I have the paper?"*
	Brian gives her the paper.
Sherry reads out loud:	*"I nervous. I want staff attention now. Staff busy."*
Sherry:	*"Then what do I say?"*
	She hands the paper back to Brian who puts it aside. Sherry takes it back.
Sherry:	*"Can you copy me?"*
Sherry, playing Brian:	*"I can wait. Nervous is OK. I not die."*
Brian:	*"I can wait. Nervous is OK. I not die."*
Sherry:	*"I can wait. Nervous is OK. I not die. What else can I say to myself? Can you remember anything?"*
Brian:	*"Calm down. Don't blow up."*
	Sherry writes this down and repeats it.
Sherry:	*"Calm down. Don't blow up. What else?"*
Brian:	*"I don't know."*
Sherry:	*"Let me see if I can think of some things. What about, 'No emergency. Staff busy. I am OK. I will not die. I can wait. Later talk staff'?"*
Brian:	*"Okay."*
Sherry:	*"Should we write that down?*
	Sherry hands him the paper. "What would you write? I'll help you."
	Sherry knows Brian can't write well and is careful not to embarrass him about this. She offers help when he seems receptive.
	Sherry is coaching a reluctant Brian through this process step by step. She prefers that Brian uses his own words, but if he is unable to come up with them, she'll offer suggestions and ask him to add to them. If Brian could not read or write at all, Sherry could still try to coach him to remember the script or look for pictures that could serve as prompts.
	Later, they role play again. Sherry again plays Brian and Brian plays George.
Sherry (as Brian):	*"I want to talk to staff now! I am mad! I am nervous!"*
Brian (as George):	*"Calm down!"*
	Sherry (as Brian, thinking out loud): "I'm supposed to read something, to talk to myself. Where is the paper?"
Brian:	*"You put it on your refrigerator."*

Sherry:	*"Oh, yeah."*
	Sherry gets the paper and starts to read the script. Then stops.
Sherry (as Brian):	*"This is stupid!"*
	By now, Brian is starting to enjoy taking on the role of George, the staff person.
Brian (as George):	*"No, read it. You don't want staff to be afraid."*
Sherry (as Brian):	*"Right. If I stay calm, staff will come see me."*
	Sherry models thinking this out loud.
Sherry:	*"Hmm, now think, Sherry, think. If I stay calm, staff feel safe, and then they come see me. I can do it. I can show them."*
Sherry (to Brian):	*"Should I add that to the paper?"*
	Eventually, over many sessions, they develop a coping script, which becomes another coping strategy for Brian. George and Sherry ask Brian to share the script with other staff working with him and with Simon, his counselor, so that all of them can work together to help Brian develop this new ability.
	The team also finds they can draw on this coping strategy at other times. For instance, they use it with Brian during his treatment planning meetings when he seems to be on the verge of becoming angry. They decide to ask Brian to begin all their meetings with a minute of deep breathing, followed by reading his coping script. They also ask him to teach the coping script to another person. The tool's usefulness, combined with other coping tools, becomes more apparent when Brian begins to use it on his own and even starts to add new phrases to it.

Bright idea 10.3: Memorizing a script may be a good starting point, but it is not a great ending point. You want people to use the script as a prompt for finding their own words. Ideally, they will adjust the script to fit the situation. Some people do best when they have a script to follow but, whenever possible, encourage people to find new, different words to accomplish the same goal. You want them to experience this as real and convincing self-talk, not just empty phrases.

Bright idea 10.4: Coping scripts can only work if they are practiced and used. Role playing is an excellent way to practice them. It often helps to start by having the client act out the staff role, coaching the staff person who pretends to need help remembering what to say. This often elicits more insight into the person's self-talk. Then, you can switch roles.

Questions to Help People Think Differently

Lessons 3, 6, and 7 focused on asking good questions to help people recognize their skills, thoughts, and behaviors. This is more effective than directing or giving advice. Good questions help people discover their own answers. And, when people discover answers on their own, they are more likely to use what they learn.

Cognitive behavioral therapists are trained to ask many questions. But, as you've learned, many standard CBT questions are based on the assumption that the person has abstract thinking abilities. Many of the individuals you serve will not have these abilities, at least initially, and sometimes ever. What follows is a set of common CBT questions. Can the people you serve readily understand these questions? If they can, great! If they can't, can you develop their ability to understand questions such as these? That's the pre-therapy work:

- Do you notice what you are thinking? And what you are feeling? How are they connected?
- When you think this way, how do you feel? When you feel that, how do you think? How do these thoughts and feelings effect your behavior?

- What kind of thinking goes along with a depressed mood? Before you harm youself, what goes on in your mind? When you talk to yourself that way, what happens?
- How much do you believe that thought that goes on in your head? How much do you doubt it?
- What evidence tells you whether or not that belief is true or helpful?
- Where did these ideas come from?
- How could you test whether or not that idea is true or helpful?
- If you were talking to a friend who said that to him or herself, how would you respond to your friend? How would you try to show your friend that his or her thinking is making things worse?
- If you think this way, how do you benefit? Is there a cost connected with thinking this way?

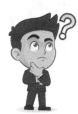 **Questions to ponder 10.4:** Is the meaning of all of these questions clear to you? Could you answer them for yourself?

Let's look at two scenarios that show how this kind of questioning is used with someone who has adequate language and thinking skills, compared with the experience of someone with language challenges in a similar situation.

Scenario 10.8

Sally was just admitted into a mental health respite program. She had thoughts of wanting to harm herself, but the emergency room worker thought she would do better with a short stay in the respite program than in a psychiatric hospital. On arrival at the respite program, Ben, a staff person, asks Sally what's been going on in her life recently.

Sally: *"I can't believe I'm here again. I'm so stupid. I should be able to handle things without having to come here or, even worse, end up in the hospital every time I'm stressed out."*

Ben: *"So you're telling yourself, 'I'm stupid because I'm here again.' Is that right? You're not saying to yourself, 'I did a good job asking for support, and I'm going to try to use this program for a few days to feel stronger.' You're not saying that. You're just saying you are stupid and, I'm guessing that you are also saying that you are a failure. Is that right?"*
Sally nods.

Ben: *"Well, I know that you struggle with depression. I wonder, when you say you're stupid, if that is the depression talking?"*

Sally: *"No. I really am stupid."*

Ben: *"You really believe you are stupid. You don't think this is depression talking. You think it is the truth. And when you think that way, you feel . . .?"*
Sally pauses before answering.

Sally: *"Depressed."*

Ben: *"Are you sure that notion that you are stupid isn't coming from the depression monster?*

Sally may be capable of considering more abstract questions, such as the ones listed earlier. But, what would happen if the person can't understand these questions?

Scenario 10.9, Part A

Alan is also in the respite program but has much more limited capacity for understanding these questions. He is depressed and hasn't been able to clearly identify his thoughts. His reading and writing skills are poor so thought bubbles or scripts would have to be limited to a few key words. When Ben, the staff person, tried to ask Alan what he was thinking, Alan responded with a blank stare.

Alan: "I don't understand. I'm stupid."
Ben: "You're thinking, 'I'm stupid.'"
          Alan nods.
Ben: "You say to yourself, 'I'm stupid.'"
Alan: "Yes."
Ben: "You're thinking, 'I'm stupid,' and you are feeling depressed. Do you think they are connected?"
          Alan shrugs and looks away.
Ben: "I want to try to act this out. OK? So, here I am, Ben, I'm talking to myself. 'Ben, you are stupid! You are the stupidest person in the world. Everyone knows you are stupid!' How do you think I feel?"
Alan: "Stupid?"
Ben: "Yeah, and what else? Happy? Sad?"
Alan: "Sad."
Ben: "Yeah. I tell myself, 'You are stupid.' Then I feel more sad, more depressed."
          Alan nods.
Ben: "What could I tell myself to feel better?"
          Alan walks away.
          Ben isn't sure what Alan understood. While Alan is in the respite program, Ben will keep looking for opportunities to help Alan notice his thoughts. He'll also try creating a depression monster with Alan and role playing the depression monster and ways to talk back to it. He'll also look for evidence of anything Alan does that shows intelligence, such as Alan's skills at working jigsaw puzzles. Ben will see if he can catch Alan working on the puzzle in the main room and then ask him, one-down, how Alan can do the puzzle if he is stupid. If Alan doesn't respond to any of this, Ben will try to help him notice other coping skills such as "walk-away" skills or "distraction with puzzles" skills. Alan may not yet be able to use a cognitive coping strategy like self-talk.

Even when a person has difficulty identifying thoughts, they will still show you what they think. In Scenario 10.9, Part A, Alan says, "I am stupid." These thoughts are symptoms of depression, as well as causes of depression. The trouble is that Alan isn't yet able to think about his thoughts. For the moment, Ben has more information about what contributes to Alan's depression than Alan does and, as a result, is looking for any avenue that may open this up for him.

Scenario 10.9, Part B

Ben takes advantage of another opportunity to work with Alan when he notices Alan using some self-talk that helps him cope. When Alan appeared to be frustrated with a peer, Alan walked away and said to another staff person, "I don't want to talk to him. I'm going to my room." Ben seizes the moment.

Ben: "I just have to tell you, you are using some good thinking skills."
          Alan shrugs.
Ben: "You seemed to be thinking. 'I don't want to talk to him. I'm going to my room.' You weren't mean or insulting or threatening. You just thought, 'I will take a break right now.' Am I right?"
Alan: "I don't know."
          Alan walks to his room.
          By asking good questions, Ben has planted the seed. This may be the best possible intervention right now. Ben should keep working on this, possibly for a long time, before he concludes that Alan isn't capable of working on changing his self-talk. However, he should also look for non-cognitive coping skills, such as sensory grounding skills, that may be easier for Alan to understand and use.

Here are some ways to ask simpler questions about thinking. Notice, again, how the simpler cognitive therapy is just about self-talk. There is little or no analysis of thinking patterns or questions about evidence. Instead, it's just about practicing different words that someone can say to themselves that help them feel better. There is a little bit of perspective taking skill involved (the monsters' perspective vs the recovery creatures' perspective). If they respond to this, we can try developing the skill using the more advanced questions:

1. What did you just say to yourself? What went on in your head?
2. Is that the depression monster or the recovery monster talking?
3. What would the anger monster say? How does the monster convince you to feel/behave that way?
4. What does the recovery/coping/helpful voice in your head say? If that voice came from a creature, what would the creature be/look like? What else would it say?

If an individual is unable to reflect on what has happened, try acting it out. Model what the person appears to be thinking and speak/or sign it to make it visible. Ask the person to do this, then ask, "What did you feel?" You also can do the same thing with scripts that promote coping and recovery.

Helping people to tune into their thinking can take a long time. But it is worth the effort! Once people can observe their own thoughts, they have more tools for coping and recovery. People who can pay attention to their own thoughts are better prepared for CBT.

Practice Exercise 10.3, Part A

1. Ask a colleague to help you with this exercise.
2. Ask the person to identify a problem emotion or symptom.
3. Ask the person to create a creature that represents the problem.
4. Ask the person to create a creature that represents recovery.
5. Ask the person to explain the self-talk that fosters the problem.
6. Ask the person to explain the self-talk that fosters the recovery.
7. Write out a recovery script that the person might use.

Practice Exercise 10.3, Part B

1. Ask the other person to role play the problem thinking related to the problem identified in Part A of this exercise.
2. Ask the other person to role play the recovery script.
3. Present the strongest argument for each position as you can.

Lesson 10 Skill Sheet

- Participant demonstrates the ability to help a person externalize a problem emotion or symptom by creating a monster that verbalizes the self-talk that creates these emotions/symptoms.
- Participant demonstrates the ability to help a person create a creature that verbalizes the self-talk associated with coping and recovery.
- Participant demonstrates the ability to help a person create a recovery script for a particular mood state.
- Participant demonstrates the ability to engage in a role play of both a problem and a recovery-oriented script.
- Participant can ask questions that help people notice healthy self-talk.

Lesson 10 Quiz

1. Samantha is a client in a program. One day, a staff person hears Samantha say, "Everyone treats me like crap! You stink, every one of you!" What mood is most likely associated with these statements?

    a. Depression.
    b. Anger.
    c. Anxiety.
    d. Satisfaction.

2. Which of the following techniques could be used to help Samantha recognize how thinking this way affects her mood and behavior? (Check all that apply.)

    a. Put the thoughts in a thought bubble and ask Samantha if that is what she is really thinking.
    b. Ask her to create a monster that thinks this way, then ask her what else the monster would say.
    c. Ask Samantha if she notices how she feels while she is saying what the monster would say.
    d. Ask Samantha to do an Internet search on cognitive distortions associated with an angry mood.

3. Which of the following techniques might help Samantha to notice and change her thinking as a way of decreasing her anger?

    a. Ask her to create an anger monster and a coping creature.
    b. Ask her what the coping creature she created would say to her to help her calm down when she is angry like that.
    c. Ask her if she is willing to write out a script to help her cope when she is really angry.
    d. Ask if she is willing to role play how to use self-talk to make her less angry.
    e. Ask her if she wants to better understand why she became such an angry person.

4. Which of the following coping thoughts could Samantha find useful? (Check all that apply.)

    a. "Well, maybe I'm exaggerating. Not everyone treats me like crap. Just some people."
    b. "If I keep getting so angry, I'm going to make myself sick."
    c. "Maybe this isn't as bad as I'm thinking.
    d. "All of you can go to Hell!"

5. Which of the following self-talk statements are most likely to promote coping well with a stressor? (Check all that apply.)

    a. "I can't stand it!"

    b. "No big deal."

    c. "Just because you have a problem doesn't mean I have to take it on."

    d. "I don't deserve to be treated any better."

Lesson 10 Questions for Discussion

1. Have you ever used the technique of externalizing to represent a mood or problem?

2. Are you aware of an inner comforting voice? Is the voice associated with a person, religious figure, or God? Have you ever used a pet to represent a comforting voice?

3. How easy is it for you to shift between the voice of the problem and the voice of the recovery? How easy is it for you to embellish each voice and present it as a convincing expression of the script for each side?

4. When you listen to another person, how much can you "hear" a script that promotes a problem vs. a script that promotes recovery?

5. Have you been part of an agency or organization, such as Alcoholics Anonymous, that promotes the use of particular slogans as a recovery strategy? Are there any slogans you already draw upon that help you cope with problems?

6. If you are part of a religious tradition, does it offer a "script" that helps you cope with your problems? Does your religious tradition also provide a script that contributes to greater emotional distress?

7. As you work with people to help them notice thoughts that promote both distress and recovery, do you see a difference in their capacity to understand and do this task?

8. CBT, especially the C or cognitive part, involves asking a lot of abstract questions. Many people with language and learning challenges have difficulty with this kind of task. However, the cognitive part of CBT also can be accomplished by focusing on self-talk and helping people learn self-talk associated with coping and recovery. Do you think this second strategy is "easier" than asking abstract questions? Can you use this cognitive strategy with all the people you serve?

9. Can you think of a time when you were in a stressful or difficult situation and you coached yourself through it? What was the situation? What did you say to yourself?

10. Are there sayings, slogans or affirmations that you use to help yourself cope with stress? What are they?

Lesson 10 Quiz Answers

1. Samantha's statements, "Everyone treats me like crap!" and "You stink, every one of you!" are most likely feeding feelings of anger. However, she might have an underlying belief that "I'm not worth being treated well." This would reflect depression more than anger. The people supporting her will need to explore whether this or another underlying belief is involved.

2. All of these interventions might be helpful. Some people find that externalizing feelings through an anger monster is helpful; others find the exercise childish. Asking Samantha to do a web search is the most intellectually demanding and academic task. This is more appropriate for people with adequate reading skills who are already inclined to search the Internet for answers. If you know that a person likes to use the web that way, you could use questions—not directions or commands—to guide the person to use their skills to research this topic.

3.   Any of the suggestions in answers *a* through *d* might help. The way that *e* is framed is problematic. You don't want to suggest that Samantha is an "angry person." That's the opposite of externalizing. In externalizing, the goal is to put the problem (anger), outside of the person so they can work on it. If you say she is an "angry person," you root the problem in her personality, making it more difficult to help her learn skills that will help her to change.

4.   Answers *a* through *c* are possible coping thoughts. Answer *d* would, quite clearly, promote angry feelings.

5.   Answers *b* and *c* would promote coping. *D* would promote depression. *A* could promote anger, depression or anxiety depending on what else the person says to him or herself.

Note

1. Externalization is a technique made popular in the narrative approach to family therapy (Freedman & Combs 1996; White 2007; White & Epston 1990).

Bibliography

The externalizing strategy comes from the "narrative therapy" work of Michael White and David Epston (1990). Matthew Selekman (1997) is one of many who describes using the technique of drawing a monster to help children externalize a problem. In their book, March and Mulle (1998) use this technique to help children cope with obsessive compulsive disorder externalize their symptoms. Donald Meichenbaum's later work, in which he uses a lot of narrative or "constructivist" techniques, focuses on asking good questions and, as he says, "plucking out" people's stories of coping, recovery, and resiliency.

Freedman, J., & Combs, G. (1996). *Narrative therapy: The social construction of preferred realities*. New York: W. W. Norton & Company, Inc.

March, J. S., & Mulle, K. (1998). *OCD in children and adolescents: A cognitive-behavioral treatment manual*. New York: Guilford Press.

Meichenbaum, D (1994). *A clinical handbook/practical therapist manual for assessing and treating adults with post-traumatic stress disorder*. Waterloo, Canada: Institute Press.

Meichenbaum, D. (2001). *Treatment of individuals with anger-control problems and aggressive behaviors: A clinical handbook*. Clearwater, FL: Institute Press.

Selekman, M. (1997). *Solution-focused therapy with children: Harnessing family strengths for systemic change*. New York: Guilford Press.

White, M (2007). *Maps of narrative practice*. New York: W. W. Norton & Company, Inc.

White, M., & Epston, D. (1990). *Narrative means to therapeutic ends*. New York: W. W. Norton & Company, Inc.

Deaf Mental Health Care and Relapse Prevention I

Introduction

Lessons 11 and 12 introduce five key counseling and teaching techniques that are particularly effective when working with persons with language and learning challenges. You'll also learn how to apply these techniques to relapse prevention, a common but advanced CBT approach. I chose relapse prevention both because it is important that all mental health workers have some grounding in it and because this approach can be particularly hard to implement with persons who have language and learning challenges. I want to illustrate how five teaching/counseling strategies commonly used in Deaf mental health care (DMHC) are helpful for making the complex topic of relapse prevention more accessible.

Five Key Strategies

These five teaching/counseling strategies are so widely used in Deaf mental health care that practitioners may not even realize that they are far less commonly used with hearing persons. The first four have been discussed and illustrated throughout this workbook; the fifth is new. These five crucial DMHC teaching and counseling strategies are:

1. Mindful attention to language and communication.
2. Using teaching stories and examples.
3. Using visual aids and art.
4. Role playing.
5. Drawing on the desire of community members to help and teach each other.

Strategies 1 and 2 are presented in this lesson. The remaining three are presented in Lesson 12.

These last two lessons will move back and forth between discussions of Deaf mental health care and discussions of relapse prevention. The goal is both to offer practical strategies to make this advanced topic easier to understand and to illustrate some contributions from Deaf mental health care. This entire workbook, while offering techniques that are helpful when working with hearing persons with language and learning challenges, is grounded in decades of my own experience and that of many colleagues in Deaf mental health care using these techniques.

Finally, hopefully you will recognize how the pre-therapy work covered in this workbook serves as a bridge to the more familiar world of CBT. The pre-therapy work presented here is somewhat like a prequel movie. For instance, *Star Wars 4, 5*, and *6*, were made, and then the prequel stories, *Star Wars 1, 2*, and *3*, were created. Too much of CBT starts at too advanced a level for many persons served in mental health and rehabilitation programs. It assumes foundational skills that may not be there so we have to construct this foundation; that is, do the pre-therapy work first. We see with each individual how far into the world of CBT they can go.

Introduction to Relapse Prevention

Scenario 11.1

Alan is trying very hard to stick to his low-calorie diet. His wife and friends support his efforts. He carefully monitors the food he takes in and allows himself cookies and pastries only once a week and, then, only in small portions. However, when he attended a family reunion, his aunt offers him a large piece of the cake she has made. His aunt says, "I made this just for you because I love you so much. I worked on it for three hours. Don't you care about all the work I put into making this for you? How can you say no to your loving aunt?" Alan doesn't want to hurt his aunt's feelings so he eats a piece of cake. Later he becomes angry with himself for letting his aunt make him feel guilty for trying to follow his diet plan.

Alan had trouble following his weight loss plan because he failed to think about situations in which he would be tempted to relapse. In other words, he didn't have a strong relapse prevention plan. A relapse prevention plan is a *self-management* plan that a person sets up for him/herself to change a specific behavior that he or she has identified. In this case, Alan recognizes that weight and food are problems *for him* and he voluntarily and skillfully sets up a plan to help him manage this problem. He has support—his wife and some friends encourage him to follow the plan. But his aunt, clearly, is not on board. Before he went to the family reunion, he should have thought through what might happen and how he would respond if she used guilt to get him to eat something that clearly is not on his diet. She's probably been doing this his whole life. But, because he didn't anticipate that happening, he wasn't ready to manage this *trigger*.

As a mental health worker, you could help Alan create a relapse prevention plan but he's the only one who can decide whether or not to follow it. Although you can't make Alan follow his diet, you can help him in other ways. For example, you could help him think about how he might respond to his aunt next time or help him to recognize and predict other kinds of trigger and high-risk situation that could prompt him to relapse. You also could help him to create a plan for avoiding these triggers. But, in the end, only Alan can decide what he will do.

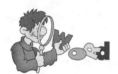

Relapse prevention

Definition 11.1: Relapse prevention: Relapse prevention refers to strategies people adopt to prevent the reoccurrence of a problem behavior, symptom or mood.

Example of relapse prevention: Chris knows he has a drinking problem and is trying to stay sober. He finds it hard to not drink wine when his friends do so he asks them if they mind not drinking when he is with them.

For a relapse prevention plan to work, the person needs:

- To "own" the problem; that is, to accept that he has a problem and he is responsible for changing it.
- To "own" the plan *and* its strategies.
- To be motivated to follow it.
- The right set of skills.
- A good set of social supports.

Any behavior that a person considers a problem can be the basis for a relapse prevention plan. Relapse prevention plans are often developed to change behaviors such as:

- Smoking.
- Eating.
- Substance abuse.

- Aggressive or self-harming behaviors.
- Problem sexual behaviors.

Relapse prevention plans also can be used to help people manage symptoms *they* don't want. For instance, symptoms of depression, mania, panic attacks, suicide attempts, and hallucinations can all be treated with relapse prevention plans, *but only if the person understands and wants to use them for that purpose.*

Skills Required for Relapse Prevention

Relapse prevention requires more complex skills than simple coping or conflict resolution skills. However, coping and conflict resolution skills are an important part of any relapse prevention plan and must already be present for a plan to work. This is one reason that pre-therapy work places so much attention to helping people recognize, label, and develop these skills. Having a vocabulary about simple, foundational skills, and an appreciation that one already has some of these skills, clears the path to CBT and then to relapse prevention.

Consider this common example of a statement that might be included in an anger management relapse prevention plan: *"I will notice I am angry and give myself a time out. I will go outside for a five minute walk."* Obviously, in order to put this plan into action, the person would need the coping skills of *noticing and labeling one's feelings* and then *removing oneself from a situation.* Social skills, such as asking for help and managing interpersonal conflicts, are also commonly used in many relapse prevention plans. For example: *"When I'm tempted to drink, I will call my sponsor."* In this case, other skills also need to be present, such as noticing the urge to drink and establishing and using a relationship with a sponsor.

Other skills that are often required for relapse prevention can be seen in Table 11.1.

TABLE 11.1 Skills Required for Relapse Prevention

Ownership of a problem	The person must believe: "This is my problem. I don't want it anymore and I will take action to prevent it." Some of the people you serve do not have this kind of understanding and motivation, nor do they believe that they can actually do something to impact their own lives (i.e., a sense of personal agency). Typically, relapse prevention plans are created with people who are actively trying to change. At this point, they are *not* engaged in pre-therapy but are well into the process of changing themselves.
Ability to predict and anticipate when problems might occur in the future and plan how they will respond	Coping skills are used in the present; a relapse prevention plan is developed for the future. The person must be able to plan for what *might* happen at a later date. The person must therefore have a strong sense of linear time and the ability to understand and imagine cause and effect (e.g., "If this happens . . . then that.") If a person's sense of linear time is weak, they won't be able to make and follow a plan designed for use at some future time. This is a particular challenge for many deaf people who have experienced extreme language deprivation.
Abstract thinking and analytic abilities	A coping plan involves things as simple as going for a walk or breathing. A relapse prevention plan requires a person to be able to understand abstract concepts, such as "triggers," "risks," and "warning signs." The individual also needs to be able to brainstorm, evaluate solutions and see patterns (e.g., the way you behave here is similar to how you behave there and requires a similar relapse prevention strategy.). These problem-solving and rational thinking abilities must already be in place.
Ability to implement the plan during times of stress	Relapse prevention plans are usually created when the person feels calm; yet, they need to be implemented at a time the person is triggered and feeling stressed. For instance, you would most likely plan how to handle a craving to drink at a time when you don't feel the craving. Later, when you do feel the craving and are at risk for relapsing, you are in a different emotional state than when you made the plan. A person's ability to carry out a plan when they are satisfied and calm is not the same as a person's ability to carry out a plan when they actually crave a drink. Many people who develop wonderful relapse prevention plans fail to use them because what they learned in one emotional state is hard to apply when they are in another emotional state.

Based on this information, you can see why relapse prevention is a CBT topic, not a cognitive behavioral *pre-therapy* topic. Relapse prevention work is typically the final stage of CBT when one is engaged in using skills to prevent old patterns from re-emerging. For example:

Example 1: An alcoholic who attends regular AA meetings, works with her sponsor, avoids her old drinking buddies, seeks out special supports at high-risk times like New Year's Eve, and has let everyone in her family know not to offer her drinks has the knowledge, skills, and supports to manage her addiction on her own. She has the skills she needs to keep herself sober.

Example 2: A man who has panic attacks while driving has developed a set of strategies to help him cope while behind the wheel. He uses slow, deep breathing and positive self-talk. He keeps packs of gum in the glove compartment because he finds the chewing motions helpful. He plans his route to be sure there are places he can stop at. He has a medication nearby that he can take if necessary. Just knowing it is there seems to be calming for him. This man is managing his problem and preventing the re-occurrence of panic attacks.

Even though relapse prevention is an advanced CBT topic, it can be made more accessible for people who are in pre-therapy. Deaf mental health care providers often adapt standard therapy practices to make them more accessible to people with language challenges. Even people with strong language skills and a solid educational background benefit from these adaptations because they can make the work more fun, interesting and engaging.

 Bright idea 11.1: Relapse prevention requires a more complex set of skills than managing internal experiences (e.g., coping or emotion self-regulation) or managing relationships with other people. It is typically introduced and worked on towards the end of CBT. However, you can make it easier and more appealing with some creative treatment adaptations.

Teaching and Counseling Strategy 1: Mindful Attention to Language and Communication

Like hearing people, every deaf person is a unique individual with different abilities, skills, interests, personalities, and talents. Yet, if any single statement comes close to being universally true among deaf people it is this: *Deaf people care deeply about communication.* They attend to it constantly. When problems occur, they often attribute the problems to poor communication and will say, *"The problem is communication and the solution is better communication."* Because deaf people are so routinely left out of conversations and the sharing of information, they develop an exquisite sensitivity to communication matters. When they are in a position to improve service delivery in programs, they almost always focus first on how to improve the communication environment for deaf people.

A hallmark of talented Deaf mental health and education professionals is the care they devote to the communication process. In general, hearing people tend not to be as attuned to the nuances of communication. Because they have always had access to at least one language, they find it hard to imagine life without a native language or living with poor language skills or a life where you must fight each day to be included in the conversation.

Unfortunately, this lack of appreciation for other people's communication struggles tends to get worse with more education. As people become better educated, their language skills become more sophisticated and complex. In time, individuals with more education may talk over the heads of less educated people, often without realizing it. Mental health professionals, as a group, are highly educated. The main tools they use are language and conversation, both of which work most easily with people who have good language skills and value self-analysis; in other words, people like themselves.

Talented Deaf counselors and teachers have something important to teach the rest of us—the value of paying mindful attention to the communication process. They do not assume that they are communicating clearly or that the people they work with understand them. Instead, they regularly check in about communication and are always on the lookout for ways to communicate more clearly.

Am I Clear?

One question that these Deaf counselors and teachers repeatedly return to—Am I clear?—needs to be asked much more often than it typically is, especially in connection with working with people who are not skilled language users. The strategy of close and mindful attention to communication, the hallmark of Deaf mental health care, is the starting point for all work with people who have language and learning challenges.

The question, "Am I clear?" is very different from the question, "Do you understand?" Deaf people are very sensitive to this difference. "Am I clear?" is a more respectful question because it puts the responsibility for good communication on the speaker, not the person receiving the message. It means "I'm responsible for communicating better." By the same token, "Do you understand?" presumes that any communication problems are the recipient's fault. Even after asking "Am I clear," skilled DMHC counselors continue to confirm that communication is successful.

Scenario 11.2

Janet is a deaf person with a moderate developmental disability who communicates using a vocabulary of approximately 25 signs. She lives in a group home with all hearing peers. She also attends a day habilitation program where she is the only deaf person. The staff who work with her are all hearing people. They attend sign language classes where they learn sign vocabulary for common objects and actions like toilet, eat, drink, help, etc. Staff members think that because Janet has a vocabulary of 25 signs, they need only a slightly larger vocabulary. They aren't that invested in helping Janet's vocabulary grow beyond a few more words for common objects and actions and think their own signing abilities are "good enough." As a result, Janet's vocabulary essentially stays the same. Janet continues to have behavioral problems that people sometimes, but not always, recognize as related to her communication difficulties. No one seems to think that the problem lies with them, that they are not clear, that they need help, and that Janet needs exposure to real sign communication experts, not people whose sign communication abilities are as limited as hers.

All babies begin life without knowledge of language. Imagine if people believed that, therefore, the child's parents only needed a small vocabulary or that when a baby knows five words, her parents only needed to know six words. It is widely accepted that it takes a person with native abilities in a language to teach a child to become a native user of that language. Unfortunately, in too many instances, people who work with deaf children think that any degree of sign language skill is "good enough." When they work with a deaf person whose sign language skills are poor, they often mistakenly believe that it is acceptable for staff to have equally poor sign language skills. The opposite is actually true. The more dysfluent and impoverished the person's language skills, the more they need to work with language experts who know how to help them develop language.

Scenario 11.3

Cindy is a Deaf woman with severe cerebral palsy (CP) who attends a day treatment program. Cindy can communicate reasonably well through finger spelling but her CP makes it difficult for her to use formal sign language. Nonetheless, she has a good receptive understanding of ASL. Cindy needs nearly total physical assistance to eat, dress, use the bathroom, and all other tasks of daily living. It can be very painful to her when a staff member moves her the wrong way. She stiffens and lashes out by biting or spitting, and then accuses the staff of abusing her.

The director of the day treatment program hired a hearing person who knows some signs to work with Cindy. This person also works with about 20 other clients. When asked how they provide Cindy with communication access, the director refers to the new staff signer. There is a day program with more signing Deaf clients and staff about 30 minutes away but, since it is "out of area," there are no financial resources to send Cindy there.

Cindy regularly complains to her mother that no one communicates with her at the day program. The staff person and program director are completely baffled. How could this be? After all, a staff person who "knows sign language" communicates with her every day. The program director proudly points out that he hired this signing staff person specifically so Cindy would have someone to talk with. He reminds Cindy's mother that the center doesn't have the resources to hire Deaf staff or interpreters for one deaf client. He believes that what he has done is good enough.

This kind of communication misunderstanding can have serious health consequences as seen in Scenario 11.4.

Scenario 11.4

One night on a psychiatric inpatient unit, something bad may have happened. While doing ward checks, Joe, a staff person, entered the bedroom of Isabel, a deaf developmentally disabled woman who had severe language deficits. Isabel appeared to be very upset. Joe asked Isabel what was wrong. She mentioned that a male patient on the unit, a young hearing man named Claude who Isabel was known to like, had pressured her to kiss him and touch him sexually. At least that's what Joe, who knew just a little sign language, thought Isabel said.

Joe was very enthusiastic about learning sign language and working with deaf people. He regularly volunteered to "interpret" for Isabel and any other deaf patients that were occasionally admitted to the unit. Isabel was distressed and Joe wanted to help, but it was hard for him to admit that he didn't really understand what she was saying.

Joe told the charge nurse that Isabel said the male patient had pressured her to have sex. The charge nurse, who couldn't communicate with Isabel, sent her for an invasive medical examination for sexual assault. The nurse wasn't clear what had happened, but felt it was her responsibility to rule out any kind of rape. During this exam, the doctor examined her private parts. When Isabel returned, she seemed even more distressed.

The next day, a Deaf social worker and expert interpreters were brought in to help Isabel and determine what should happen next. The first thing they learned was that it was not at all clear what exactly had happened. There were numerous communication errors and staff had jumped to several conclusions. Nobody involved understood Isabel's communication abilities and nobody explained to her, in a way she could understand, why she was going to a hospital and why a doctor was examining the private parts of her body.

It actually took the social worker and interpreters several hours to get a clearer version of the story from Isabel. To do this, they used role playing. They used toy human figures. They drew pictures. They used simple sign language and gestures that matched Isabel's sign communication abilities. They knew that Isabel had difficulty telling a story, with a clear beginning, middle, and end, and using time references. She often was not clear about who did what to whom. She also wasn't always able to clearly separate what actually happened from what she hoped or feared might happen. The interview required both linguistic and clinical sensitivity.

The medical evaluation did not show evidence of physical penetration or damage. Yet, even with all the communication resources that were brought in, it was impossible for the team to be confident about what actually happened. They knew that Isabel was frightened, perhaps as much by the way staff responded as by whatever has occurred. They took steps to protect and help her.

It's easy to assume that the people you serve easily understand the words you use every day. In fact, many times they can't and don't. It's also can be easy to assume this even when you speak the same language.

Scenario 11.5

Simon is a staff person whose been asked to run an "anger management group" for people in the group home where he works. Simon and all the residents of the home are hearing people. He approaches two residents with particularly explosive tempers. He announces that he is starting a group "for people who have problems with anger" and that it's called an "anger management group." He explains that they will be learning about triggers and coping skills and ways to recognize and change thinking errors. He asks if they want to join.

Both residents stare at him blankly. They don't have a clue what he's talking about.

Simon hadn't considered whether the residents would understand the psychological jargon that was used in the anger management workbook he is using. He also hasn't considered that some residents won't be able to read or understand much of the book. Simon is frustrated that none of the house members is showing interest in this new group even though they continue to show aggressive behaviors.

Even really competent language users may have reasons for not understanding what a health professional says as Scenario 11.6 illustrates.

Scenario 11.6

Lucia has a doctorate in European medieval studies. She is a highly intelligent and accomplished scholar. However, she's just been diagnosed with what appears to be a malignant brain tumor and is in emotional shock. Her doctor is talking to her in highly technical language about her treatment options. She stares at him and doesn't take in anything he's saying. After he describes the options, he gives her a few brochures and leaves the examination room. When she arrives home, Lucia tells her wife, Sue, that she has a malignant tumor. Sue asks her questions, but Lucia can't recall anything else the doctor said.

As this scenario illustrates, the problem of poor communication in human services is widespread and isn't confined to mental health services for minority language users. Poor communication can be a problem even when working with highly intelligent, competent language users like Lucia. When deaf people are served in treatment programs, their communication skills and needs are often poorly understood and the resources to create inclusion may not be secured. Interpreters may be part of the resources needed, but are interpreters sufficient? How well prepared are the interpreters to work with this particular client? Skillful communication assessments of the deaf person's spoken and sign language abilities are rarely done. The treatment providers usually don't know the right questions to ask and probably don't know what effective communication *with this person* looks like.

It is important to understand the individual's actual language abilities and to consider how well an interpreter can help bridge the gap. Can the communication be clear if the people receiving services don't understand the concepts being discussed or the communication process is rapid and confusing with many people interrupting each other? An equally important issue is whether or not anyone even questions the effectiveness of the communication process.

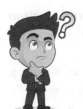

Questions to ponder 11.1: Have you ever talked to a health professional and not understood them well? Have you had similar experiences elsewhere, such as talking with tradespeople or anyone who uses jargon particular to their field?

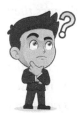

Questions to ponder 11.2: Are you making assumptions about what the people you work with understand? Do you ever ask, "Am I clear?" Do you question whether the communication resources you have available are sufficient?

Bright idea 11.2: It's common to assume you are communicating effectively when you aren't. Checking out whether or not you are clear, asking for feedback, and asking for help when needed are all hallmarks of good practice. This is always important, but when you are working across a language barrier, it is essential.

Unclear Communication and Relapse Prevention

Relapse prevention has its own terminology and most of the concepts are abstract. We saw in Scenario 11.4 how language deprivation and unclear communication can make it very hard to determine what happened to someone who may have been sexually victimized. In the next scenario, we see how language deprivation and unclear communication makes it difficult to treat the abuser.

Scenario 11.7

Bart is a 25-year-old Deaf male who was raised in a country where he had no formal education until he moved to the United States when he was 10 years old. At that time, he was placed in a Deaf residential school where he had his first exposure to ASL. His language development started then and, by age 19, he could communicate in very simple ASL. However, his language gaps and limited knowledge of the world were still huge problems. Just as important, he had very little experience using language to express his feelings and almost no vocabulary that he could use to help describe his inner world. While in school, he was offered counseling, but most of it had to be focused on language development. He drew and did games with his counselor. In the process, the counselor tried to help Bart learn to express himself with signs, and Bart made some progress.

Bart always had behavior problems, especially aggression, but his behaviors improved as he developed language skills. He became accustomed to the structure of the residential school he attended, but when he graduated he was unprepared for adult life. There were no resources to support him, like a group home, so he returned to living with his grandfather, the only available family member. There was very little meaningful communication between them. With nothing to do, Bart roamed the streets, got involved in petty theft, and started drinking heavily and visiting prostitutes. Bart didn't always pay them, and he got into some physical fights with the women and, once, with a man who may have been a pimp.

One day, Bart was arrested by the police. A woman had accused him of sexual assault. The police came to his home to arrest him, and they found him drunk, confused, and angry. They couldn't communicate with him. Feeling bad for him, the police brought him to a psychiatric emergency program rather than to jail. From there, after many days of searching for a placement, he was committed to a state psychiatric hospital which had had some experience working with deaf people. Bart was referred to a non-signing hearing psychologist who arranged for an interpreter. The counselor hoped to work with Bart on a plan to address drinking, aggression, and sexual assault.

The psychologist knew about treatment for addicts, sexual offenders, and persons with anger control problems but he knew nothing about language and cognitive development in deaf people. He assumed the interpreter would bridge the language barrier.

The psychologist started interviewing Bart with the interpreter, but they seemed to be making no headway. The psychologist wasn't clear why, and he asked the interpreters for a consultation about Bart's language skills. He learned they were much poorer than he thought. The psychologist, with Bart's permission, also contacted the school to talk with his previous counselor. Eventually, the psychologist learned some of the challenges they faced:

a. *Bart's language skills were at, perhaps, a first grade level. He had no words or signs for body parts (he just pointed), and certainly has none of the vocabulary needed for relapse prevention. Concepts like "relapse," "trigger," "warning sign," "coping skills," "relapse prevention," and "risk" would go completely over his head and would not be easily learned. Neither would Twelve Step concepts like "powerlessness over alcohol" and "higher power." The psychologist wasn't sure he could even explain what "addiction" meant.*

b. *Bart had had very limited sex and substance abuse education in ASL. The school had tried, but his language delays made this difficult even for them. There were no written treatment materials on either subject that Bart could use. The school did have some pictures, dolls, and toys they had used in their "life education" classes. Even treatment materials developed for children were too advanced for him.*

c. *Bart lacked both the vocabulary and relevant experiences for talking about his feelings. Bart knew he was in trouble, but he denied any drinking problem and blamed the woman for lying about him. Bart's main complaint was that he had no money.*

    Bart was a long, long way from developing any kind of relapse prevention plan. Before he could develop such a plan, he needs to have a basic vocabulary for coping skills. He would need to be able to recognize and name what he felt, and he needed to have some plan for managing these feelings. He would also need some basic social skills such as "expressing self safely," "asking for help," "conversational turn-taking," "listening," and "responding when people say 'no.'" In addition, of course, he'd need to recognize that he had some problems which he was responsible for managing.

    The psychologist began to feel overwhelmed. The hospital administration and insurance providers were expecting a treatment plan with a goal like sobriety, anger management, or, at the least, practice of some simple coping skills. They were expecting progress within a few days or, at worst, weeks. Interpreters were provided for the treatment sessions (although not for most of the day during milieu treatment times). If Bart was not making progress, would they assume this was because the psychologist wasn't competent?

    The psychologist and his team started looking for places they could refer Bart to.

 Bright idea 11.3: If you are working with signing Deaf people and you don't sign, it is easy to assume that all you need to bridge the communication challenges is a qualified interpreter. Remember, interpreters work best with people who have fluent and clear language skills and roughly comparable world views. If one or both parties are very dysfluent, and/or each party's "fund of information" is widely different, interpreters may not be able to bridge this gap. Talk with your interpreters about what can be done to bridge gaps in language, fund of information and life experience.

 ## Practice Exercise 11.1, Part A: Am I clear?

The next time you are working with someone who is upset about something, ask the person to tell you the story of what happened. Pay attention to the story the person is telling. Ask yourself:

1. Is the story clear?
2. Does it have a clear beginning, middle, and end?
3. Is it clear who in the story did what to whom? If it isn't clear, can you help the person tell their story more clearly?

When people have language problems, the first and principal challenge may be helping them tell their stories more clearly. When working with deaf people who have been language deprived, an early and key therapeutic task is often simply helping people develop and use language. Does this make sense in your clinical setting?

 ## Practice Exercise 11.1, Part B

1. Identify an abstract concept that you want to teach or explain to a client. It might be a word you use every day like "symptom," "treatment," or "recovery" or jargon from the mental health field, such as "anger management," "coping," or "relapse prevention."
2. Ask the client to participate in this exercise.
3. Ask a colleague to observe your discussion with the client.
4. Explain or illustrate the concept. Use examples.

5. Check in with the person. Ask, "Am I clear?" See if the person can repeat back to you what you just said.
6. Check out whether your client understands the concept. Don't ask whether or not they understand but ask them to explain the idea back to you. How confident are you that they understood?
7. Ask your colleague whether or not he or she thinks you were clear. If you are a new signer and you are practicing this with a deaf person, it is especially important to get good feedback on how clearly you are communicating.

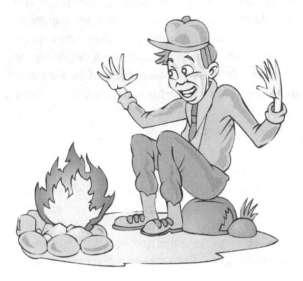

Figure 11.1

©iStock.com/FeralMartian

Teaching and Counseling Strategy 2: Using Stories and Examples

The Magic of Story Telling

If a counselor is meeting a Deaf client for the first time, a culturally friendly way to begin is to say, "Can you tell me the story of what happened to you?"

Stories appeal to nearly everyone. The human brain seems wired for stories. When we are having difficulty explaining something, a good story usually helps. Deaf people are no different than hearing people in this regard. Using stories to engage and teach seems to be a particularly culturally affirmative way of working with Deaf people, especially if the stories are well signed. Stories are also a wonderful way to engage and teach people with other language or learning challenges. Indeed, helping them to tell their stories, as part of their language and cognitive development, is an appropriate and excellent therapeutic goal.

Sometimes you can find teaching stories on the web and other places. TV shows or movies can also provide useful stories[1] and can be very helpful in engaging people or illustrating points you are trying to teach.

The movie *The Woodsman* (Kassell 2005), starring Kevin Bacon, is about a newly released child sex offender who is trying to start a new life. Searching for a job and an apartment, he faces prejudice and discrimination. Many people he meets make assumptions about him and loathe him without knowing him. He also struggles with his continuing attraction to young girls. The tension in the movie is over the question of whether or not he will relapse and molest another child. It is a powerful topic, told very sensitively, that illustrates all the major concepts involved in relapse prevention:

- What triggers him?
- What risky places should he avoid?
- How, because of errors in his thinking, does he give himself permission to re-offend?
- What does his offense cycle look like?
- What skills and supports enable him eventually to break this cycle?

Sometimes showing movies like this can be a powerful and effective way to start a relapse prevention discussion.[2] Of course, you have to consider the appropriate time to bring in a story, and the story you choose must match the audience. *The Woodsman* is a great teaching story for staff and others with intact language and cognitive abilities who are learning about sexual offending and relapse prevention.

You don't need to be a professional writer or storyteller or use well-known fairytales or media to engage people through storytelling. It's more a matter of recognizing that people are always telling stories. If you listen well, you can use a person's stories therapeutically.

Scenario 11.8

       Barry, a client in an outreach program, calls Steven, his outreach worker.

Barry: "I'm mad at you."

Steven: "You're mad at me? Really? Why?"

Barry: "You keep telling me how worried you are about me. You keep telling me you are worried I'm going to hurt somebody. You don't trust me. You keep talking about the past. This makes me mad."

Steven: "You're mad at me because I told you I'm worried that you will hurt somebody and I keep talking about it? You think I don't trust you."

Barry: "Yes!"

Steven: "Wow. I have to thank you."

       Barry is confused.

Barry: "What?"

Steven: "I have to thank you. You're giving me really good feedback. You're telling me exactly what I did that bothers you. You aren't insulting or threatening me. You are just asking me to behave differently. I think that is really good communication. That's using 'I-statements.' Remember we talked about that? I appreciate you telling me directly how you feel in such a clear way."

Barry: "Oh, OK. You're welcome."

       At a later session, Barry starts talking about something else that is bothering him, but this time he makes insulting comments to Steven. He calls him a jerk and an asshole.

Steven: "Barry, remember the last time you got mad at me? Last week, when we spoke on the phone? Remember what you said?"

       Together, they reconstruct the story of the last phone call.

Steven: "So, last week you gave me really good feedback using I-statements. It was very skillful. Are you doing that now?"

Barry: "No."

Steven: "You did it before. You have the skill to express yourself without making me feel bad. Can we try again?"

Steven is reminding Barry of his own previous success using skills. He reminds him of the story of how he used these skills previously. He recaps that story. If you pay close attention to the persons you serve, you will come across story after story about skills and strengths. Each story is a gem ready to be polished. You just have to notice it and store it away until you need it. Then, bring out the story of their success, reconstruct the story together and use it as a guide for moving forward.

    As you'll recall, in Lessons 9 and 10, you learned about how people always have at least two stories about their lives. One is the story of problems (e.g., a person is bothering them, something is unfair, other people are jerks, they feel sad, angry, or nervous). They also have stories of how they coped and survived in spite of these problems. Now, you are noticing and telling the story of the person's success back to them. You're reminding them of skills they have shown, no matter how undeveloped, and marveling out loud at these abilities. Doing this in a story format is engaging and no story is more engaging to someone than the story of something they did well.

Scenario 11.9

Justin, a 21-year-old deaf male, has his first job, stocking merchandise at a department store. He wants to do a good job so he can be promoted. However, he has a supervisor who, from his perspective, is giving him a hard time. The supervisor was upset with him for being late, for taking long breaks and using the bathroom too often. Justin tells Sam, his outreach worker, that his supervisor is a jerk and he's ready to quit.

    Sam responds by telling Justin the story of his own experience with a difficult supervisor. Sam tweaks the story slightly to fit Justin's situation. Simon says he was also working at his first job and had a supervisor who seemed to criticize him no matter what he did. He thought about quitting many times, but then thought about the consequences.

He needed the money. He really wanted to be successful at the job so he could get other jobs. He didn't want a bad reference. He had only been working there a short time, and he could put up with it for a while longer. And also, maybe the supervisor had some good points about how he could do better. Sam worked hard to have a good attitude, even with the difficult supervisor. After three months, he was able to transfer to a different department where the supervisor was easier to work with. Looking back, he was really happy he didn't quit, Sam said.

Justin listened to Sam's story. In their next meeting, Justin told Sam that he was trying hard to keep cool.

Sam: *"What did you do to keep cool?"*

Justin: *"I just nodded my head, took a deep breath, and went back to work. I remembered your story."*

Sam: *"Wow. Do you see the skills you're using?"*

Sam used his own story to teach Justin. This was much more effective than lecturing Justin on good behavior or telling Justin to "use his coping skills." Just as important, Sam helped "pull" Justin's story of how he was coping, in spite of a difficult supervisor. Sam was trying to help Justin construct a story about his own abilities to cope and survive even when things don't go his way.

Throughout this workbook, stories have been used to teach important concepts. These stories all come out of real-life situations that I experienced directly or know about. All of these stories are now teaching tools. Remember the story of my experiences zip lining in Costa Rica from Lesson 1 that I used to introduce the topic of coping skills? As part of my coping self-talk at the time, I told myself that *if I just get through this ordeal, in the end I'll have a good teaching story!*

Bright idea 11.4: Stories appear to be the most universal teaching strategy that exists. Consider how central stories are to the main texts of every religion. Think about *The Big Book* of Alcoholics Anonymous, which is essentially a collection of stories. Think about how Twelve Step meetings are organized around storytelling. Search for stories that illustrate powerfully the points you want to convey.

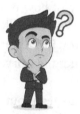

Questions to ponder 11.3: What stories have been really important to your own development? What stories do you keep returning to? What stories can you draw on now in your therapeutic role?

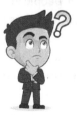

Questions to ponder 11.4: When you listen to people, can you hear both the story of the problem and the story of the recovery? Can you help someone attend to the elements in their story that point to their own skills, strengths, and resiliency?

ASL and Building from Specific to Abstract

Now we are going to shift the focus from stories and relapse prevention to Deaf mental health care and learn something about American Sign Language (ASL) that has practical implications for the way you work with deaf and hearing people who have language and learning challenges.

ASL and English have very different grammatical structures. For instance, as with Spanish, adjectives in ASL often follow the noun (i.e. ASL "HOUSE RED" is the equivalent of English "red house"). As with German, verbs in ASL often come at the end of the sentence (e.g., ASL "BOOK YOU I-GIVE" is the equivalent of English

"I give you the book"). As with Hebrew, there are no to-be verbs in ASL (e.g., ASL's "I HAPPY" is the equivalent of English "I am happy"). As with Mandarin Chinese, verbs in ASL don't change form to indicate tense. Instead, tense is indicated by the context or with a time marker like YESTERDAY or PAST. For example, the sign "GO" does not change in ASL from YESTERDAY I GO to TODAY I GO. Rather, tense is established through the time markers YESTERDAY and TODAY.

ASL also differs from English in the way that many abstract categories are formed. This profoundly influences the way abstract ideas are discussed in a sign language conversation. Consider the following examples of what are called "superordinate categories"—that is, collections of specific items: tool, crime, jewelry, vehicle, and musical instrument. There is no way to express these concepts in one sign, unless one has been developed recently or is used locally. These concepts are created by putting together a string of specific examples, often followed by a sign for "etc." In ASL, these concepts are conveyed roughly as follows:

- Tool: HAMMER SAW SCREWDRIVER ETC.
- Crime: KILL STAB RAPE ETC.
- Jewelry: RING BRACELET NECKLACE ETC.
- Vehicle: CAR MOTOCYCLE BICYCLE ETC.
- Musical instrument: CLARINET PIANO GUITAR ETC. (Klima and Bellugi 1979)

There are grammatical rules in ASL for the way vocabulary for abstract categories is created. In ASL conversations, there is a much stronger tendency than in English to give a number of specific examples as a way to convey abstract ideas. ASL *punctuates* reality differently than English by putting more emphasis on details and specifics. In addition, a simple ASL sign like EAT may pack more information in it (i.e., be more highly inflected) than the English word. That is, a Deaf ASL user signing EAT may also be conveying whether they eat fast, slow, carefully, sloppily, a lot, etc. based on how they modify or inflect the sign and use accompanying facial grammatical features. There are commonly more details packed into an ASL conversation than a user of spoken English would convey.

This tendency in ASL to attend to details has contributed—wrongly—to the idea that deaf people are more concrete thinkers than hearing people. People with language and learning challenges, both deaf and hearing, are likely to be concrete thinkers. This doesn't mean that most deaf people have difficulty with abstract thinking. Many are articulate language users of one, two, or even several languages. Deaf people work in professions requiring the highest levels of education. There are deaf philosophers, and deaf people without high levels of education have conversations without difficulty about highly abstract topics like the meaning of life.

In day-to-day conversation, ASL's tendency to build from specific to abstract has profound implications for counseling and teaching. This tendency often results in interpreting or clinical challenges. For example, consider the interpreting challenges posed by these questions often used in a mental status exam (Table 11.2).

TABLE 11.2 Abstract Questions in the Mental Status Exam

What has your mood been like in the last two weeks?	There is a new sign for "mood" that many deaf people use. Usually the concept is conveyed by giving examples of different emotions. An ASL translation might be: YOU UP-TILL-NOW TWO-WEEKS, ANGRY, SAD, NERVOUS, TEND WHAT?
Is there a history of mental illness in your family?	The concept of "mental illness" would have to be explained with examples. The idea of family history would also be explained with examples.
Do you sometimes hear voices giving you messages when no person is present?	The problem here is not just that "hearing voices" has the more familiar meaning for deaf people of whether or not you can hear speech sounds. It's also that people with limited life experiences and vocabularies may not know the concept of hallucination or be able to clearly distinguish it from related concepts such as thinking, day dreaming, and dreaming. In addition, "hallucination" is another subordinate category. In ASL, one would tend to be more specific, distinguishing between voice, visual and tactile hallucinations (Glickman 2007). Each would be signed differently.

Even concepts such as "touch" and "hurt," which do have signs, are used differently in ASL than in English. The sign TOUCH is usually located in the place the touch occurred, complicating translation of a sentence like "Did he touch you?" Likewise, the sign HURT is usually located on the body where the pain occurred. Headache and stomachache use the same sign for HURT but are located on different parts of the body. When you sign IMPROVE, you indicate how much you have improved by how large the movement of the sign is. In each case, a sign refers to something more specific than the English word. Similarly, concepts like "assault," "attack," or "abuse" often have to be "unpacked," as interpreters say, to specify exactly what kind of assault, attack, or abuse occurred. In ASL, you would provide examples of assaults, abuse, attacks, etc. to get to the abstract meaning.

As you can see, ASL conversations tend to be more detailed and specific. This is something that many counselors need to take into consideration, especially when teaching and counseling deaf people with language and learning challenges.

One way to do so is to follow the lead that ASL provides. That is, teach through examples and move from examples to abstraction, not the other way around.

Coping and conflict resolutions skills, for instance, are defined by giving lots of examples, as in Lessons 1 and 2. This is why Lesson 1 begins with a story, and why this workbook relies so heavily on teaching stories. To engage people in the process of learning skills, begin in a strength-based way by helping them notice and label specific skills they already have. For instance: *"You noticed you felt angry. You thought about it. You decided to go to your room and watch TV. You used 'stop and notice' skills, 'thinking' skills, and 'calm down with TV' skills."* Using specific examples helps establish a schema for the abstract concept that "we get better by learning skills." It sets the stage for asking the question, "What other skills do you want to learn?"

Teaching Abstract Concepts

There are two different ways to teach abstract concepts. The first way is to start with a definition and then provide examples. This is much more common among English-speaking hearing people, especially those with high levels of education. It *moves from abstract to specific*. For instance:

"Coping skills are strategies people use to regulate emotional states and manage environmental stressors. All human beings need coping skills because life is filled with stressors and unpleasant experiences. Indeed, the true measure of psychological health is not how happy and content one feels, but how well one manages the unpleasant emotional states (anger, sadness, anxiety) that are natural parts of the human condition. Some examples of coping skills are deep breathing, exercise, and positive self-talk. What are your coping skills?"

The second approach starts with examples and then proceeds to abstract concepts. This approach is considered more Deaf friendly because it better fits the structure of ASL discourse. For instance:

"When I am sad, I do a number of things to feel better. I seek out friends to talk to. I go to my yoga class. I play with my dog, Baxter, who never tires of my attention. When I am angry, I need to go to my room, to stay away from people, until I am calm. Sometimes I'll sit and meditate but other times I'll just distract myself by surfing the Internet. Eventually, I calm down, and I can deal with people again. These are some of my coping skills. Everyone has coping skills. When people have many coping skills, they can stay calm and in control no matter what happens to them, no matter what they feel. This makes them more psychologically healthy. What are your coping skills?" (Glickman 2013, p. 209)

The first approach moves from abstract to specific; the second moves from specific to abstract. Neither approach is perfect for all circumstances. Both approaches involve abstract thinking. Standard education usually promotes the first style even when the second style may be more effective, especially when communicating with people who have language and learning challenges.

Concrete examples and stories are generally clearer and more engaging than abstract principals. Have you ever gone to a lecture where the presenter spends most of his or her time talking in a very abstract realm, saving one or two examples for the end? Or, even worse, have you experienced a time when the presenter run out of time and didn't even get to the examples? Have you ever wished for more examples or that the examples came earlier in the presentation? If you have, you are asking for a more Deaf-friendly teaching style. Placing more emphasis on examples and stories often leads to better teaching and counseling for hearing people also. Deaf mental health care specialists often do this naturally and easily. It turns out, this a very effective teaching and counseling style to cultivate and use more widely.

Back to Relapse Prevention

We've seen that the world of relapse prevention is filled with abstract concepts. In fact, relapse itself is an abstract concept. A common sign for "relapse" in some places literally means *fall down*. Hearing people, like myself, can learn this sign for relapse without realizing that it is metaphorical; falling down is a metaphor for relapsing. I clearly recall working with a Deaf young man with anger management problems for over six months. During that time, I constantly was signing RELAPSE PREVENT. One day, he became so exasperated with me that he signed and mouthed: WHO FELL DOWN? That was one of many wake-up moments. I hadn't been clear.

We need to teach core recovery concepts, such as the Twelve Steps, though multiple examples. For example, Step 1 is "We admitted we were powerless over alcohol and that our lives had become unmanageable." *Powerless* can be conveyed with the signs POWER NONE but a skilled teacher or counselor would first provide a number of stories or examples to illustrate the concept. The same is true for the concept *unmanageable*. Indeed, Twelve Step meetings are often composed mainly of people telling stories. People will illustrate how their own lives became unmanageable, and use examples of their own lived experience to explain how they became powerless over alcohol or other drugs.

The different conversational styles of spoken and signed languages is one of many reasons why placing an interpreter in a meeting often does not create communication inclusion. As we've noted, many abstract concepts have to be *unpacked* with examples, and the fast pace of spoken conversations may not allow time for this. This is why, again, it is so crucial periodically stop to ask "Am I clear?"

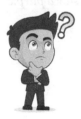

Questions to ponder 11.5: Think about a therapeutic concept you want to teach. Talk to sign communication experts about how that concept is conveyed in your country or region's sign language. Is there a recognized sign that closely matches the English word? Are the interpreters "unpacking" the concept by providing examples? Do they need you, therefore, to provide more examples and check in as to whether or not your client really understands what you mean? Does this suggest that you might have to work differently with this client?

Stories Are Examples

The idea of teaching through examples is crucial for complex topics like relapse prevention that consist of many abstract ideas, such as relapse, warning sign, trigger, risk, cycles, etc. Remember, stories are simply examples that provide concrete instances that teach particular points. Good stories are teaching gems. One of the best things that you can do, as a professional and a person, is to share stories that have helped you in your work and in your life.

As you'll recall, the movie *The Woodsman* illustrates many principles that are central to relapse prevention. Let's examine a scene from this movie to see how you can use examples to teach abstract concepts, such as risk and risk management, that are so central to relapse prevention. One way to explain a concept is to break it down into different examples. In this case, you can identify different kinds of risk—risky places, risky behaviors, risky emotions, and risky thoughts.

Scenario 11.10

Walter, the character played by Kevin Bacon, is the convicted sex offender who is newly released from jail and trying to start a new life. He is battling his demons, including his continuing attraction to pre-adolescent girls. In one scene, he gets off a bus and follows a young girl into a park. He first makes the decision to not get off the bus at his usual stop. He waits till the girl gets off and then follows her. Then he walks into the park and starts a conversation with the girl who is looking at birds in a tree.

Walter:	*"Hi."*
Girl:	*"Hello." She sees Walter staring at something.*
Girl:	*"What are you looking at?"*
Walter:	*"Up in that oak tree, there's a nest."*
Girl:	*"Where?" (She looks up in the tree with her binoculars.)*
Walter:	*"Up there. A little higher."*
Girl:	*"The little chicks. You want to see."*
Walter:	*"Sure."*
	The girl hands Walter her binoculars. "They're starlings."
Walter:	*"Is that right?"*
Girl:	*"I don't like starlings."*
Walter:	*"Why not?"*
Girl:	*"They're extremely aggressive birds, plus their habits are pretty filthy."*
Walter:	*"Their mother must have her hands full."*
	He returns the binoculars.
Walter:	*"You always carry these with you?"*
Girl:	*"When I go bird watching."*
Walter:	*"It's just a city park."*
Girl:	*"You'd be surprised how many different kinds of birds you find here. Last week, I saw a purple martin, and the week before that, I saw a solitary vireo. That's rare."*
Walter:	*"Solitary vireo. I like that."*
Girl:	*"Their sound is really musical."*
	She looks at Walter with suspicion.
Girl:	*"Are you a bird watcher, too?"*
Walter:	*"Me, no, I'm more of a . . . people watcher."*
	The girl looks concerned.
Walter continues:	*"The way you were staring up at the trees, I thought you were going to take off and fly."*
	The girl steps away to leave.
Girl:	*"I should go now."*
Walter:	*"You come here a lot?"*
Girl:	*"My daddy likes me home before dark."*
Walter:	*"Well, it's good to listen to your daddy."*
Girl:	*"Bye."*
	Walter watches her walk away.

Many risk factors are illustrated here:

- Walter has gone to a high-risk place (a park with few people).
- He has put himself in a high-risk situation (talking with a girl he's attracted to in an isolated area).
- He's engaging in high-risk behaviors that are preparing a potential victim, often referred to as "grooming."
- We can guess at the high-risk feelings (loneliness, boredom, depression, sexual lust).
- We can guess at high-risk thoughts ("This girl is lonely. She needs a friend. She wants company. I can help her.")

Later, we discover that Walter has indeed found a girl who is very vulnerable to sexual abuse as he continues to groom her for sexual contact.

This scene can be used to help illustrate that there are many types of risk. It also can lead to discussions of different types of risk (see Table 11.3).

TABLE 11.3 Breaking "Risk" Down into More Concrete Components

Risky places	<ul><li>A bar is a risky place for an alcoholic.</li><li>A schoolyard is a risky place for a child sexual offender.</li><li>A casino is a risky place for someone addicted to gambling.</li></ul>
Risky situations/behaviors	<ul><li>Hanging out with former drinking buddies is a risky situation for an alcoholic.</li><li>Going to a shopping mall is a risky situation for someone who doesn't manage money well.</li><li>Going to the "all you can eat" buffet is a risky situation for someone on a diet.</li><li>Watching pornography can be a risky behavior for a sexual offender, as can allowing oneself to masturbate to violent sexual fantasies.</li></ul>
Risky emotions	<ul><li>In AA, there is the idea of HALT (hungry, angry, lonely, and tired) to point out the four emotional/physical states that can trigger drinking.</li><li>Risky places and situations can be avoided. Risky emotions may be unavoidable. They have to be recognized and managed.</li><li>For sexual offenders, sexual lust may be a risky emotion. So might anxiety or anger. For other people, depression, anxiety and other emotions may trigger problem behaviors.</li></ul>

Risky Thoughts

Lesson 9 discussed how thoughts can create emotional states and trigger certain behaviors. Risky thoughts are well illustrated in this scene, which appears late in the movie.

Scenario 11.11

Walter has been waiting for the girl in the park. She arrives and they talk. He learns her name is Robin and he tells her his name is Walter. Eventually, in the movie's most important moment, he asks her, "Robin, would you like to sit on my lap."

	Robin looks puzzled.
Robin:	*"What?"*
Walter:	*"Would you like to sit on my lap?"*
Robin:	*"No, thank you."*

Walter:	"Okay, it doesn't matter."
Robin hesitates before responding:	"Do you want me to sit on your lap?"
Walter:	"Yes, I would enjoy that . . . I know this place that is quiet except for the sounds of these tiny little birds."
Robin:	"They sound like finches."
Walter:	"Yeah, they might be finches. Do you want to see?"
Robin, after a long pause:	"My daddy lets me sit on his lap."
Walter:	"Does he?"
Robin, weakly:	"Yes."
Walter:	"Do you like it when he asks you?"
Robin:	"No."

The camera closes in on Walter's face and his changing facial expressions. We read this expression change and know that he's realizing something very important. He thought Robin wanted to sit on his lap. He was talking himself into molesting her by telling himself that she wanted it. Suddenly, he realizes she doesn't want it. She doesn't like sitting on her father's lap and she doesn't want to sit on his lap. He had imagined, and told himself, that she would enjoy this sexual contact. Now he realizes his thinking was wrong. This challenge to a core belief that supports his molesting behavior is shattering to him.

Walter:	"Why not?"
	Robin starts to cry.
Walter continues:	"Are you two alone when he asks you? Does he say strange things? Does he move his legs in funny ways?"
	As he watches Robin crying, Walter realizes that she has been abused by her father and it has hurt her, and he was about to do the same thing.
Robin:	"Walter, do you still want me to sit on your lap? I will. I don't mind."
	We can see Walter badly wants for her to do it. Instead, he answers very quietly and unconvincingly: "No. Go home, Robin."
	Robin hugs him and leaves.
	This moment was pivotal for Walter because it is only when his core belief that "she wants this" is shattered that he is able to make a breakthrough in his recovery.

Teaching about thinking errors is inherently abstract. Does this story and example make the concept clearer for you?

 Bright idea 11.5: Stories can be an excellent tool for teaching very abstract ideas. The next time you struggle to explain something difficult to someone, search for or create a story that can illustrate the concept. Some of your favorite movies and television shows might provide examples.

Stories Are Everywhere

The story in *The Woodsman* is quite sophisticated and subtle. Therefore, it may not be suitable for persons with language and learning challenges. Some people will not be able to connect the risk factors that Walter faces to the risk factors they may face in other domains, such as with alcohol or aggression. If you are deaf, understanding this story requires the ability to read the captions. It's a challenge to find movies and videos that can be used by people who are deaf and cannot read well.

In most cases, the best examples and stories come directly from the people you serve. Are the people you work with doing something to manage risk even when they don't understand the abstract concept? Can you teach them about risk in a strength-based way by finding instances in which they are managing risk and, through these examples, give them words/signs for what they are doing?

Scenario 11.12

Daryn is a Deaf 40-year-old male who uses ASL at a very simple level. His signing is often unclear and his thinking is very concrete. He can't define a concept like "risk" or give clear examples. His risky behaviors have to do with inappropriate sexual touching of pre-adolescent and adolescent males. He understands the rules that sexual partners should say "yes" to sex and must be adults. Those are concrete ideas. However, he misreads other people's facial expressions and body language, and misunderstands what they say, so he thinks they are consenting when they aren't. He also thinks that some of the young men he's attracted to want to have sex with him and that they should be able to even if they are under 18. He has been arrested before and he doesn't want to go to jail or get in trouble.

Daryn lives in a group home. When he goes into the community, staff accompany him. One day, he was in a store with staff person, Arnold, when a young attractive boy, who was about 12, entered the store. Arnold saw that Daryn noticed the boy and was watching him closely. Daryn saw Arnold watching him, then Daryn asked to leave the store. When they talked about it later, Daryn said he was uncomfortable being near the boy who, he said, had smiled at him. Daryn left the store because he didn't want to get into any trouble.

Daryn and Arnold talked about this story many times. The story provided an example of how Daryn was actually managing his risk of sexual offending. Arnold tried to teach Daryn about risk by pointing out the risky situation (being near a boy in a public place), asking Daryn what he felt and trying to learn what he thought. Daryn could say he felt nervous but not that he felt attracted to the boy. He could say he felt afraid he would get in trouble. Arnold pointed out that there was a "risk" that he would get in trouble if he did "risky behaviors" like talk to the boy so, instead, he did safe behaviors like leaving the store and talking to staff. Over many conversations, this story and others helped Daryn to understand what "risk" meant and that he was working with staff to decrease risk and increase safety. Eventually, when the concepts are clear enough, Daryn may be able to understand this as "risk management" or even "relapse prevention."

 Practice Exercise 11.2 Part A

1. Go to your own collection of TV shows, movies and books.
2. Find one story that you think you could use to teach a skill to another person.
3. Discuss with at least one other colleague how you'd like to use this story.
4. Share relevant stories with each other.

 Practice Exercise 11.2, Part B

1. Consider a topic you want to identify the people you serve (e.g., symptom management skills for anger or anxiety or depression management).
2. Brainstorm with your team to create teaching/counseling strategies that will be more effective in working with people with language and learning challenges.

Practice Exercise 11.2, Part C

1. Identify examples/stories that indicate that the people you serve are already doing some type of relapse prevention. The stories are about examples of skills they already used.
2. Use these examples to teach a relapse prevention concept like risky behaviors, situations, emotions or thoughts.

 Practice Exercise 11.2, Part D

1. If you are working with Deaf people with language and learning challenges, consult with your communication experts on how these abstract concepts are conveyed in the sign language used in your area and how the concepts may need to be "unpacked" for the people you are working with.
2. Consider whether the person has enough language ability to learn these concepts at this time. It might be that the person isn't ready for this particular topic or kind of treatment work.
3. Ask yourself: "Where is the person in the pre-therapy to therapy continuum?"

Summary

In this lesson, you learned some things about American Sign Language and Deaf mental health care that have bearing on teaching and counseling practices for deaf and hearing persons with language and learning challenges. You learned about the importance of paying very close, mindful attention to communication and to whether or not you are communicating clearly. You also learned about the importance of checking to be sure the person understands what you are communicating. You learned not to assume you are communicating well but to ask and test out understanding.

You also learned about the value of being concrete and specific and that people often learn best from examples and stories. Learning to communicate with details and stories makes you a better teacher or counselor for persons who have language and learning challenges and, quite possibly, with most people. This becomes very important in trying to help people understand abstract ideas such as relapse prevention and symptom management.

In the final lesson, you'll learn three more core Deaf mental health care strategies that can contribute to excellent counseling and teaching of people with language and learning challenges.

- Participant assumes a humble attitude regarding communication skills as demonstrated by a willingness to ask and explore, "Am I clear?"
- Participant assumes a humble attitude regarding communication skills as demonstrated by a willingness to ask for and receive feedback.
- Participant illustrates the concepts of "relapse" and "risk" using examples and stories.
- Participant takes an abstract idea and searches for examples or stories that illustrate the idea.

Lesson 11 Quiz

1. Which of the following are reasons that relapse prevention is considered a complex set of skills? (Check all that apply.)

   a. Relapse prevention concepts are abstract.

   b. Relapse prevention plans require that basic skills, such as coping skills and social skills, are in place at least to some degree.

   c. Relapse prevention plans are self-management plans and, therefore, require a high level of "buy-in."

   d. Relapse prevention plans require a person to have a strong sense of linear time so they can imagine problems that might occur in the future.

   e. Relapse prevention plans require some strong foundational problem-solving skills.

   f. Relapse prevention plans are often made in one emotional state but must be carried out when a person is in a different emotional state.

   g. There is no way to communicate the concept of relapse in sign language.

2. Which of the following are reasons why it is important to continually ask "Am I clear?" when working with people with language and learning challenges? (Check all that apply.)

   a. You may not be communicating as clearly as you think you are.

   b. When working with people who use a different language, you may not be aware of how concepts are presented and organized in that language.

   c. The interpreting process is more complex than it seems and interpreters often need to "unpack" or reorganize concepts as they move between languages.

   d. The people you work with probably have much less vocabulary and simpler ways of using language than you do.

   e. In the process of becoming educated, language skills develop and you can get used to communicating in a more complex way than people who have not had the benefits of this education.

   f. If you have a good interpreter, you don't need to ask that.

   g. Asking whether you are clear is a way to take responsibility for the communication process and not blame the client for not understanding.

3. Which of the following are ways that stories can be effective tools for teaching or counseling?

   a. Stories provide powerful examples of concepts that one wants to teach.

   b. Most people love a good story. The human brain seems wired to take in information well through stories.

   c. Most, if not all, religions and cultures use stories to teach ideas that are important to that culture. Storytelling is as close as we have to a universal means of teaching.

d. People are drawn into stories in a way that they often are not when people just lecture to them.

e. Storytelling is useful for children but not adults.

4. The following paragraph teaches the concept of anger management by going from abstract to specific ideas.

> Anger management is a set of strategies for recognizing and handling angry feelings and aggressive behaviors. Anger management problems result in violent and anti-social behaviors. Many relationships have been ruined because the individuals involved could not handle their angry feelings without becoming aggressive and hurting other people. Anger management work often starts with helping a person stop and notice when angry feelings occur and how they manifest in the person's body, thoughts and behaviors. Then the person is taught skills, such as taking a time out, diaphragmatic breathing, progressive muscle relaxation, or mood logs, that help them respond to angry feelings more effectively.

Write or sign a brief lecture that teaches the concept of anger management by going from *specific to abstract*. *Hint: Start with examples or stories and build to the concept through these examples.*

_____

_____

5. Look at the example you wrote for Question 4 or the one provided in the Quiz Answers section. Compare that with the example of moving from abstract to specific. Which way of explaining the concept is easier for you to understand?

Lesson 11 Questions for Discussion

Think about a person you serve that you have difficulty communicating with. Discuss questions 1 through 3 with at least one other person, being mindful of the confidentiality guidelines in your setting:

1. How well do you understand the language and communication abilities of the person?

2. How well does this person read and write? How much does your program depend on the abilities of people you serve to read and write well? Is it possible that people are acting out in order to cover up their embarrassment at not being able to read or write well?

3. What are some of the difficult words or jargon that are used in your program? For example, do you regularly use terms like "coping skills," "trigger," "anger management," "treatment, "relapse," "higher power," "recovery," "self-regulation," "mindfulness," etc.? Does the person you are working with understand these terms? How do you know?

4. Who are the best communicators in your program? How do you know?

5. Do you feel like you have permission to say when you need help communicating with someone? If you use sign language, are you able to acknowledge when you don't understand someone or when someone doesn't understand you? If you acknowledge that you are having trouble communicating with some clients, will your job be in jeopardy?

6. If you are working with deaf people through sign language interpreters, how much do you understand about the language skills of the deaf consumer? How much do you understand about how the interpreter works? For instance, do you think that the interpreter is just substituting signs for words? Have you talked with the interpreters about what is going on in the interpreting process? Have you asked the interpreters if there are ways you can help to create greater communication inclusion for the deaf person in a hearing setting? If you haven't had these conversations with the interpreter, why haven't you?

7. Can you promote a discussion of whether the staff members in your program or service are able to communicate clearly with the people you serve and what additional supports are needed?

8. The playwright George Bernard Shaw is supposed to have said "the single biggest problem with communication is the illusion that it has taken place." Do you see applications of this saying in your workplace?

9. Another well-known saying is "A little knowledge is a dangerous thing." Do you have enough knowledge about communication dynamics with the people you serve to be confident that you understand where communication barriers exist?

10. What kind of language or communication problems do you find commonly in the *hearing* people you serve? Do you see similar language or communication problems in the staff?

Lesson 11 Quiz Answers

1. Answers *a* through *f* are all true. The concept of relapse can be communicated in ASL in a variety of ways. There is a commonly used sign but it can also be communicated through examples and stories.

2. Answers A through E and Answer G are all good reasons to ask whether you are clear. F is not. It is a mistake to assume that the presence of interpreters solves all communication challenges. A good practice is to engage the interpreter in a discussion of language and communication challenges.

3. Answers *a* through *d* are true. Is *e* true for you?

4. Here's one possibility:

When Sean gets angry, it affects how he holds his body, walks, and even breathes. He gets all puffed up. He clenches his teeth. He moves like he's imitating the Hulk. His breathing gets short and shallow. He then gets very close to people and uses his large frame to tower over them and scare them. Often he proceeds from there to yelling, insulting, threatening, pushing, and, sometimes, punching.

His wife has told him he has an anger management problem. She said that if he doesn't see a counselor and learn some better ways to manage his angry feelings, she will leave him. The next time they argued, he blamed her, called her a "bitch," and threw a plate on to the floor. She packed up and left that afternoon.

Sean doesn't realize that his behavior with his wife is an example of an "anger management problem."

Notes

1. While writing this workbook, the Pixar movie *Inside-Out* was released. This movie is a brilliant teaching tool for helping people connect thoughts to emotions. It also provides an excellent example of the techniques of externalizing and using stories to teach psychological principles.
2. If the persons you are working with are deaf, they need to be able to read the captions. If one cannot hear or read well, the number of TV shows and movies available is much fewer.

Bibliography

Burns, G. W. (2001). *101 healing stories: Using metaphors in therapy*. New York: John Wiley & Sons, Inc.

Burns, G. W. (2005). *101 healing stories for kids and teens: Using metaphors in therapy*. Hoboken, NJ: John Wiley & Sons, Inc.

Glickman, N. (2007). Do you hear voices?: Problems in assessment of mental status in deaf persons with severe language deprivation. *Journal of Deaf Studies and Deaf Education* 12(2): 127–147.

Glickman, N. (Ed.). (2013). *Deaf mental health care*. New York: Routledge.

Kassell, N. (2005). *The Woodsman*, New Market Films.

Klima, E., & Bellugi, U. (1979). *The signs of language*. Cambridge, MA: Harvard University Press.

Wedding, D., Boyd, M. A., & Niemiec, R. M. (2010). *Movies and mental illness: Using films to understand psychopathology*. Cambridge, MA: Hogrefe Publishing.

Deaf Mental Health Care and Relapse Prevention II

Introduction

In Lesson 11, you learned how to teach relapse prevention by drawing on two strategies common in Deaf mental health care (DMHC) (Glickman 2013):

1. Paying close, mindful attention to the communication process.
2. Teaching abstract concepts using examples and stories.

In this final lesson, you will learn how to apply three other common DMHC strategies:

3. Use of pictorial aids and drawing.
4. Role playing.
5. Empowering people receiving services by placing them in roles where they help and teach others.

Teaching and Counseling Strategy 3: Using Pictorial Aids and Drawing

As the saying goes, "a picture is worth a thousand words." People turn to art when they don't have strong language skills or cannot read or write. Using pictures is optional with people who read well; it's essential when people don't read well and have other language and learning challenges. Thus, when you want to teach something to individuals with these challenges, ask yourself, "Can we draw or find a good picture for it?"

The Internet has many options that make this task much easier.

This workbook uses many photographs that were obtained through commercial stock photo companies or drawn by Deaf artist Michael Krajnak. You can find a CD with these drawings accompanying the author's 2009 book, *Cognitive behavioral therapy for deaf and hearing persons with language and learning challenges.* These drawings can also be found at the Routledge website for this workbook. (http://routledge.com/9781138916937. Click on the E-resources tab for this book.) Michael is especially good at drawing pictures illustrating psychological symptoms. These pictures can be used for psychoeducation regarding mental health and illness and as part of self-monitoring to help someone evaluate whether or not they are improving. For example, here is a pictorial self-monitoring form that has been used to teach persons with language and learning challenges about the symptoms of depression. Note that in standard CBT for depression, clients may be asked to complete a tool such as the Beck Depression Inventory regularly as a way of measuring progress in treatment. The pictorial self-monitoring form in Figure 12.1, even though it hasn't been validated through research for this purpose, could also be used by the client to give a rough measure of progress.

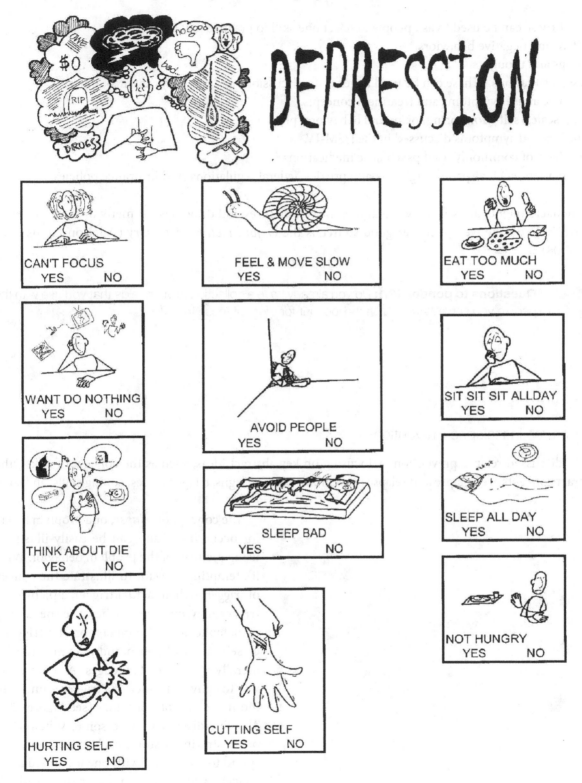

Figure 12.1 Pictorial self-monitoring form for depression symptoms

At the Westborough Massachusetts State Hospital, where these pictures were developed, the value of the pictures spread from the Deaf Unit to the hearing adolescent units to the adult psychiatric inpatient units. The pictures are still (2016) widely used at the Worcester Recovery Center and Hospital, where Deaf inpatient services are currently located. On Michael's CD and the Routledge website, there are pictures that represent:

1. Skills. (These can be used to ask people to select one skill to practice that day.)
2. Positive and negative behaviors.
3. Feelings and thoughts.
4. Stressful situations. (These can be used to generate discussions and role plays about skill use.)
5. Substance abuse symptoms and treatment concepts.
6. Rating scales, self-monitoring forms and behavioral plans.
7. Disorders and symptoms discussed in the DSM-IV.
8. Side effects of commonly used psychiatric medications.
9. Legal matters, such as patient rights, health proxies, federal regulations, and insurance policies.

While Michael's talents are still very much in demand, pictures and drawings for many of these issues are widely available on the web. Another good source is the *Oxford picture dictionary* (Adelson-Goldstein & Shapiro 2008).

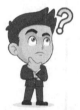

Questions to ponder 12.1: Do you already have a collection of visual aids that you use with the people you serve? Are you on the lookout for more of these tools?

Using Pictures in Relapse Prevention

Lesson 11 discussed relapse prevention by focusing on key abstract ideas, such as the concept of risk. Other key abstract concepts are: relapse and relapse prevention, warning signs, trigger, cycles, coping skills, and social supports.

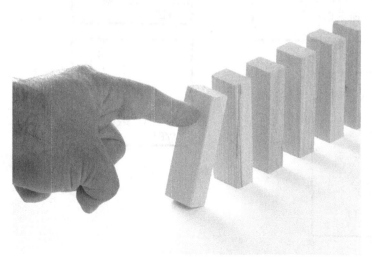

Figure 12.2 One picture for "trigger"

©iStock.com/Ljupco

The concept of *relapse*, or a problem behavior occurring again, can be easily illustrated using pictures of the problem behavior. While it's tempting to want to illustrate the concept of *trigger* with an actual trigger, a picture of a trigger may not be clear because the concept is metaphorical. The metaphor of a trigger is closely tied to English and may not translate literally into other languages. A more useful way to convey the idea of a trigger is one domino in a chain of dominoes (see Figure 12.2). This was discussed in Lesson 6. When telling or illustrating a story, each event can correspond to a domino, with one identified as the trigger. Alternatively, a finger that sends the dominoes cascading can be described as the trigger.

A trigger also can be portrayed with a series of pictures that illustrate a relapse cycle. In Figure 12.3, a person with a drug addiction is triggered by seeing people using drugs or by having people invite him to use with them. This picture can also illustrate a relapse "cycle."

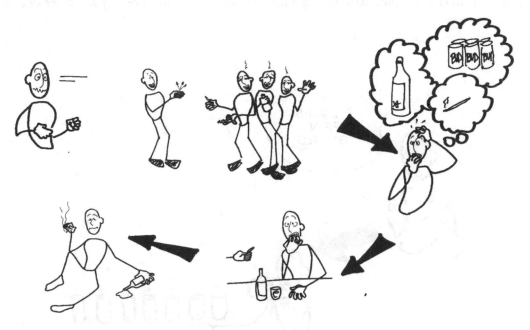

Figure 12.3 Picture depicting relapsing and a cycle

In Figure 12.4, an argument and a memory can both be considered triggers for self-harming behaviors.

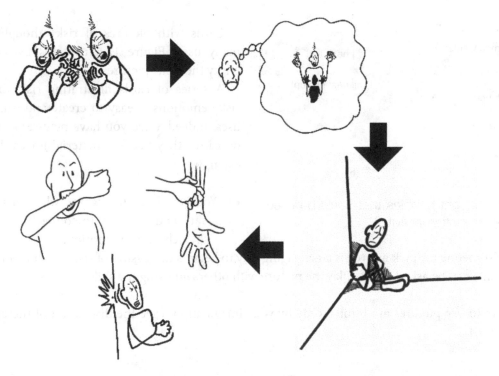

Figure 12.4 Picture depicting trigger, cycle, and relapse of self-harming behaviors

As mentioned in Lesson 11, the concept of *risk* can be made somewhat more concrete by breaking it down into types of risk, particularly risky emotions, thoughts, and behaviors. Each can be illustrated with examples and stories, as well as with pictures. The most abstract concept to explain is *risky thoughts*. Thought bubbles can be used, with thoughts followed by the risky behaviors. In Figure 12.5, the thought "I'll just have a few beers," coupled with the sign for "It's nothing," is followed by a picture of a person having many beers.

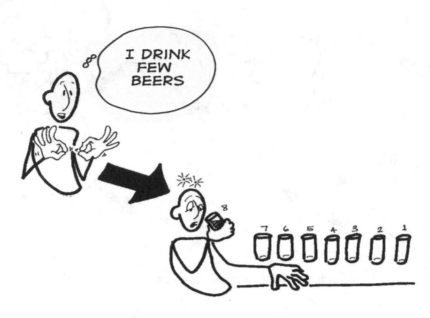

Figure 12.5 Picture depicting "risky thoughts"

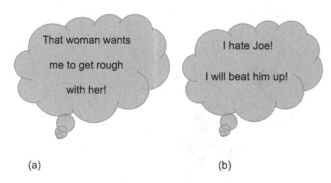

(a)   (b)

Figure 12.6 Thought bubbles that could be used in a relapse prevention activity

Cards with pictures of risky thoughts can have many uses. Figure 12.6 contains two examples of "risky thought" pictures:

A series of cards illustrating risky behaviors or risky emotions is easy to create and can have many uses. Indeed, once you have pictures of any concept on cards, they become material for card games. For example:

- You could create a game where a person picks a card and then has to connect the thought to a risky behavior or emotion.
- Inviting someone to "pick a card" is an engaging way to begin a discussion of the concepts on the card.
- Participants can be asked to role play the picture with others guessing the skill or concept.

Creative ways to use pictures are limited only by your imagination! (See the discussion of therapy games in Glickman 2009.)

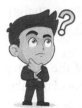

Practice Exercise 12.1

1. Read each of the following concepts in Table 12.1.
2. Consider how you might represent each concept in a picture.
3. Identify resources where you can find pictures to illustrate each.
4. Write your ideas in the spaces provided.

You can find examples of how these concepts have been turned into pictures on Michael's CD-ROM or at the Routledge link given earlier.

TABLE 12.1 How Could You Represent These Concepts with Pictures?

Concept	Representations	Resources
Mania		
Symptoms of mania: Racing thoughts, a grandiose sense of self, impulsive and reckless behaviors, decreased need for sleep, poor attention span, extreme talkativeness		
Paranoia		
Example of paranoid thinking: Imagining people are saying negative things about you when they aren't		
Medication side effects		
Most of these are very concrete and easily illustrated with pictures. Examples: Weight gain, blurred vision, low blood pressure, and dizziness		
Communication skills		
Examples: Listening, repeating back what you heard, showing appropriate non-verbal behaviors, etc.		

Role Shifting in ASL

The Internet, and YouTube in particular, provides a venue for training and information sharing in ASL. Deaf culture has a rich "oral" storytelling tradition, and many wonderful ASL storytellers can be found on the web. One such storyteller is Keith Wann (have a look at the website http://www.youtube.com/watch?v=1ePOq_S04p8). The YouTube clip shows him giving a masterful rendition of Eric Carle's story, *The very hungry caterpillar*. The story is far more entertaining in ASL than it is in English.

In the story, Keith shifts between the roles of narrator and the caterpillar. He tells the story of the hungry caterpillar eating one apple, two pears, three plums, four strawberries, five oranges, one piece of chocolate cake, one ice cream cone, one pickle, one slice of Swiss cheese, one slice of salami, one lollipop, one piece of cherry pie, one sausage, one cup cake, and one slice of watermelon. By shifting his body and using wonderful facial expressions, he becomes the caterpillar as it eats each item and gets fatter and fatter. He then shifts his body to become the narrator talking to the caterpillar, the narrator's cat, and the other people in the room. When the caterpillar is ready to make a cocoon, Keith becomes the caterpillar building his cocoon, wrapping himself in toilet paper and going to sleep. Finally, as a very full and large butterfly, he breaks his way out of the cocoon and flies off, as Keith, the narrator with a stomachache, rushes off to the bathroom.

When you watch master ASL storytellers like Keith in action, it's easy to see how ASL creates a narrative in which the narrator becomes each character. In everyday ASL discourse, this is routine—though less dramatic. The person telling a story does not say, "He said, she said." Rather, he or she uses body posture and, often, facial expression and body movements, to become each participant of a story. This ASL grammatical feature is called "role shifting." It's one of the dramatic features of ASL that makes it such a captivating language.

ASL also makes use of spatial properties. A dialogue between an adult and a child, for instance, is represented by having the adult look and sign down while the child looks and signs up. Describing what happened at a doctor's visit, an ASL signer is likely to shift body posture and manner to assume the roles of the doctor, nurse, patient, people in the waiting room, etc. In addition to role shifting, the signer will likely reference each speaker in different parts of the signing space. Many ASL signs, such as HELP, TEACH, GIVE, INFORM, and COUNSEL, are directional. The movement of the sign shows who is acting on whom. Articulate signers make their stories come alive through their ability to act out the postures, expressions, and behaviors of various characters as well as use space and movement to create visual pictures.

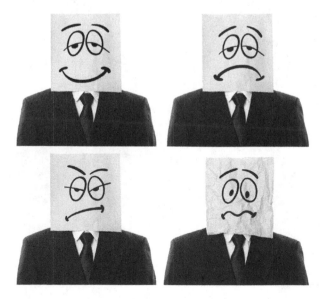

Figure 12.7 Role playing

©iStock.com/ZoneCreative s.r.l.

From Role Shifting to Role Playing

It's a small step from role shifting in a dialogue to role playing as a teaching or counseling technique. Perhaps this is why role playing is used so often in DMHC. While some hearing counselors use role playing when working with hearing people, it is common practice among DMHC practitioners. It is especially common when working with deaf people who have language and learning challenges.

Role playing is a form of active learning. Counselors who use role playing to teach concepts and skills are already doing the skill building associated with CBT. ASL *pulls for* role playing, just as it *pulls for* use of examples and details. These grammatical qualities of the language *pull for* teaching and counseling strategies where one acts out the concepts and skills one wants to learn. They *pull for* a concrete, immediate, active learning style that has broad relevance beyond Deaf individuals or persons with language and learning challenges.

Scenario 12.1

Abigail and Thomas are two deaf staff members working with Ted, a deaf resident of a group home. Ted is large and stocky and likes to get very close to women, often invading their space and frightening them. He has a reasonably good relationship with Thomas. Recently, he got much too close to Abigail and she had to keep moving backwards until she was cornered against a wall. Thomas is trying to help Ted understand the impact of his behavior and find more skillful ways to get what he wants. Thomas is about Ted's size.

Thomas (to Ted):	"Let's role play. I'm going to be you. Okay? I want you to be Abigail."
Ted, who is used to role playing:	"OK."
Thomas, thinking out loud:	"I want Abigail's attention. What can I do? I'm going to go up to her now."
	Thomas approaches Abigail (played by Ted) in an aggressive manner, getting much too close.
Ted (as Abigail):	"No. Get back!"
	Thomas continues to get closer and closer, in a threatening way.
Thomas:	"Will you talk to me? Will you talk to me?"
Ted:	"You are too close! Get away!"
Thomas:	"OK."
	Thomas moves away and stops the role play.
Thomas:	"What happened? How did you feel when I got too close to you like that?"
Ted:	"Not comfortable. Nervous."
Thomas:	"How do you think Abigail felt when you did that to her?"
Ted:	"Nervous."
Ted, to Abigail:	"I'm sorry."
Abigail:	"Yes, I feel very nervous when you approach me like that. I feel like I don't want to talk to you. I want to get away."
Ted:	"Sorry."
Thomas:	"Do you want Abigail to quit her job? Do you want her to stay so she can keep working with you?"
Ted:	"Stay."
Thomas:	"Well, if you want her attention, what can you do?"
Ted:	"Ask her."
Thomas:	"Let's role play that."

This kind of work is very common in Deaf mental health care. To teach a point, people act it out. This technique is often used to help people appreciate how their behavior affects other people. It is also used to learn skills.

Scenario 12.2

In a coping skills group, participants are practicing coping in various situations that can trigger stress. They are using cards with pictures of common stressful situations that require coping, called "situation cards[1]." One picture shows a person putting money into a candy machine. The candy machine takes the money, but the candy bar never comes out. The group leader asks one member to role play the person who has lost his money. Someone else gets to role play the withholding machine, a fun assignment. A third person takes the role of skills coach, helping the person whose money was taken think through his response. Then, the next person picks another card, and the group role plays coping with this new stressor.

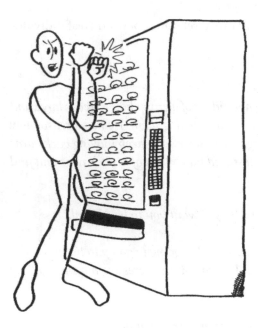

Figure 12.8 A "situation card"

The most direct way to teach a skill is to break it down into parts, and then model and practice it. The basic steps of skill building are:

1. Explain the skill by breaking a skill down into components.
2. Model it.
3. Practice it in role plays.
4. Give feedback, especially on what the person did well.
5. Practice some more.
6. Have the person teach the skill to someone else. (This last point is often overlooked and will be discussed shortly.)

Role playing is the best way to practice. For instance, the "red, yellow, and green traffic light" coping skill, presented earlier, is a useful, pictorial way to represent a variety of coping skills. The red light represents the "stop and notice" moment. The yellow light represents doing something to calm down, such as taking a break or diaphragmatic breathing. The green light represents positive self-talk or some other problem-solving skill.

Scenario 12.3

Johan and Sam are two staff members in a residential program. They are helping David, a resident, practice the "red, yellow, green light" coping skill. Johan role plays a staff person setting a limit such as, "I can't talk with you right now. Can you wait?" Sam helps David stop and notice his feelings, take a few deep breaths, and then repeat comments such as "Johan is busy. I can wait." They switch roles, with David becoming the coach for Sam, who is stressed because Johan is not available. David decides to hang the picture of the traffic light on the wall of his room as a reminder to use this skill.

Bright idea 12.2: To learn a new skill, one has to practice it. Talking about how you would handle a situation is not nearly as powerful as acting it out. Role playing is one way to practice.

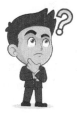

Questions to ponder 12.3: How often do you use role play in your counseling work? How comfortable are you with this technique? Do you see benefits to using role play in many counseling situations, not just people with language and learning challenges?

Role Playing and Relapse Prevention

In Lesson 6, you explored questions that are commonly part of a behavioral analysis. In a behavioral analysis, one tries to understand why a problem behavior happened by asking about the events, thoughts and feelings that came before, during and after the problem behavior. As you'll recall, in its simplest form, a behavioral analysis may have just two or three parts. A simple behavioral analysis might be:

My brother picks on me ⟶ I feel angry ⟶ I hit him

Ideally, you would like to create a more complex behavior analysis, including, at the least, how the person thought. However, it isn't always possible to get to that level of complexity when working with people with language and learning challenges. In most cases, it is possible to do a simple three-step analysis focusing on what happened (the trigger), the emotion, and then the behavioral response. We might also search for a fourth factor by asking what happened next. After "I hit him," for example, did that behavior get me something I wanted?

A relapse prevention plan will usually start with identifying some coping or social skills that can be used to handle a stressor. A coping skill might be taking deep breaths and counting to 10; a social skill might be telling one's brother how his behavior makes you feel and how you plan to respond in the future. The discussion between the counselor and the person receiving services focuses on the stressors (triggers) that provoke an emotion and how the person responds to them.

The counselor's goal is to help the client understand that the brother's behavior, however obnoxious, did not cause the assault. Rather, the brother's behavior provoked anger, and the person handled this anger by hitting. Although the person doesn't necessarily feel like he made a choice, he actually did because, obviously, there are other ways to respond to provocation besides hitting.

In a role play, the counselor playing the part of the client asks the client to play the part of the brother. The counselor shows that no matter how much the brother teases and insults him, he uses his "shield," takes deep breaths, talks to himself to remind himself that his brother wins if he blows up, and then walks away. Then they reverse roles, with the counselor playing the role of the obnoxious brother. The client practices some of these coping or social skill responses and the counselor provides supportive feedback. If the client is ready, the counselor can increase the stress to make the practice more real.

Scenario 12.4 illustrates how role play can be used in relapse prevention.

Scenario 12.4

Nathan, a counselor:	*"Kal, you've done a great job of using your 'shield' skill. I teased you and you put up your shield and walked away. Now, can we make this a little harder?"*
Kal:	*"What?"*
Nathan:	*"Before I just teased you a little. Now I'm going to tease you a lot. Maybe I'll say some insulting words. I will try harder to make you mad. Is that okay with you?"*
Kal:	*"Oh, okay."*
Nathan:	*"Let me ask you, should I be a little bit meaner or a lot meaner."*
Kal:	*"Just a little bit."*
Nathan:	*"OK. I'll be a little bit meaner, and we'll practice some more. Are you ready?"*

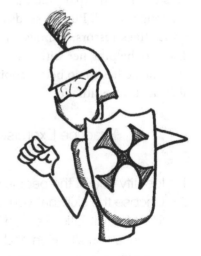

Figure 12.9 The shield skill

A very common problem in role playing any kind of coping, social, or relapse prevention skill is that a person talks about and practices a coping skill that he or she doesn't need at the moment. For instance, the person practices coping with anger when he isn't feeling angry. Then the person isn't able to access the skill when it is needed (for instance, when he really is angry) because the earlier practice didn't make any impact. Impatient staff may then respond by criticizing the person, saying, "Why didn't you use your coping skills? We practiced this before!" This is unskillful work from the staff.

Consider a relapse prevention plan designed to help someone cope with a craving. It's easy to avoid overeating when you are full. It's easy to avoid drinking alcohol if there is nothing triggering you to want a drink. It's easy to avoid problematic sexual behavior if you are not sexually aroused. Problems arise when it comes time to use the skills that are in your plan when they are actually needed.

To make skill plans real, two things must occur. First, the skills must be practiced and the practice situations must approximate real-life situations. Role playing is one way to practice. Role playing your response to increasingly challenging stressors, with the person's permission, makes a skill more likely to be actually learned.

Second, when the person does use a skill in a real-life situation, the staff must stop and notice and help the person celebrate this accomplishment no matter how imperfectly the person used the skill. All the foundation work discussed in Lessons 1 through 3 on noticing and labeling skills pays off when it is applied in relapse prevention as illustrated in Scenario 12.5.

Scenario 12.5

Lucille has a really difficult time handling what for most people would seem to be very small stressors. She has difficulty processing even simple language. When she doesn't understand, Lucille starts to cry and complain that nobody likes her. Staff can see that she becomes easily overwhelmed when she doesn't understand what is happening, and they have worked with her on stopping and noticing, breathing slowly, and saying, "I don't understand."

Stopping and noticing is the most difficult part for Lucille. She can't yet notice when she is overwhelmed but staff help her recognize when this happens. They stop and notice, look down and take slow deep breaths to cue Lucille to do the same. Then they ask Lucille, "Am I clear? Should I repeat more slowly?" When Lucille says "Yes," staff responds by saying, "Great job stopping, breathing, saying you don't understand, asking me to repeat."

It takes many sessions before Lucille starts to do this on her own. One time, she just stopped, started to breathe, and then began to cry. Staff, responded, "Great work. You stopped the conversation. You took slow breaths. What's next?"

Another time, Lucille said, "You sign too fast!" Staff responded, "Thank you for telling me. Great job communicating about a problem. Let's stop, breathe together, and start again more slowly."

This can be slow, painstaking work, especially when it feels like getting to a genuine relapse prevention plan is a long way off. But the seeds of a relapse prevention plan are already being planted. Staff are helping Lucille notice the stressors, feelings and, perhaps at some point in the future, the thoughts that precede a meltdown. They are helping her with very basic coping and social skills. The concept of "relapse" hasn't been introduced yet. Lucille has to do better coping in the moment of stress before she can work on how she might cope in an abstract future situation.

 Practice Exercise 12.2, Part A

1. Identify one of the people you serve who needs to work on a coping or social skill.
2. Choose the skill that you will focus on.
3. Identify a situation related to that this skill that you can role play with this individual.
4. Discuss this situation and ground rules for the role play with the client.
5. Decide who will play each role. *Hint: It is often easiest for you, as the counselor, to start playing the role of the stressed person so you can model effective coping.*
6. Role play the situation.
7. Discuss what happened during the role play.
8. Reverse roles.
9. Discuss what happened during the next role play.

Increasing Stressors When Role Playing

In CBT, stressors can be intensified as a person becomes more capable. For instance, if the stressor is exposure to alcohol, this can be done by first talking about alcohol, then viewing pictures of people drinking, then watching video clips about drinking behaviors, and eventually going into a liquor store, or being exposed to people encourage the person to join them in drinking.

It is very important that the client control the pacing and intensity of any exposure experience. This can be visualized as turning a dial or moving up a level in a game. Before increasing the intensity of the exposure, the counselor asks, "What would the next level be?" and "Are you ready to try that?" This kind of work should be done in consultation with a mental health professional because it carries a risk of re-traumatizing the person if it is not done carefully. *The client must be able to understand fully and consent to this kind of treatment.*

If you and the people you serve are doing this kind of work, you are well beyond pre-therapy and have moved into the CBT world. If the people you are working with are not ready for this, it can still be helpful to know that the foundation skill building you are doing is setting the stage for more complicated work at a later time.

Practice Exercise 12.2, Part B

1. Decide if you think the person you were working with in the first part of this exercise is ready to role play a more intense stressor.
2. If you think the client is ready, ask permission to repeat the role play with more intense stressors.
3. If the client agrees, repeat the situation that was the focus of the role play in Part A. This time, increase the intensity of the stressor. For example, if the person was teased lightly in the first role play, teasing should become harsher and more provocative in Part B.
4. You should play the client role. Be sure to model good coping strategies.
5. Discuss what happened in the role play.
6. Switch roles and repeat the role play.
7. Discuss what happened in the role play.

Teaching and Counseling Strategy 5: Have the People You Serve Become Helpers and Teachers

The foundation of the final teaching strategy is recognition that the people receiving services can sometimes be the best teachers and supporters for their peers experiencing similar challenges. To understand this concept, it's important to understand a key aspect of Deaf culture and Deaf people.

The single most important difference between a culturally Deaf and a culturally hearing perspective can be summarized in two expressions:

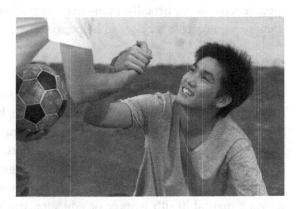

Figure 12.10 Turning people receiving care into helpers and teachers

©iStock.com/PeopleImages

- Culturally hearing people understand deaf people as "suffering" from a "hearing loss."
- Culturally Deaf people understand Deaf people as enjoying what a recent book refers to as "Deaf gain" (Bauman & Murray 2014), the opposite of "hearing loss."

When Deaf people enter a hearing mental health setting, the hearing professionals working with them often hold unexamined prejudices that stem from a belief that deaf people are disabled and that it is terrible to be deaf. These prejudices may seep into psychiatric diagnoses when these professionals assume that a person's current problems are a by-product of deafness. For example: "This person is depressed because she is deaf," or "The person is paranoid because he is deaf." These prejudices also may seep into the outlook the professional holds about the individual's potential for recovery (e.g., "The person can't cope because she is deaf"). They may presume that the person is more disabled than they are or that the person can't do something because he or she is deaf. The limitations deaf people face in life are overwhelmingly those placed on them by other people, not by the fact of hearing loss itself.

Deaf people often hold the opposite belief towards each other. They are predisposed to see each other's strengths, and to assume, as they often say, that "Deaf people can," for several reasons:

- They understand Deafness in relation to language and culture.
- They often enjoy rich, nuanced communication with one another.
- They see one another's abilities.

Bauman and Murray's book, *Deaf gain*, is part of a movement that appreciates how aspects of the Deaf experience, especially sign languages, are not only positive for Deaf people, but offer contributions to the hearing world. This is true of the Deaf mental health care pre-therapy work that has been the focus of this workbook. The five teaching and counseling strategies from DMHC offered here have much broader relevance. It may well be that what is sometimes called "Deaf-friendly" teaching and counseling is also "hearing friendly."

Effective DMHC offers an additional, critically important lesson: Disability may well be in the minds of the beholder. People who are considered disabled may actually be *multiply-abled*, although their abilities may not be obvious to outsiders. Appreciating this difference leads to recognition that a multi-abled individual can be engaged more effectively in treatment by placing them in helper or teacher roles. "Deaf gain" questions this "disabled" belief and reorients therapy towards seeing what people with profound life challenges *can* do. When you see people's abilities, you can invite them to help and teach others—including you!

In Lesson 3, you learned the difference between a strength-based and problem-based focus. The ASL sign for this radical difference in perspective can be literally translated as "turning your head around." (See Figure 3.6.)

If you are hearing, you need to turn your head around by consciously looking for the abilities that Deaf people have. More broadly, many helping professionals need to turn their heads around by seeking ways to put people who receive services in helper or teacher roles.

Learning by Teaching

Sometimes the best way to learn something is to teach it. Sometimes the best way to engage people in the process of learning is to invite them to help others by teaching what they know. In order to teach something, you have to find the words/signs to explain it to another person. You have to find a way to make something clear. The process of searching for those words/signs, for the way to explain something well, can cement your own understanding. It can also create for you the belief that "I can learn and I can teach." With this sense of personal agency, you may become motivated to learn more. A taste of success can be tantalizing.

As a mental health worker or educator, you must become a good student before you can become a good teacher. To learn how to teach, you must learn how to learn. Good teachers know how to learn and know how to help others learn. When people are invited to help or to teach, they often become more invested in learning. When people have learned something, they can strengthen what they have learned by teaching it to others. This is reflected in the twelfth and last step of the Alcoholics Anonymous tradition: "Having had a spiritual awakening as the result of these steps, we tried to carry this message to alcoholics, and to practice these principles in all our affairs."

Thus, a powerful avenue for engaging someone in the process of skill development can be to invite them to help or teach others what they know. The typical power dynamics can be reversed and therapeutic opportunities created when hearing clinicians humbly ask deaf clients to help or teach them. Staff members who approach the people they serve and say, "Help me, teach me," with regard to some skill or strength the person has, often find new opportunities for building relationships and developing skills.

This may be a new idea for professional helpers, but it isn't a new idea for Deaf and other minority communities. They are very used to turning to each other for help. Sometimes they have to fight against professional helpers who, whatever their intentions, can seem more concerned with control than with empowerment. The strategy of turning to each other for support was discovered by Deaf and other minority communities long before there were professional helpers such as mental health providers.

We listed common steps for learning a skill. The last step, teaching the skill to someone else, is often overlooked. Donald Meichenbaum and Andrew Biemiller, in their 1998 book *Nurturing independent learners*, emphasized this part of the learning process (Meichenbaum & Biemiller 1998). Their book explores "helping students take charge of their learning" by engaging students and helping them develop critical learning skills. In a mental health context, the comparable challenge is helping people discover that they can do something to make their own lives better such as learning important life skills. This pre-therapy process of helping people discover how they can grow and learn brings them into the world where education and mental health care practices, like CBT, make sense and seem useful. In this pre-therapy process, as they develop a sense of personal agency ("I can do it"), the teaching or counseling process not only becomes easier. It becomes possible.

This approach is illustrated in Scenario 12.6.

Scenario 12.6

Jason was a 20-year-old deaf male admitted to a psychiatric inpatient unit because others believed that he was suicidal. He was recently diagnosed with diabetes and refused to follow his new diet or monitor his insulin levels. His parents are medical professionals who bombarded him with information about diabetes care. Jason wanted none of it. He was just entering adulthood and experiencing some independence and freedom for the first time; he wanted to eat and do what he pleased. Because he wouldn't follow these new rules for living, he experienced a serious medical crisis and was hospitalized. In the hospital, his health stabilized, but he still refused to follow any new diabetes rules. As a result, he was transferred to a psychiatric unit.

In a psychiatric inpatient setting, the usual treatment for this kind of problem would be psychoeducation about diabetes self-management, but Jason had already made it clear he had no interest in this. An astute nurse took a different approach. She explained to Jason that **she** *had a problem and wondered if Jason could help her. She explained that the unit served many people with diabetes, but her staff knew very little about the subject. She wondered whether Jason,* **because he knew about diabetes**, *would be willing to help her train her staff.*

Jason responded very enthusiastically to this idea. The nurse then invited him to work with her to prepare a diabetes "seminar" for her staff. They met a number of times to review all the basics of diabetes and plan the seminar. The process of planning this seminar provided, of course, the psychoeducation that Jason needed. Because it was presented to him as a way to draw on his own expertise to help others, he was open to it. Eventually, he and the nurse created the seminar and invited the staff and outside providers, including his astonished parents, to attend. When Jason got up to speak, he didn't really provide much diabetes education. Instead, he told his story. At some point during the process of preparing for this seminar and telling his story, something shifted in him. The story he told was about how he learned to accept and manage his diabetes. That was, of course, the real goal of this skillful pre-therapy intervention.

The toolbox of every mental health professional should include strategies for engaging consumers as helpers and teachers. One of the more helpful questions to ask about your work with the people you serve is: *"Can I engage them more effectively in the process of developing skills if I invite them to step out of the role of a person receiving help to, instead, become a peer or helper of others, including me?"*

Learning from Others with "Lived Experiences"

The entry of "people with lived experience" into professional helping roles is another way the mental health field is turning its head around. In the substance abuse recovery field, people in recovery have long led treatment efforts. Twelve Steps programs such as AA and NA are peer run. People in recovery bring the wisdom of the Twelve Steps to peers who are also struggling with recovery from addiction. Although well established in the addiction field, this is a relatively new idea for mental health providers. Increasingly, people with lived experience are providing services and helping mental health care workers to be more welcoming and respectful of the people we serve.

People receiving services can be engaged on a smaller scale by inviting them to help and teach others, including staff. This was introduced in Lesson 5 as a one-down strategy of "asking for help." Here are some other ways that the people you serve can become therapeutic helpers and teachers:

- Ask someone who is particularly good at a skill to demonstrate it to other people.
- When you catch someone using a skill, ask him or her to explain it to you or to someone else. If needed, help them do this but give the person all the credit.
- Invite people to participate in seminars where they model and teach something. Ideally, pay them for their time and expertise.
- Invite people to share teaching stories about how they learned something important.
- Ask the people you serve to help plan the day's activities (e.g., as part of a morning community meeting). Conflicts, such as when people want to do different things, can be presented as problems to be solved by the group. Ask for help. Admit you can't solve this challenge without their input. What do they suggest?
- Ask people if they are willing to create teaching videos of something they are good at. Pay them for this work if possible.
- Invite the people you serve to co-present at conferences, such as those presented by the United States Psychiatric Rehabilitation Association or state chapters of this organization.
- Ask people for their opinions. This very simple intervention isn't done often enough. For example, "I need your help. I'd really like your opinion about this. I want you to be honest. Would you be willing to tell me what you think?"
- When you, as a staff member, are stuck, "share the dilemma." For instance, *Terrence isn't following his service plan. He's refusing to let staff accompany him into the community and he's approaching women in a way that previously got him into trouble. Staff has no authority to impose tighter supervision, so they share their dilemma. They are worried about choices Terrence is making. They don't want to control him but they are worried because he is doing the things that previously got him in trouble. What does he think? Can he help them?*
- Ask the people you serve for regular feedback on how well you are doing helping them. This can also be an opening to asking them to evaluate their own progress towards goals.
- Work to elevate the voices of people, often former patients, who want to make the mental health system less about power and control and more about choice and collaboration on shared goals.

Have Recipients of Services Help and Teach Relapse Prevention

The relapse prevention approach began in the world of addiction treatment where people in recovery helping one another is the norm. One of the main ways that people in recovery help one another is by telling their personal stories and using themselves as examples for other people who are struggling as they have. By telling their stories and offering to help others, they demonstrate the sense of personal agency that is so central to any personal development and recovery.

Promoting the competencies of people receiving services takes both humility and an understanding that sometimes it is best to get out of the way and let them step to the front of the line and be recognized as helpers.

Scenario 12.7

Betsy runs a relapse prevention group at the partial hospital program. She wants to be able to talk with participants about how to anticipate and avoid problem behaviors or symptoms. She often finds, however, that participants have little interest in this topic; and some don't seem to understand it. One day, she observed during a session that several members of the group offered helpful suggestions to Jerome, a peer, who was often aggressive, and who exhibited what everyone called "blow-ups." He was talking about how staff didn't listen to him or support him. Alicia, one of Jerome's peers, suggested that he use the "red, yellow, green" coping skill. With Alicia's help, Betsy was able to engage Jerome in a role play. Alicia played the staff person doing something Jerome didn't like. Scott, another member of the group, played a skills coach. Scott coached Jerome through the red, yellow, green skills. This resulted in about 10 very productive minutes in the session, after which Betsy knew to "stop and notice" the skills people were already using. She commented on how Alicia and Scott had helped and on Jerome's willingness to practice the skill. She wondered if they'd be willing to help anyone else learn this skill.

Alicia, Scott, and Jerome seemed intrigued so she continued. Would they be willing to invent a few more role plays and then film them, so the role plays could be shown to other people? They agreed they would. Suddenly the group had a mission. They spent a number of sessions practicing "red, yellow, green" and other coping skills, and eventually made a film of it. The film was used in new sessions, with Scott, Jerome, Alicia, and others introducing and explaining their work. At these times, Betsy sat quietly in the back, enjoying how the group members were taking ownership of their own achievements.

As more and more people with lived experience of mental illness are brought into the recovery process, not just as clients but also as colleagues and providers of direct helping services, more roads to recovery will appear. Sometimes a person who is a peer can accomplish much more than a licensed professional with advanced graduate education as you'll see in Scenario 12.8.

Scenario 12.8

Three deaf members of a group in a partial hospital setting are struggling with recovery from substance abuse. Only one of the three, Benny, has actually stayed sober for more than a month. The other two members, Sally and Craig, are still using their drugs of choice. The program has hired a peer specialist, Steve, who is deaf and in recovery from addictions also. Steve tells them his story, which is powerful, but even more powerful for the group is the fact that the agency has hired Steve. He's on staff, getting paid, and is really no different than the rest of the staff. He's a living example of how recovery is possible. Craig is especially inspired by Steve's story and seeks him out for individual support. Craig starts to talk about his own goal of becoming a peer specialist.

With Steve's encouragement, all three members agreed to tell their own stories on film. Steve welcomed that but noted that people needed to hear about how they got better in order to feel some hope for themselves. Of the three, only Benny could claim that he has actually gotten better; but all three of them had had periods in their lives when they lived drug free. All three decided to talk about those sober periods. They also agreed that if they could all get two months of sobriety, they'd make the video and include this message of hope. With Steve as a role model and the goal of creating a video to help others, the three became more engaged in their recovery efforts. This was more powerful than anything the professional staff had been able to devise.

Another way to assist people with relapse prevention is to draw out their healthy side and encourage them to become their own advisors. Relapse prevention is about anticipating problems before they happen. However, it's no secret that many people who create wonderful relapse prevention plans don't use them. How can you help them prepare for a moment when they might ignore their relapse prevention plan? Some options might be have them write letters to themselves (if they have the writing skills) that they can read at those moments, or even better, creating a brief film of them offering themselves advice on following their plans.

Scenario 12.9

Marcello is a deaf man who has struggled with addiction to cocaine and heroin. He understands what relapse prevention means and says he wants to stay sober and straight, but he isn't able to follow his own recovery plans when he craves substances. Staff in his program invited him to make a video in which he talks to himself. Marcello liked the idea that he would be his own coach. In the video, he reminds himself of all the reasons he has for not getting high and the plan he worked out for these moments when he craves. The process of preparing for the video filming took a few weeks of counseling sessions. The process of creating this script also developed his self-talk and self-coaching abilities.

In the video, Marcello greets himself. He said, "I'm you, and I'm here to remind you to stay straight." He goes on to review all the troubles that drugs have got him into: Loss of jobs, ruined relationships, arrests, jail time, and serious illness. He reminds himself of what he promised he'd do: Go to an NA meeting, talk to his sponsor, stay with his sober friend, Kirk, and stay with his dog. At the end of the video, Marcello looks himself in the eye and signs, SHOOT HEROIN, SNORT COKE, WILL DIE!

For Marcello, the many sessions that led to development of the video script were just as important as the video itself. Preparing the script was a concrete activity. Marcello didn't write well, which was another reason why rehearsal was so crucial. The process of rehearsing the script was also critical to developing—and actively practicing—the stronger self-talk that supported recovery. In the end, he had much more difficultly ignoring warnings and advice that came directly from himself.

In your day-to-day work, you will find abundant opportunities to invite the people you are serving to help you or others, *if* you stop and notice them.

Practice Exercise 12.3, Part A

One simple way to recognize the expertise of another person is to ask for their opinion. People who are receiving care are rarely asked for their opinions, especially if they have language and learning challenges:

1. Identify a person you are serving who has been difficult to engage.
2. Ask this person if they would be willing to share their opinion on something that is a real concern and of interest to the individual.
3. Ask the person something like: *"I'm wondering if you can help me. I'd really like your opinion on something. I want you to tell me what you really think. Would you be willing to do that?"*
4. Thank the person for offering this valuable opinion, regardless of what the person says, even if it is off-point or impractical. Be sure that your manner and attitude shows that you consider him or her to be an important person who has worthwhile things to say.
5. What kind of reaction did you get? Write your answer in the space provided.

_____

_____

_____

Practice Exercise 12.3, Part B

The people you are serving have many life experiences and skills that others might benefit from. There are many ways you can tap into this expertise. For example, you can ask if they might:

- Be willing to tell their stories to illustrate something about coping or recovery.
- Be willing to role play a skill they have learned to teach another person.
- Be willing to offer their advice or opinion on a topic.

- Consider making a teaching video of some kind.
- Be willing to give you, or your team, some structured feedback on a regular basis.
- Be willing to evaluate their own coping, communication, conflict solving, and other skills.

In this exercise, you will ask the people you serve to share their expertise to help and teach others.

1. Think about the people served in your program.
2. Identify possible opportunities to have them use their own experiences to help other people (including you) or teach others something.
3. Talk with them about what they do well and explore if they would be willing to help others with this skill.
4. Work to create opportunities for them to do so.
5. Who might you start this process with? What areas would you want to discuss with that person?

_____

_____

_____

_____

_____

Lesson 12 Skill Sheet

- Participants are able to draw, create, or find a picture for many of the concepts they wish to teach.
- Participants work on developing their comfort using role playing with people they serve.
- Participants search for opportunities to invite the people they serve to help someone else, including staff, especially with regard to skills they already have or are developing.
- When participants are stuck and unable to convince someone to change a problem behavior, participants practice "sharing the dilemma" and asking for help.

Lesson 12 Quiz

1. A staff person is looking for a way to use a picture to convey the abstract concept of "risk." Which of the following might help him do so? (Check all that apply.)

   a. Break the abstract idea of risk into more concrete examples, then find pictures of these concrete examples.

   b. Find a picture of someone doing something risky or dangerous.

   c. Search the Internet for "pictures of risk" to see what you find.

   d. Think about the kinds of risk that the person you are working with faces or engages in and look for pictures that represent them.

   e. Risk is too abstract an idea to convey in a picture.

2. Which of the following situations might lend themselves to role playing in a counseling context? (Check all that apply.)

   a. Person needs to cope with urges to smoke.

   b. When anxious, a person tends to send out dozens of emails to the same person.

   c. When Joe becomes angry, he starts swearing and insulting everyone he is with.

   d. Sarah is thinking about how she will handle her urges to drink wine when she is out at a restaurant with her friends.

   e. George tends to be very passive when talking to his doctor and often leaves without understanding what the doctor wants him to do.

3. What are some of the ways in which ASL and Deaf culture might influence the counseling process with Deaf persons? (Check all that apply.)

   a. Deaf people are concrete thinkers so the counseling process should always occur at a concrete level.

   b. The way in which ASL discourse is often more detailed and specific than discourse in spoken English, and the way in which ASL forms abstract categories, can "pull" for more use of examples in counseling.

   c. ASL lacks signs for certain concepts so these concepts can't be conveyed in ASL.

   d. Role shifting and the use of the signing space can pull for role playing as a counseling technique.

   e. Because ASL is a visual language, counseling in ASL should use pictures.

4. What are some benefits of asking people to whom you are providing services to help other people or help you?

   a. It can lower defensiveness about engaging in services.

   b. Sometimes the best way to learn something is to teach it.

   c. It can foster a different attitude about recovery.

   d. Peers sometimes do a better job of helping each other than professionals do of helping them.

e. It's insulting to a professional to ask a person receiving services to be the helper. It takes extensive training to do this work well.

5. What are some ways in which people with lived experience can be brought into the treatment and recovery process as helpers? (Check all that apply.)

    a. They can run peer-based recovery groups, such as Twelve Steps meetings.

    b. They can serve as advocates for people in recovery or as liaisons with professional, licensed helpers.

    c. They can offer support or concrete advice.

    d. They can tell their own recovery stories to provide hope to others.

    e. They can assist professional helpers to recognize how their personal attitudes and behaviors may be interfering with their ability to develop therapeutic relationships with the people they serve.

Lesson 12 Questions for Discussion

1. What kinds of visual aids are used in your program or service? Are there areas where you'd like to have more pictorial tools? Where could you go to find them?

2. Do you, or some of the people you serve, have any hesitancy using pictures in your work? How would you respond to a person who feels insulted and says that says the use of pictures is childish?

3. Besides pictures, do you regularly invite people to draw? Does your program/service encourage the people they serve to draw? How do you handle the common responses that "I can't draw" and that "drawing is for children?"

4. How comfortable are you personally with role playing?

5. Do you agree that role playing is commonly used in DMHC? If you agree, why do you think this is true?

6. Give some examples of situations in which you have found role playing helpful.

7. Beyond role playing, are you familiar with any other drama therapy techniques? Is this something you'd want to learn more about?

8. What other active teaching and counseling strategies have you discovered that seem to work well with persons who have language and learning challenges?

9. Do you think ASL *pulls for* visual teaching and learning techniques? What would be examples of this? Could hearing people benefit from this style of teaching?

10. Have you ever gained knowledge or skill through a game? Do you ever try to teach new knowledge or skills through games?

11. Do you agree that the structure of ASL, such as its way of creating abstract categories or its use of role shifting, actually influence the way teaching and counseling with signing Deaf people should occur?

12. If you know another language besides English, does use of that language effect how you would teach or counsel someone?

13. How might a person's language and culture *pull for* certain kinds of therapeutic intervention?

14. How comfortable are you letting someone you serve help or teach you? Do you think that you are more or less skillful when you take this kind of one-down role?

15. Consider the people you serve. What skills do they have that you might help them to develop further by putting them in the role of a helper or teacher? How do you think they would respond to this approach?

16. In Lessons 11 and 12, it was argued that DMHC often draws on these strategies:

    • Humble and mindful attention to the communication process.

    • The tendency to draw upon specific examples and stories.

    • Use of pictures and visual aid.

- Use of role playing.
- Encouraging people who receive help to act as helpers and teachers.

Do you agree with this? Would you add or take away any other characteristics of DMHC that you think are representative of this work?

17. What other techniques that DMHC specialists routinely use do you believe can be helpful to counselors working with hearing people?

18. If you are part of the controlling or more powerful group (that is, whites as opposed to racial minorities in the United States and Europe; men with regard to women; heterosexuals with regard to persons with different sexual orientations or transgender people; non-disabled as opposed to people with identified disabilities), have you personally benefited or gained when the less powerful group becomes stronger? For example, if you are a man, have you benefited from feminism? If you are non-white, have you benefited from the civil rights struggles of racial minorities? If you are hearing, have you benefitted personally from interaction with strong, culturally Deaf people?

19. Is there a "gain" for hearing people in Deaf mental health care?

Lesson 12 Quiz Answers

1. Answers *a* through *d* are useful approaches for illustrating abstract concepts, such as "risk."

2. All of these situations lend themselves to role playing. In answer *a*, the person practices skills for managing urges to smoke. In *b*, the person practices skills for managing anxiety. In *c*, the person practices skills for managing anger. Answer *d* practices a relapse prevention skill. Answer *e* practices a communication skill, such as assertiveness.

3. Answer *a* is false. You cannot and should not generalize about deaf people. The techniques in this workbook are designed for deaf *and* hearing people with language and learning challenges, not only deaf or only hearing people. We argued in favor of *b* and *d* in both Lessons 11 and 12. Answer *c* is not true. Because a specific sign for a concept doesn't exist does not mean that the concept can't be conveyed in the language. For example, even though it takes two words to represent the concept "brown rice" where another language might do it in one word, the concept is still clear. Answer *e* is an overgeneralization. Deaf people, even Deaf signers, are not necessarily visual thinkers. ASL can be used by deaf-blind people through tactile strategies. Not all Deaf signers like the use of pictures.

4. Answers *a* through *d* are all benefits of asking for help. Answer *e* is a common attitude among mental health professionals who at times might feel threatened if they think that someone who has not had their level of training can be just as effective a helper, or even more so.

5. People with lived experience have been brought into the mental health and substance abuse recovery process in all of these ways.

Note

1. You can find situation cards on Michael's CD or at the Routledge website www.routledge.com/9781138916937.

References

Adelson-Goldstein, J., & Shapiro, N. (2008). *Oxford picture dictionary*. Oxford: Oxford University Press.

Bauman, H.-D. L., Murray, J. J. (Eds.). (2014). *Deaf gain: Raising the stakes for human diversity*. Minneapolis, MN: University of Minnesota Press.

Glickman, N. (2009). *Cognitive-behavioral therapy for Deaf and hearing persons with language and learning challenges*. New York: Routledge.

Glickman, N. (Ed.). (2013). *Deaf mental health care*. New York: Routledge.

Meichenbaum, D., & Biemiller, A. (1998). *Nurturing independent learners: Helping students take charge of their learning*. Newton, MA: Brookline Books.

Printed in the United States
by Baker & Taylor Publisher Services